WITHDRAWN FROM STOCK

D1556500

5 044 100 0

COMPUTER MODELLING
OF BIOMOLECULAR PROCESSES

ELLIS HORWOOD SERIES IN MOLECULAR BIOLOGY

Series Editor: Dr A.J. TURNER, Department of Biochemistry, University of Leeds

COMPUTER MODELLING OF BIOMOLECULAR PROCESSES

J.M. GOODFELLOW and D.S. MOSS
Department of Crystallography, Birkbeck College, London

ELLIS HORWOOD
NEW YORK   LONDON   TORONTO   SYDNEY   TOKYO   SINGAPORE

KEELE UNIVERSITY
LIBRARY

2 4 JAN 1994

B/26048

First published in 1992 by
ELLIS HORWOOD LIMITED
Market Cross House, Cooper Street,
Chichester, West Sussex, PO19 1EB, England

A division of
Simon & Schuster International Group
A Paramount Communications Company

© Ellis Horwood Limited, 1992

All rights reserved. No part of this publication may be reproduced, stored in a retrieval system, or
transmitted, in any form, or by any means, electronic, mechanical, photocopying, recording or
otherwise, without the prior permission, in writing, of the publisher

Printed and bound in Great Britain
by Redwood Press, Melksham

British Library Cataloguing in Publication Data

A catalogue record for this book is available from the British Library

ISBN 0–13–161944–6

Library of Congress Cataloging-in-Publication Data

Available from the publisher

Table of contents

1

Computing and molecules

J.M. Goodfellow, D.S. Moss, and I.J. Tickle
Department of Crystallography, Birkbeck College, Malet Street,
London WC1E 7HX

1. INTRODUCTION

Many of the exciting insights in molecular biology over the last 40 years have come from the elucidation of molecular structures. Perhaps the most spectacular and well-known is the modelling of the DNA helix by Watson & Crick. During this period, we have also seen the experimental determination of over 500 protein structures by X-ray diffraction from crystals, and we are beginning to see the determination of solution structures of a number of proteins and nucleotide fragments from 2D NMR spectroscopy.

It is no coincidence that the solution of protein structures from X-ray crystallography has gone hand in hand with the development of ever more powerful computers, whether for the initial determination of the electron density map by using Fourier transform techniques or for the refinement of the protein structure against the experimentally determined structure factor amplitudes. Software for such calculations now exists on many types of computer from personal computers (PCs) to supercomputers such as the CRAY. One of the new problems for the computer user is to decide which machine or perhaps range of machines is best suited for a given application. This is non-trivial, given the rate at which new machines are appearing.

Computers dedicated to molecular structure determination are now obligatory, as they are used not only in data collection and data processing but also in generating the electron density map, displaying the map, and building amino acids into electron density, as well as for the final refinement processes. However, there has also been a massive increase in the computational techniques used to model macromolecular structures in terms of their conformations, dynamics, and interactions. It is this modelling or simulation of macromolecules that is the primary subject of this book.

The reasons for the rise of modelling techniques are quite clear. First, that the experimental data from crystallography are limited so that frequently very little information is available on the dynamics of molecules. Can simulation techniques such as molecular dynamics, originally used to study fluids by physical chemists, be used to study much larger and more complex macromolecules? Secondly, DNA cloning techniques have led to the elucidation of more than 20 000 protein sequences. In contrast, only around 500 3D protein structures are known. Can we predict the structure of proteins from their sequence? Can we use information on homologous proteins, or can we use databases of structural information on all proteins whose structure is known, to build a likely structure? Thirdly, even if an enzyme structure has been determined experimentally, the structure of an enzyme/substrate complex might not be available. Can we use docking techniques based on simple energy calculations to find a possible ligand binding site? In electron microscopy, can the experimental data be processed to produce clearer images?

Chapters in this book directly describe the background, assumptions, and applications of a number of modelling techniques which are in current use.

2   MACROMOLECULES

It is not the intention of this book to describe molecular structures in detail but to outline some of the essential points about a few important structures. It should be remembered that some of the techniques such as computer graphics can be used to display small molecules, atomic, or ionic structures as well as macromolecules. Enjoyable textbooks on structures in general include *Molecules* by P.W. Atkins (1987) Scientific American Library and *The Cambridge guide to the material world* by R. Cotterill (Cambridge University Press, 1985). Biochemistry textbooks with a structural bias include *Biochemistry* by L. Stryer (Freeman, 1988). More advanced textbooks concerned with specific macromolecular structure include the excellent reviews by G.E. Schulz & R.H. Schirmer on the *Principles of protein structure* (Springer-Verlag, 1979) by W. Saenger on the *Principles of nucleic acid structure* (Springer-Verlag, 1983) and *An Introduction to Protein Structure* by Branden and Tooze.

2.1   Databanks
Two of the main sources of structural data on biomolecules are the Brookhaven Protein Databank (Bernstein *et al.*, 1977) and the Cambridge Structural Databank. Both are available at Daresbury Laboratory for academic users via SEQNET initiative.

3.   COMPUTERS

Which computer to use is often an important decision. The answer will depend on what machines are already available or the sum available to buy new machines. The following is an attempt to describe briefly what can be achieved on various categories of machine.

3.1   PCs, workstations, and networks

The personal computer (PC) and the personal workstation are both designed to be used on the scientist's desktop or laboratory workbench, and there are also portable PCs available. They are usually connected to other users' machines, normally within the same or adjacent buildings, via a local area network (LAN). Also connected in the LAN may be 'server' computers; these are set up for some specific type of operation. For example, a compute server provides computational power, a disk server provides centralized on-line storage of programs, data, documentation, etc., a print server provides hardcopy capabilities, a boot server downloads a copy of the operating system to 'diskless' machines on power-up or at the user's request, and a mail server acts as the interface for communications via wide area networks (WANs) to users and machines on other LANs in different buildings, cities, or countries. This is the 'client-server model' of provision of computing resources, whereby the 'client' machines which require specific services are separated physically from the 'server' machines which provide those services (and which may also be in separate locations from one other), and each server may service many clients.

PCs are used for a variety of tasks, perhaps most commonly for word processing (for example in the preparation of scientific reports and papers), as well as for software development and for testing and running programs with cut-down data, for example as a teaching aid. Simple but effective 3D molecular graphics can be done on a PC, provided that the number of atoms is not too great (100 or fewer). Spreadsheet and statistical and graph-plotting programs are available for processing limited quantities of data obtained, for example, by data acquisition directly from a laboratory instrument. Workstations generally possess more powerful processors, and are able to provide much more sophisticated plotting capabilities, such as 3D macromolecular model building in real time. They are also quite powerful general purpose computers in their own right.

The operational system used on PCs is either DOS (disk-operating system) which provides very basic facilities for program and data file manipulation, or Unix, which is much more sophisticated and is becoming generally recognized as the 'universal' operating system, now available on PCs, workstations, mid-range computers, and supercomputers. However, the uninitiated user needs to be aware that the implementations of DOS and Unix currently available do not adhere to any universally recognized standard, which means that although the commands by which the user requests the operating system to perform specific actions may appear on first sight to be identical on different machines, there are very likely to be commands and command qualifiers which are not in common, or which perform different actions. This situation can be more confusing than having to learn two completely different sets of operating system commands.

A piece of software commonly associated with DOS or Unix is a 'windowing' system, such as X-windows. This provides the user with a mode of working which frees him/her from having to wait for the computer to complete one task before issuing the command to start another, and just as importantly to retain the environment in which the original command was issued, so that all the relevant information is always available on the display screen. For example, one might want to break off in the middle of writing a report to perform a calculation, plot the results, and then return to writing the report, using the plot as a diagram in the report, and perhaps doing this several times.

3.2   Supercomputers

Supercomputers such as the Cray X-MP or the Convex C3800 are available in the UK for academic users at the national supercomputer laboratories in London, Rutherford, and Manchester. Although the Cray machines have more than one processor, they are not often used in parallel mode. Optimization of sequential code to take account of the machines' vector abilities provides significant increase in the speed of many calculations. One of the main modelling applications which takes full advantage of such a supercomputer is that of molecular dynamics. Vectorized code is available for the AMBER and GROMOS software packages (see the chapter on computer simulation). Although the dynamics of small proteins *in vacuo* may be simulated on less powerful computers, large-scale simulation of solvated proteins, estimation of free energy calculations, and the use of path integral methods to simulate quantum particles in classical molecules are frequently undertaken on a supercomputer. A related area which makes similar use of the power of supercomputers is that of quantum chemistry, and packages such as GAMES, CADPAC, QUEST, and GAUSSIAN can all be run on the Cray. A wide range of applications with specific use of the power of supercomputers in the UK is given in a review of Supercomputer Assisted Research (ULCC, 1989).

3.3   Parallel architecture machines

The idea that the speed of sequential computers is inherently limited has led to the development of computers with parallel architecture. These include machines such as the DAP, Intel hypercube, and transputer based hardware such as the Meiko Computing Surface. In the UK, there are a number of centres for parallel computing including those at Edinburgh and Southampton. Parallelized code has been written for some applications relevant to computer modelling of biological molecules, but in general it is very labour intensive.

REFERENCES

Atkins, P.W. (1987) *Molecules*, Scientific American Library.

Bernstein, F.C., Koetzle, T.F., Williams, G.J.B., Meyer, E.F., Brice, M.D., Rodgers, J.R., Kennard, O., Shimanouchi, T. and Tasumi, M. (1977) The Protein Data Bank: a computer-based archival file for macromolecular structures, *J. Mol. Biol.*, **112**, 535–542.

Branden, C. and Tooze, J. (1991) *Introduction to Protein Structure*, Garland Publishing, London.

Cotterill, R. (1985). *The Cambridge Guide to the Material World*, CUP.

Saenger, W. (1983) *Principles of Nucleic Acid Structure*, Springer-Verlag, New York.

Schulz, G.E. and Schirmer, R.H. (1979) *Principles of Protein Structure*, Springer-Verlag, New York.

Stryer, L. (1988) *Biochemistry* (3rd edn) W.H. Freeman, New York.

2

Molecular geometry

David S. Moss
Department of Crystallography, Birkbeck College, Malet Street,
London WC1E 7HX

1. INTRODUCTION

This chapter introduces the reader to the most useful mathematical techniques used
in the description, manipulation, and display of molecular structures on a computer
system.

2. NOTATION

Molecular geometry calculations are often expressed in terms of vectors and matrices.
It is assumed that the reader already has an elementary understanding of vector and
matrix manipulation and also understands determinants and matrix inverses.

In this chapter the following conventions are used. Scalar quantities are designated
by italicized letters such as x. Vector quantities and matrices are expressed as bold
lower case letters such as $\mathbf{a}$. Rectangular or square matrices are represented by
uppercase bold symbols such as $\mathbf{A}$. Primed symbols represent transposed quantities
so that $\mathbf{x}$ represents a column matrix and $\mathbf{x}'$ denotes its transpose.

3. COORDINATE SYSTEMS

The positions of atoms in space are determined in terms of coordinate systems.
Coordinate systems may be classified as *internal* or *external*. In *internal coordinates*
only the relative positions of the atoms are determined by the coordinates. Thus a
molecule might be described in terms of bond lengths, bond angles, and torsion
angles. In external coordinates, the position of each atom with respect to a frame of

reference in space is denoted by three numbers called *external coordinates*. Cartesian coordinates and spherical polar coordinates are examples.

4.   EXTERNAL COORDINATES

The most appropriate general purpose external coordinates are those where the position of each atom is described by three numbers. Formally these three numbers (x, y, z) are the components of a position vector $(\mathbf{r})$ of the atom which expresses the atomic position in terms of three *base vectors* $(\mathbf{a}, \mathbf{b}, \mathbf{c})$ emanating from an origin O. In terms of these vectors the position vector can be expressed as

$$\mathbf{r} = x\mathbf{a} + y\mathbf{b} + z\mathbf{c}$$

By convention the base vectors are always chosen to form a *positive triad*. Mathematically this means that **a.bxc** is chosen to be positive. To see when this is

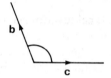

Fig. 1. Base vector convention looking along positive direction of **a**.

so, look along the positive direction of **a**, and **c** should follow **b** in a clockwise sense. This is illustrated in Fig. 1.

In crystallography base vectors are used which define a parallelepiped in the crystal called the *unit cell* and the coordinates are then known as *fractional coordinates*. Fractional coordinates are often used in crystallography because the coordinates of symmetry-related molecules can be generated in the crystal by simple transformations.

An important matrix associated with the base vectors of a coordinate system is the *metric matrix* $(\mathbf{G})$. This matrix is required when molecular geometry calculations are carried out by using fraction coordinates. The elements of the metric matrix are the scalar products of the base vectors as shown in (1)

$$\mathbf{G} = \begin{bmatrix} a^2 & ab\cos\gamma & ac\cos\beta \\ ba\cos\gamma & b^2 & bc\cos\alpha \\ ca\cos\beta & cb\cos\alpha & c^2 \end{bmatrix} \tag{1}$$

where a, b, and c are the lengths of the base vectors and α, β and γ are the angles between the pairs of vectors $(\mathbf{b}, \mathbf{c})$, $(\mathbf{c}, \mathbf{a})$, and $(\mathbf{a}, \mathbf{b})$ respectively. By using this matrix it is possible to calculate interatomic distances from the fractional coordinates of the atoms. If $\mathbf{x}_A$ and $\mathbf{x}_B$ are two column matrices containing the fractional coordinates of atoms A and B, then the interatomic distance is given by

$$l^2 = \mathbf{x}'_{AB}\mathbf{G}\mathbf{x}_{AB} \tag{2}$$

where

$$x_{AB} = x_A - x_b \tag{3}$$

The unit vectors and right angles in the cartesian base mean that the associated metric matrix is a unit matrix. This can be seen by making the appropriate substitutions in (1). Thus if x_A and x_B contain cartesian coordinates, then (2) simplifies to

$$l^2 = x'_{AB}x_{AB} \tag{4}$$

This is simply Pythagoras' Theorem in three dimensions. Thus the use of cartesian coordinates results in a simplified expression for the distance that does not include metric matrix coefficients. The same is true for other molecular geometry calculations, therefore it is usual to transform fractional coordinates to cartesian coordinates before carrying out geometrical calculations.

5. FRACTIONAL TO CARTESIAN COORDINATE TRANSFORMATIONS

To carry out this transformation, the directions of the cartesian base vectors (i, j, and k) must be chosen relative to the unit cell vectors (a, b, and c). This may be done in an infinite number of ways, and there are several conventions for their relative orientation. The convention presented here is that adopted by the Brookhaven Database for the transformation of macromolecular fractional coordinates to the cartesian coordinates which are stored in the database. In this convention i lies along

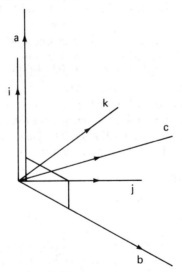

Fig. 2. Brookhaven vector convention.

a, j lies in the ab plane, and k completes the right-handed triad. This is illustrated in Fig. 2. A column x containing the fractional coordinates of an atom can be transformed to cartesian coordinates in a column x_0 by the matrix transformation

$$x_0 = Rx \tag{5}$$

where

$$\mathbf{R} = \begin{bmatrix} a & b\cos\gamma & c\cos\beta \\ 0 & b\sin\gamma & (c[\cos\alpha-\cos\beta\cos\gamma]/\sin\gamma) \\ 0 & 0 & V/(ab\sin\gamma) \end{bmatrix}$$

Sometimes it is necessary to transform cartesian coordinates back to fractional coordinates. This might arise in the study of intermolecular contacts in a crystal when it might be necessary to regenerate the fractional coordinates in order to compute the coordinates of symmetry-related molecules in the crystal. For this transformation we require the inverse of the matrix R.

$$\mathbf{x} = \mathbf{R}^{-1}\mathbf{x}_0 \tag{6}$$

where

$$\mathbf{R}^{-1} = \begin{bmatrix} 1/a & -\cos\gamma/(a\sin\gamma) & bc(\cos\gamma\cos\alpha - \cos\beta)/(V\sin\gamma) \\ 0 & 1/(b\sin\gamma) & ca(\cos\beta\cos\gamma - \cos\alpha)/(V\sin\gamma) \\ 0 & 0 & ab\sin\gamma/V \end{bmatrix}$$

In the above matrix, V is the volume of the crystallographic cell (which is the square root of the determinant of **G**) and is

$$V = abc\,(1-\cos^2\alpha-\cos^2\beta-\cos^2\gamma + 2\cos\alpha\cos\beta\cos\gamma) \tag{7}$$

6. BOND ANGLES

In the rest of this chapter it will be assumed that atomic coordinates are cartesian. A frequent calculation is that of a bond angle. Given three atoms A, B, and C as

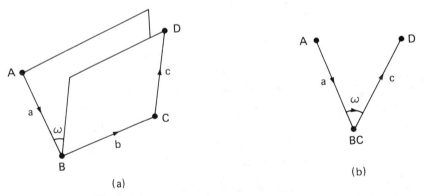

Fig. 3. Calculation of bond angle and torsion angle.

shown in Fig. 3(a) then the angle θ between the vectors **a** and **b** can be calculated from the dot product.

$$\mathbf{a}.\mathbf{b} = l_{AB}l_{BC}\cos\theta \tag{8}$$

so that

$$\theta = \arccos(\mathbf{x}'_{AB}\mathbf{x}_{BC}/(l_{AB}l_{BC})) \tag{9}$$

The bond angle will be in the range $0 < = \theta < 180$ degrees, and arccos is available as the function acos in Fortran or C.

7. TORSION ANGLES

Given four atoms, A, B, C, and D, as shown in Fig. 3, the torsion angle ω associated with the torsion axis BC is the angle between the planes ABC and BCD. If the four atoms are non-coplanar, then when viewed along the torsion axis, as in Fig. 3(b), there will either be a clockwise or anticlockwise sense of screw when moving from atom A to atom D. By convention the torsion angle is positive for a clockwise screw and negative if the screw is anticlockwise. If the four atoms are reflected in a mirror the sense of screw will change, hence the torsion angle is sensitive to the chirality of the molecule. Unless a molecule possesses an improper symmetry operation, it will be physically distinguishable from its mirror image and the molecule and its mirror image will have torsion angles of opposite sign. To calculate the torsion angle, we require the the vectors **a**, **b** and **c** which are shown in Figure 3(a). In terms of these vectors the $\cos\omega$ is given by

$$\cos\omega = \frac{(\mathbf{a} \times \mathbf{b}) \cdot (\mathbf{b} \times \mathbf{c})}{|\mathbf{a} \times \mathbf{b}| \, |\mathbf{b} \times \mathbf{c}|}$$

To find the sign of ω, the triple scalar product **a.(bxc)** is calculated by evaluating the determinant of the matrix

$$\begin{bmatrix} a_x & a_y & a_z \\ b_x & b_y & b_z \\ c_x & c_y & c_z \end{bmatrix} \tag{10}$$

where the rows of the matrix are the components of the vectors. The sign of the determinant is the sign of the torsion angle.

Details of the torsion angle calculation may be seen in the computer program in the Appendix to this chapter.

8.   LEAST SQUARES PLANES AND LINES

Frequently it is required to find the 'best' plane or line through a set of N atoms. This is done by setting up the 3×3 variance–covariance matrix C of the set. The elements of this symmetric matrix are given by the equations

$$C_{11} = (\Sigma x^2)/N - (\Sigma x/N)^2 \tag{11}$$

$$C_{12} = C_{21} = (\Sigma xy)/N - (\Sigma x \Sigma y)/N^2 \tag{12}$$

and analogous equations for the other four matrix elements. The next step is to find the three eigenvectors(v) of **C** and the corresponding eigenvalues(λ). The eigenvectors are (3 × 1) column matrices and the eigenvalues are scalar quantities. They satisfy the equation

$$\mathbf{Cv} = \lambda \mathbf{v} \tag{13}$$

Subroutines to solve these equations are widely available, and they usually return the eigenvectors as the columns of a (3 × 3) array. The columns are usually normalized so that the sum of the squares of the elements is unity. Each column therefore contains the coefficients of a unit vector which defines a direction in the molecule. The interpretation of these vectors and the associated eigenvalues is as follows.

The smallest eigenvalue corresponds to the mean square deviation of the atoms from the least squares plane and the corresponding eigenvector is perpendicular to the plane. The 'best view' of a molecule, which gives rise to minimum overlap of atoms, is obtained by viewing along this eigenvector. To plot the coordinates (x_p, y_p) of the atoms as seen in this projection the scalar products of the cartesian coordinates $(\mathbf{x}_0)$ with the two smallest eigenvectors $(\mathbf{v}_1, \mathbf{v}_2)$ are

$$x_p = \mathbf{v}_1' \mathbf{x}_0 \quad y_p = \mathbf{v}_2' \mathbf{x}_0 \tag{14}$$

Sometimes the least squares line is of more interest. For example, the atoms may form the backbone of an α-helix, and it may be required to find its axis. In this case the largest eigenvalue corresponds to the eigenvector which lies along the axis of the helix. This is the direction of the least squares line. The mean square distance of the atoms from the helix axis is given by the sum of the two smallest eigenvalues.

9. INTERNAL COORDINATES

Molecular geometry may be specified completely in terms of bond lengths, bond angles, and torsion angles. These are *internal coordinates* because they do not relate the molecule to any frame of reference outside itself. Cartesian coordinates are external because they refer the positions to an origin point and they specify an orientation for the molecule. Fractional coordinates are also external because they specify the molecular orientation and/or position with respect to crystal symmetry elements.

It requires $3N$ external coordinates to specify the geometry of a molecule; that is, three for each of the N atoms. It requires only $3N$-6 internal coordinates to specify molecular geometry because six coordinates (three translational and three orientational) are not required for locating the molecule within its frame of reference.

10. Z-MATRIX

To specify the $3N$-6 coordinates, consider the molecule shown in Fig. 4. Atom 1 does not require any internal coordinate. Atom 2 requires a bond distance l_1. Atom 3 requires both a bond distance l_2 and a bond angle θ_1. Atom 4 requires a bond length

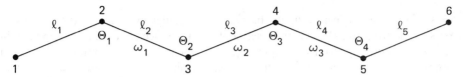

Fig. 4. Internal coordinates of a schematic molecule.

l_3, a bond angle θ_2, and a torsion angle ω_1. Subsequent atoms all require a bond length, bond angle, and torsion angle. These requirements can be specified in a matrix which is known as a Z-matrix. The Z-matrix shown below specifies the geometry of the molecule in Fig. 4.

$$
\begin{bmatrix}
l_1 & 0 & 0 \\
l_2 & \theta_1 & 0 \\
l_3 & \theta_2 & \omega_1 \\
l_4 & \theta_3 & \omega_2 \\
l_5 & \theta_4 & \omega_3
\end{bmatrix}
$$

11. ROTATION ABOUT A BOND

Sometimes it is required to rotate selected atoms of a molecule about a bond. This may arise when the energy of a molecule is required as a function of some of its torsion angles. To rotate the atoms round the bond through an angle ϕ, it is first necessary to compute the components of a unit vector along the bond which is to be the rotation axis. If the two atoms of the bond have coordinates $\mathbf{x}_A$ and $\mathbf{x}_B$, the column matrix containing the components of the unit vector is formed by calculating

$$\mathbf{x}_{AB} = \mathbf{x}_A - \mathbf{x}_B \quad \mathbf{n} = \mathbf{x}_{AB}/\mathbf{x}_{AB} \tag{15}$$

The components of n are then used to form the rotation matrix $\mathbf{R}$ in which θ is the angle through which the atom is to be rotated. Clockwise rotations are expressed by positive θ and anticlockwise rotations be negative θ.

   The coordinates of an atom in the column matrix $\mathbf{x}_C$ are rotated about the bond by premultiplication by the matrix $\mathbf{R}$ to yield the rotated coordinates in the column matrix $\mathbf{x}_D$:

$$\mathbf{x}_D = \mathbf{R}\mathbf{x}_C \tag{16}$$

The matrix $\mathbf{R}$ is shown on page 75.

12. STRUCTURAL COMPARISON OF MOLECULES

A measure of the geometrical similarity between two molecules may be obtained by superimposing the molecules over each other so as to minimize the sum of the squared distances between corresponding atoms. For example, the two molecules may be proteins which show some topological similarity. In this case the main-chain atoms of the two molecules might be chosen for superposition. First, the pairs of atoms to be fitted together must be selected from the two molecules. In the protein example, it may be possible to match every main-chain atom in one molecule with a topologically equivalent atom in the second molecule. In other cases deletions may be required in one sequence before the atoms can be meaningfully paired. When this has been done, the sum of the squared distances (M) between the corresponding pairs of atoms can be minimized. M can be calculated using a three-dimensional Pythagorean formula

$$M = \Sigma(x_1 - x_2)^2 + (y_1 - y_2)^2 + (z_1 - z_2)^2 \tag{17}$$

where the subscripts 1 and 2 refer to molecules 1 and 2 and the summation is carried out over all pairs of atoms selected for the superposition. The minimum of M always occurs when the centroids of the molecules are superimposed over each other, and therefore we can consider the above coordinates to be referred to the centroids of their respective molecules as origin.

Many methods have been proposed for finding the rotation that minimizes M. The literature has been reviewed by Diamond (1988). The simplest methods require the computation of the eigenvectors and eigenvalues of a 4×4 matrix. If $x_m = (x_1 - x_2)$ and $x_p = (x_1 + x_2)$ with similar definitions for y_m, y_p, z_m, and z_p then the symmetric matrix

$$\begin{bmatrix} \Sigma(x_m^2 + y_m^2 + z_m^2) & \Sigma(y_p z_m - y_m z_p) & \Sigma(x_m z_p - x_p z_m) & \Sigma(x_p y_m - x_m y_p) \\ \Sigma(y_p z_m - y_m z_p) & \Sigma(y_p^2 + z_p^2 + x_m^2) & \Sigma(x_m y_m - x_p y_p) & \Sigma(x_m z_m - x_p z_p) \\ \Sigma(x_m z_p - x_p z_m) & \Sigma(x_m y_m - x_p y_p) & \Sigma(x_p^2 + z_p^2 + y_m^2) & \Sigma(y_m z_m - y_p z_p) \\ \Sigma(x_p y_m - x_m y_p) & \Sigma(x_m z_m - x_p z_p) & \Sigma(y_m z_m - y_p z_p) & \Sigma(x_p^2 + y_p^2 + z_m^2) \end{bmatrix} \tag{18}$$

has its smallest eigenvalue equal to the minimum of M (Kearsley 1989). The corresponding normalized eigenvector is what is known as a *unit quaternion* and has components

$$[\cos(\theta/2), l\sin(\theta/2), m\sin(\theta/2), n\sin(\theta/2)] \tag{19}$$

where θ is the rotation about an axis with direction cosines (l, m, n) that will give the least squares superposition of molecule 2 upon molecule 1.

The square root of M divided by the number of atom pairs is then quoted as the root mean square (rms) difference between the two molecules. When quoting rms differences it is important to make clear how the comparison has been carried out. For example, when comparing protein molecules, a higher rms difference will generally result if all atoms are used rather than main-chain atoms only.

13. DISTANCE PLOTS

The chain fold of a protein molecule can be represented by a distance plot, which is a map of the interatomic distances in the protein represented in a square matrix. In its simplest form the rows and columns of the matrix may correspond to the alpha carbon atoms of the protein, and a non-blank entry may appear in the matrix at each position where the corresponding alpha carbon atoms are greater than a certain distance apart. Figure 5 shows a distance plot using every fifth alpha carbon atom in apo-lactate dehydrogenase. The circles are printed at positions where the inter-atomic distance is less than 160A. More sophisticated presentations of these matrices use contour maps where each contour represents a certain distance.

Different features of secondary structure give rise to particular patterns in these maps. Alpha helices, for example, give rise to short distances close to the diagonal. The domain structure of a protein may also be revealed by these plots. In Fig. 5 the four domains of apo-lactate dehydrogenase are clearly seen as four clusters of circles along the diagonal.

Another useful plot is the difference distance plot, which is simply the difference between two distance plots from different proteins. It can reveal the regions where two structurally similar proteins differ. For example, if the two proteins each contain similar domains but in different relative orientations, then the difference distance plot will show up only the inter-domain distances.

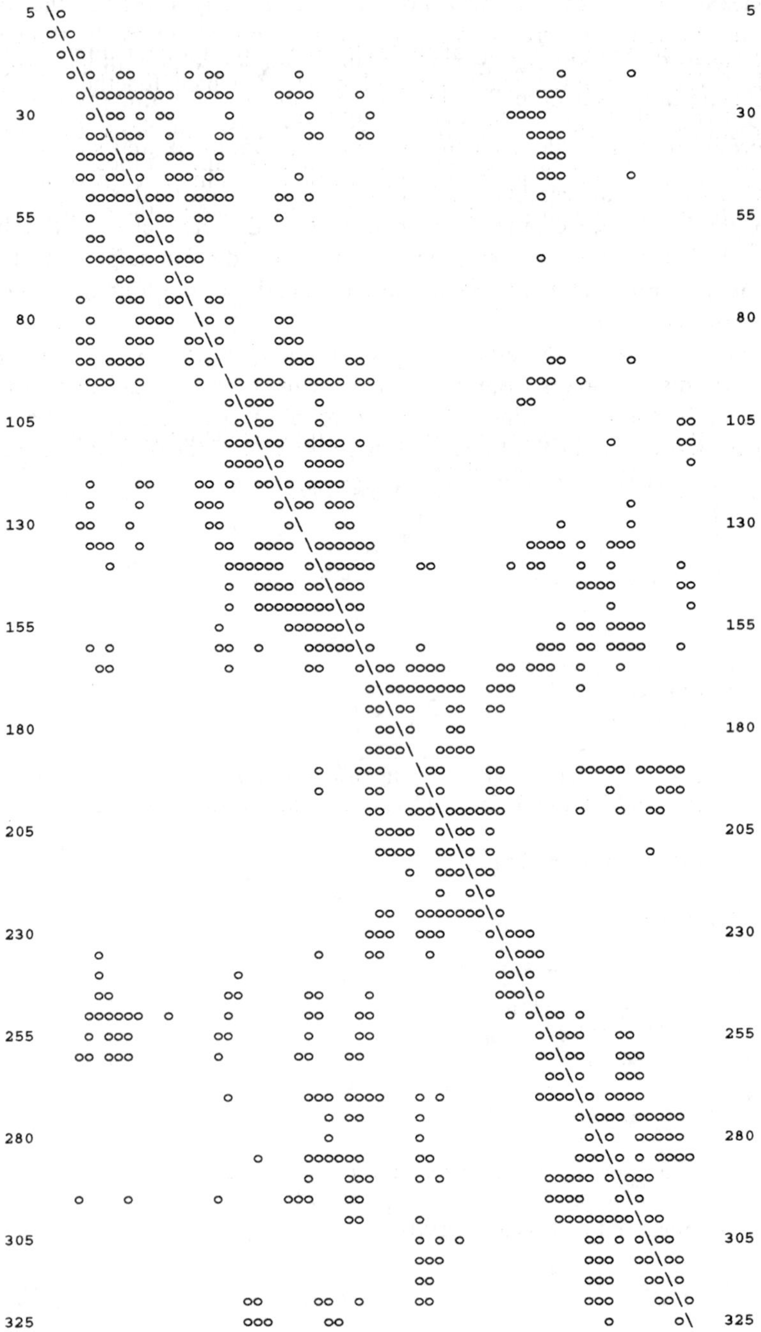

Fig. 5. Distance plot of a chainfold of an apo-lactate dehydrogenase. The numbers down the sides are residue numbers and four similar domains are shown by the repeating pattern along the diagonal.

APPENDIX

The following computer program calculates the main chain torsion angles of a protein molecule. It is written in the programming language C which, together with Fortran, is widely used in modern biomolecular computing.

The program reads a file from the Brookhaven Databank and stores the names of the residues and coordinates of the main-chain atoms in an array of structures. A function torsion is then called once for each torsion angle and the results are printed in a table.

```
/* program to calculate torsion angles from the main-chain atoms
   of a protein from a Brookhaven file
                        D S Moss  1991
*/

/* preprocessor directives */

#include <stdio.h>
#include <stdlib.h>
#include <string.h>
#include <math.h>

#define MAXATS 1000     /* dimension of atom array */
#define RADDEG 57.2958  /* converts radians to degrees */

/* external variables */

typedef struct
        {
        char resname[4];
        char resnum[7];
        float xyz[3];
        } Atom;

float torsion(Atom *pt[]);

/* main program to read Brookhaven file and call function torsion */

void main(int argc, char *argv[])
        {
```

```
int i, j, k, natoms;
char brkfile[20], line[100], field[9],
        *atom_name[3] = {"N ","CA","C "};
Atom atom[MAXATS], *pt[4];
FILE *fptr;

/* check that file name has been supplied */
if (argc!=2)
{
        printf("Data file name required\n");
        exit(1);
}

/* construct path name of Brookhaven file */
strcpy(brkfile,"\\brk\\");
strcat(brkfile,argv[1]);
strcat(brkfile,".brk");

/* check that Brookhaven file can be opened */
if ((fptr=fopen(brkfile,"r")) == NULL)
{
        printf("File %s cannot be opened\n",brkfile);
        exit(1);
}

/* search Brookhaven file for atom records
   check for no of atoms exceeding MAXATS */
i=0;
while(fgets(line,100,fptr) != NULL && i<MAXATS)
        /* is it an ATOM record? */
        if (strncmp(line,"ATOM",4)==0)
                for(k=0; k<3; k++)
                        /* is it N, CA or C ? */
                        if (strncmp(line+13,atom_name[k],2)==0)
                        {
                                /* extract residue name */
                                strncpy(atom[i].resname,line+17,3);
                                atom[i].resname[3]='\0';
                                /* extract residue identifier */
                                strncpy(atom[i].resnum,line+21,6);
                                atom[i].resnum[6]='\0';
                                /* extract x, y and z */
                                field[8]='\0';
                                strncpy(field,line+30,8);
                                atom[i].xyz[0]=atof(field);
                                strncpy(field,line+38,8);
                                atom[i].xyz[1]=atof(field);
                                strncpy(field,line+46,8);
                                atom[i].xyz[2]=atof(field);
```

```
                                 i+ +;
                                 break;
                         }
        natoms = i;
        printf("\n\n*** Main-chain torsion angles of %s                ***",argv[1]);
        printf("\n\n%d main-chain atoms read\n\n",natoms);
        fclose(fptr);

        printf(" Residue\n");
        printf("Name Number   phi    psi    omega\n");
        printf("%4.3s%8.6s        ",atom[0].resname,atom[0].resnum);

        /* loop over the atoms */
        for (i=0; i<natoms-3; i+ +)
        {
                k=i+1;
                if (k%3= =0)

printf("\n%4.3s%8.6s",atom[k].resname,atom[k].resnum);
                /* set up pointers to atoms in torsion angle */
                for (j=0; j<4; j+ +)
                        pt[j]=atom+i+j;
                /* call function to calculate torsion angle then
                 print it */
                printf( "%8.1f",torsion(pt));
        }

}


/* function to calculate a torsion angle from the
   Cartesian co-ordinates of four atoms */

float torsion(Atom *pt[])

/* pt is an array of pointers to structures containing
   the co-ordinates of four atoms A, B, C and D */

{
        int i,j,k;
        float len_ABC,len_BCD,scalarprod,absangle,tsprod,
                vec[3][3],perp_ABC[3],perp_BCD[3];

        /* find the components of the four bond vectors */
        for (i=0; i<3; i+ +)
        {
                for (j=0; j<3; j+ +)
                        vec[i][j]=pt[i+1]->xyz[j]-pt[i]->xyz[j];
        }
```

```
/* calculate vectors perpendicular to the planes
   ABC & BCD */
len_ABC=0.0;
len_BCD=0.0;
for (i=0; i<3; i++)
{
        j=(i+1)%3;
        k=(j+1)%3;
        perp_ABC[i]=vec[0][j]*vec[1][k]-vec[0][k]*vec[1][j];
        len_ABC+=perp_ABC[i]*perp_ABC[i];
        perp_BCD[i]=vec[1][j]*vec[2][k]-vec[1][k]*vec[2][j];
        len_BCD+=perp_BCD[i]*perp_BCD[i];
}
len_ABC=sqrt(len_ABC);
len_BCD=sqrt(len_BCD);

/* normalise the vectors perpendicular to ABC & BCD
   by dividing by their lengths */
for (i=0; i<3; i++)
{
        perp_ABC[i]=perp_ABC[i]/len_ABC;
        perp_BCD[i]=perp_BCD[i]/len_BCD;
}

/* find the scalar product of the unit normals */
scalarprod=0.0;
for (i=0; i<3; i++)
        scalarprod+=perp_ABC[i]*perp_BCD[i];

/* find the absolute value of the torsion angle
   in degrees */
absangle= RADDEG*acos(scalarprod);

/* find the triple scalar product of the three
   bond vectors */
tsprod=0.0;
for (i=0; i<3; i++)
        tsprod+=vec[0][i]*perp_BCD[i];

/* torsion angle has the sign of the triple scalar
   product */
return (tsprod > 0.0) ? absangle : -absangle;
}
```

REFERENCES

Diamond, R., (1988) A note on the rotational superposition problem. *Acta Cryst.* **A44**, 211–216.

Kearsley, S.K., (1989) On the orthogonal transformation used for structural comparison. *Acta Cryst.* **A45**, 208–210.

3

Analysis of molecular geometry

P. Murray-Rust
Glaxo Group Research, Greenford, Middlesex, UB6 0HE

1. INTRODUCTION

The determination of molecular structure, especially by X-ray crystallography, yields a remarkable quantity and quality of high-grade numerical information. Perhaps more than in most other sciences this information is directly comparable between different experiments in different laboratories. Moreover, each experiment produces a very large amount of information which is complex and whose interpretation depends on comparison with many other similar molecules. Also, for many years, the World community of crystallographers has archived its results in machine-readable form, so that the computer-aided analysis of molecular geometry is a valuable research activity in its own right.

This chapter will outline the sources of this information and will describe some of the techniques for analysing it. Statistical methods will be described, but they should be used with common sense. A good guideline is that statistical analysis should lead to a re-presentation of the data, so that the conclusions are clear and unambiguous. Graphical presentation is especially valuable here.

After this introduction, the tools and techniques will be described, followed by some detailed case studies selected to give a comprehensive illustration of the methods.

1.1 Rationale for analysing molecular geometry

There is a fundamental assumption that the chemical variation between molecules often reveals itself in the details of the geometry. This is a theme throughout Pauling's classic *The nature of the chemical bond* (1935, 1960) where molecular geometry is used as a touchstone for the bonding processes within molecules and the interaction between them. Pauling had, perhaps, access to less than 0.01% of today's molecular geometry, but his ideas on structure and bonding have stood the test of time. More recently, Dunitz, in *X-ray analysis and the structure of organic molecules*, shows the great amount of reliable structural information available from crystallography (primary of small molecules), and his book forms a valuable reference for many of the ideas later in this chapter.

The analysis of the geometry of 'small' molecules can be highly relevant for biomolecular processes. Many of the substrates in biochemical reactions or receptor agonists or antagonists have been studied by crystallography. Two typical references from meetings organized by the crystallographic community are *Molecular structure and biological activity* (Griffin & Duax) and *X-ray crystallography and drug action* (Horn & De Ranter). These give a good account of the directed X-ray crystallography carried out by medicinal chemists and biologists, and it is now accepted that three-dimensional structure is one of the fundamental determinants of the biological activity of small molecules. Because of this, important classes of biomolecules are almost always well represented in the crystallographic data files (see below).

The three-dimensional structure of macromolecules is the main determinant of their function and action, and the comparative approach is clearly fundamental. Understanding the overall geometry of biomolecules can be thought of as a taxonomic process, but there are many other clues to the function and specificity hidden in their structures. The importance of particular conformations, interactions, or distortions can be assessed only by comparison with similar molecules.

The value of geometrical information for a given molecule is greatly increased by statistical techniques:

(a) As with any experiment, there are errors in crystallography, and these are not always obvious in a single analysis. They are most serious for macromolecules, where there are often serious uncertainties or errors in parts of the structure, especially the loop regions and chain termini. Statistical analysis can often show a 'signal' emerging over the noise of the error.

(b) A molecule in a crystal is distorted from its gas-phase or solvated equililbrium structure by 'crystal-packing forces'. The importance of these is often exaggerated, but they are clearly responsible for low-energy deformations. It has been difficult to quantify the effect for any exception the simplest molecules (hydrocarbons, with a few other functional groups). It is common for torsion angles to be affected by packing forces, as for skeletal deformations (ring pucker, out-of-plane, bending of rodlike and planar molecules). An analysis of a large number of common organic groups suggests that maximum deformation energies rarely exceed 0.3 kcal/mole. Where ionic forces are present (e.g. coordination to metals), distortions can be greater.

Although for a single structure this effect causes worries about the value of the geometry, it can be valuable when several structures involve the same molecule. Distortions from packing forces will show the most likely deformations of the molecule, and these deformations may well be those involved in the biological action.

(c) The transferable functional group approach is fundamental to organic chemistry, and to molecular mechanics. Functional groups (e.g. amides) are frequently found in widely different molecules, and geometrical comparison is a crucial test of whether they are altered by their chemical environment. The reactivity of a group is affected by the neighbouring ligands, and this can sometimes be seen in small changes in geometry.

(d) Force fields for molecular mechanics rely on a large amount of accurate structural information. Anyone wishing to add or edit a functional group in a force field should routinely analyse data from the Cambridge data file.

(e) The intermolecular forces in biomolecules are assumed to be similar to those in small molecules. In particular the analytical form of the interactions is modelled on the same functional groups and atom-based potentials. Organic crystal structures therefore provide an essential source of information on the geometrical aspects of intermolecular interaction, and multivariate statistics are an important technique.

The emphasis on this chapter will be on the strategy of comparing molecules and the methodology, rather than on a comprehensive review of results.

2. DATA

The importance of archiving crystallographic data was foreseen by Bernal (1965) who wrote:

> However large an array of facts, however rapidly they accumulate, it is possible to keep them in order and to extract from time to time digests containing the most generally significant information while indicating how to find those items of specialized interest. To do so, however, requires the will and the means.

The crystallographic datafiles (Brookhaven, Cambridge, and Inorganic) are now becoming more available in individual laboratories. They are of enormous value, and any criticisms below are minor and will disappear.

It is not always straightforward to carry out searches and statistical analyses. This is in part due to the lack of generally available software, although many laboratories have their own in-house programs for search and analysis. The present situation is roughly as outlined below.

2.1 Protein Data Bank (Brookhaven)

This file contains coordinate data for all published protein structures, where the authors have deposited them. There is a growing consensus of the need for comprehensive deposition, but many existing structures are not in, and some recent ones have a delay on the release on data.

Brookhaven is very widely available as flat ASCII files, and is almost certainly present in any macromolecular laboratory. There is no software supplied for searching or analysis. A common problem in the deposited data is that authors often differ slightly in the types of data deposited, the nomenclature, and the usage of the fields (e.g. in the ATOM records). The 'PDB' files read and written by modelling systems and crystallographic packages may also show slight variations, so that users cannot always rely on atom, residue, or chain nomenclature to describe connectivity. Ligands and other prosthetic groups are also not always consistently described. For this reason, most comparison of macromolecules has up to now been done within graphics packages or with local programs.

There are several hopeful signs of more widely useful software. The Protein Engineering Club research at Birkbeck led to a prototype database originally based on the relational model (BIPED). A major benefit of this was that the Birkbeck group standardized the individual PDB files into relational tables, and defined the basis of the information (e.g what is a 'helix', 'salt bridge', etc). These tables were accessible under the relational database management system (RDBMS) ORACLE. Searches can be carried out on a hierarchical set of concepts developed by the group (e.g. STRUCTURE, CHAIN, RESIDUE, ATOM properties) which, through the relational, model, can be very powerful. As an example, consider the question:

'How likely is a potentially glycosylatable Asparagine to be buried?'

With the properties provided in the RESIDUE table (there are over 250 column names) this apparently complex question can be answered by using the query language SQL as shown in Table 1.

The query not only retrieves the appropriate residues, but also prints out ordered numerical information (in this case the accessibility). In many cases the RDBMS is coupled to tools to analyse these data, for example by producing a histogram. Up till now, however, the installation and operation of RDBMSs has generally been expensive and complex, so that it has mainly been available through central facilities such as SEQNET at Daresbury (UK).

To surmount the overheads of the RDBMS system, an alternative to BIPED was developed, 3D-SCAN (now developed into IDITIS). This uses an SQL-like query, and uses a smaller set of the columns in the tables. In addition it is able to deal with protein sequence in an efficient manner instead of the APn fields of BIPED.

With BIPED and IDITIS there is great scope for research into protein structure, provided that precautions are taken. It is extremely important to understand the errors in the data. Firstly a (very) few structures have gross errors due to misinterpretation of the electron density maps, whilse many will have dubious regions, especially in loops and at lower resolution than about 2.5 Å. Residues and groups are sometimes disordered and one or two conformers may be present. In almost all structures some element of constraints or restraints will have been used during refinement, so that groups will have been forced to conform to a specified mean geometry and variance. (Bond lengths and angles, along with planarity of rings, are almost certain to reflect the constraints rather than the 'true' values').

Perhaps the most serious limitation of the software is that questions can be asked only about proteins. Nucleic acids have not been included, nor have any liganded molecules. For example, it would be impossible to analyse metal coordination or the geometry of sugars.

2.2 Cambridge Crystallographic Data File

This has been set up over two decades and it contains all published organic/organo-metallic crystal structures. Most journals now routinely require deposition of

Table 1

Using BIPED to answer the question: 'How likely is a potential glycosylatable asparagine to be buried?'. This question can be answered solely from the RESIDUE table. The glycosylation site is $NX(S, T)$ and requires the use of the AP columns which give the one-letter symbols for the 20 residues following the current residue. The accessibility of the residue (RRESQ) has been pre-calculated for the protein (in the quaternary structure).

To aid the interpretation of the results, they are sorted on the accessibility.

The SQL query (newlines are solely for readability and /*...*/ are comments):

```
/* Select all glycosylatable Asn and report secondary structure */
SELECT
        UNIQID,         /* Unique ID for residue */
        RRESQ,          /* Fractional accessibility */
        STRK,           /* Secondary structure (e.g. H for helix */
        SEQID,          /* Residue ID, usually from the author */
FROM                    /* which table to use */
        RESIDUE         /* the RESIDUE table */
WHERE                   /* relational operators */
        NAME = 'ASN'    /* residue name = Asparagine */
AND (
                AP2 = 'S' /* Serine at position i + 2 */
        OR
                AP2 = 'T' /* or a Threonine */
        )
AND RRESQ < 20.0        /* 20% exposed */
ORDER BY RRESQ DESC /* Sort by exposure in descending order */
```

Typical results are:

UNIQID	RRESQ	S	SEQID
1SIC.E.0123.0.0.0.0.0	19.2		123
2CPP.0.0149.0.0.0.0.0	19.1	E	149
....			
1GPD.G.0146.0.0.0.0.0	0.0	B	146
4CTS.A.0242.0.0.0.0.0	0.0	H	242
1HMG.E.0038.0.0.0.0.0	0.0		38

100 records selected

Note the UNIQID column which defines every residue in the database uniquely (protein.chain.residue__number).

coordinates. Considerable effort goes into each entry, including checks for typographical errors and other data corruption. The CCDC group add a machine-searchable record of the chemical connectivity. The coordinate data and the chemical connectivity are now matched for most entries in the file, so that it is possible to identify chemical entities in the crystal structure. Software for searching is available with the file, and it allows retrieval by textual, chemical, or numerical data.

This was the first file which it was possible to search for molecular geometry and to analyse the results. The program GEOSTAT (Motherwell + Murray-Rust & Raftery) (now called GSTAT) allows the user to define a set of atoms with chemical and geometrical constraints and to produce an ordered table of the results (independent of the authors' numbering or the chemical nature of the entry). GEOSTAT can require that atoms are bonded, but this is not essential. It is therefore straightforward to search for more general assemblies than functional groups such as hydrogen bonds or metal coordination, or even groups which are not bonded at all. GEOSTAT is thus an extremely useful tool for analysing the geometry of molecular interactions.

2.3   Inorganic Datafile (ICSD)
The inorganic crystallographic datafile is the least widely distributed of the three. It contains a substantial amount of the published inorganic and mineralogical information, which may be relevant to some biomolecules. It is often accessed on-line at a central location, using software based on a large number of search keys. Searching on a combination of elements is straightforward, but there is no chemical connectivity.

2.4   General considerations when using datafiles
Although the quality of data in the files is high, users should spend a considerable time browsing through them with simple search queries. Often there is a preponderance of multiple entries for certain classes of molecule. Problems can occur with crystallographic symmetry. Often, if a molecule lies on a crystallographic symmetry element only the asymmetric units of the data are given, so that a search may fail. In this case it may be necessary to expand the coordinate data to include symmetry-related molecules or parts of molecules; this is an option in GEOSTAT, but not in the other software. For the analysis of intermolecular interactions this expansion will be essential.

Users should be aware that the datafiles will contain 'outliers'. These are structures significantly different from the others, possibly because they represent a so far unique type, but also because they may have serious errors. It will often be necessary to exclude these structures before an analysis. Where a large number of very similar molecules are included in the datafiles, the statistics will be biased, and users should be careful not to draw fallacious conclusions. For small molecules it can be useful to exclude structures with poor R-factors (say above 0.08) or which have not been determined recently, but in general the quality of modern small-molecule structures determined on diffracometers with modern software is consistently high and independent of laboratory.

2.5   Other sources of data
A number of proteins have been studied by high-field NMR and are being deposited in Brookhaven. The emerging convention is often to describe these as a family of structures, derived from molecular dynamics or distance geometry techniques. The

statistical methods I shall describe are also extremely useful for analysing the results of molecular dynamics calculations; in fact it is difficult to see how these can be fully appreciated without computer analysis.

Molecular structure can also be calculated by empirical methods (molecular mechanics) or quantum mechanical calculations of various degrees of accuracy, and there may be times when comparison of geometrical properties is valuable.

3. COMPARISON OF MOLECULAR GEOMETRY

The question of how similar one molecule is to another will normally entail a subjective choice of method and reference criteria. Many different approaches have been developed to relate the biological activity of molecules to their three-dimensional structure. Geometrical properties used include molecular volume, van der Waals surface, moments of inertia, and topological indices derived from the connection table. These are often coupled with properties calculated by quantum mechanical methods, such as charge density, electrostatic field and potential, dipole and higher moments, energies of frontier orbitals, and many others. Some of these require the molecules to be aligned or superimposed by, for example, maximizing the overlap betwen the charge distributions. These approaches have often been coupled with multivariate statistical techniques to look for patterns or clusters in the data.

Here the comparison is restricted either to identical molecules (from different experiments or in different environments) or to identical groups (e.g. amides) in different molecules. It is assumed that there is an objectively defined one-to-one correspondence of the atoms in the groups or molecules. Either internal coordinates (bond length, angles, torsion angles, interplanar angles, pseudorotation pucker, etc.) or the cartesian coordinates can be used as the variates.

If the cartesian coordinates of molecules are to be compared, the molecules must be superimposed. For 2 molecules, the squared difference between the fitted molecules is minimized. Representing each molecule of m atoms as $3m$ matrices $x1$ and $x2$, we have:

R and **t** are the rotation and translation required to fit the molecules

$$\mathbf{x2'} = \mathbf{R}.\mathbf{x2} + \mathbf{t}$$

$$\Delta = (|\mathbf{x1} - \mathbf{x2'}|)^2.$$

then minimize so that $\delta\Delta/\delta\mathbf{R} = \delta\Delta/\delta\mathbf{t} = 0$.

For several (n) molecules the problem is less straightforward. GEOSTAT uses an iterative procedure where each molecule is individually fitted to a reference molecule (arbitrarily the first) to produce a 'mean' molecule:

$$\bar{\mathbf{x}} = \Sigma(\mathbf{x}_i)/n.$$

The process is then iterated with the mean molecule as the reference until convergence, where the n $3m$-vectors are distributed about the origin. It is important to realize that the mean molecule may be physically misleading and should be used with caution. Its internal coordinates are not the mean internal coordinates of the n molecules. (For example, if two enantiomeric molecules are fitted by this method, the 'mean' molecule will be planar!).

When several molecules are superimposed, especially if only part is flexible, or there is an interaction with a second molecule, graphical display is useful, especially if the flexible part is 'smeared' and contoured (see below).

Getting a representative 'average' molecule for, say, a fragment library will normally require careful data analysis. If there is a large spread of points the average is physically meaningless, as also is the molecule constructed with the average internal coordinates (often impossible). The only satisfactory answer is to describe the data, if possible, as consisting of various clusters (usually of conformations) and find representative points close to the centres of each.

A molecule with m atoms can be described by $3m$-6 parameters ($3m$-5 if the molecule is linear), so that the $3m$ cartesian coordinates contain redundancy (an arbitrary origin and orientation). We shall normally take the origin at the centre of mass of the molecule, and orient its inertial axes with the cartesian axes.

For many problems it is simple and appropriate to use internal coordinates for comparison, torsion angles in peptides (ϕ, χ, ψ, ω) being a good example. For molecules with rings, however, the choice is less clear. The pucker in a ribose ring can be described by 5 torsion angles, but only 2 of these are formally independent. Choosing 2 of the 5 arbitrarily may bias the way the problem is analysed, so that it is useful to create new internal coordinates, in this case the phase and puckering amplitude of the ring.

In more complex cases, or where there are isolated atoms, internal coordinates should be replaced by cartesian coordinates of fitted molecules. This has the advantage that the choice is objective, and also that the statistics can be simply related to the known experimental errors since the cartesian coordinates, not internal coordinates, are the primary results from X-ray crystallography.

The data for the comparison and statistics will therefore normally be a vector of independent internal coordinates p or a $3m$ vector of fitted cartesian coordinates $\mathbf{x}$. There is, of course, no reason why other geometrical or non-geometrical quantities cannot be included, but they should be formally independent. The description of statistics that follows is therefore not restricted to geometrical parameters.

4.   STATISTICS FOR MOLECULAR GEOMETRY

Rutherford said that if statistical methods are necessary to justify an experimental conclusion then a better experiment was needed. The statistical techniques described here should allow the researcher to understand multivariate data better and to present it in such a way that pattersn can be seen to the best advantage. Graphical presentation is always strongly recommended where possible.

In making experimental observations we are sampling one or more populations. We are attempting to discover the underlying populations and their variances. If we are successful, the populations can be identified with existing or new chemical/biochemical concepts or phenomena. The variances result from a number of causes. There is always an element due to the experimental method, part of which can sometimes be estimated through error analysis. There will be additional experimental variance when comparing different techniques (e.g. crystallography and NMR) which is very hard to quantify. There will be variance ('unique') which is intrinsic (e.g. in measures of a biological population or in radioactive decay) where there is, at present, no underlying explanation.

In multivariate analysis, we can include covariance where one variable covaries with another, and is said to 'explain' some of the total variance. Explanation of covariance represents a lowering of the dimensionality of the problem, which is useful for several reasons. Ideally the covariance will correspond to a known effect and can labelled (e.g. 'inductive effect', 'electronegativity'). If not, it may be possible to identify a new effect and create a useful label. Even if the result cannot be easily described, the dimensionality reduction may still, for example, be useful for correlating parameters in forcefields.

4.1 Univariate statistics

A probability function $f(x)$ expresses the probability of finding a member of a population in a small interval dx as:

Probability of observation in $x - dx/2$ to $x + dx/2 = f(x).dx$.

A convenient way of characterizing such a function is by its moments, where the nth moment is defined as:

$$m_n = \int_{-\infty}^{\infty} x^n f(x).dx.$$

The zeroth moment is normally set to 1 by normalizing $f(x)$, and we shall assume hereafter that:

$$m_0 = \int_{-\infty}^{\infty} x^n f(x).dx = 1.$$

Of the other moments, the first (average or mean) is:

$$m_1 = \mu = \int_{-\infty}^{\infty} x.f(x).dx.$$

The higher moments are not normally used directly; central moments taken about the mean are more useful;

$$\mu_n = \int_{-\infty}^{\infty} (x - \mu)^n.f(x).dx.$$

The most important of these is the second moment or variance:

$$\mu_2 = \int_{-\infty}^{\infty} (x - \mu)^2 f(x).dx.$$

The square root of the variance is the standard deviation of the distribution:

$$\sigma = \sqrt{\mu_2}$$

(Crystallographers often use the estimated standard deviation (e.s.d) as a measure of the experimental uncertainties in a quantity. This is derived from the refinement process and it relies on the central limit theorem. This should not be confused with the standard deviation of the parameter, which can be obtained only by observing the variance in a parameter through multiple experiments.)

Sometimes the probability distribtution is known theoretically (as for photon counting) but normally it has to be estimated. The most direct way of doing this is to sample the distribution by taking repeated measurements of a quantity. We can derive the sample mean as:

$$\bar{x} = \Sigma x_i / n$$

and the sample variance as:

$$s^2 = \Sigma (x_i - \bar{x})^2 / n$$

which is the square of the standard deviation of the sample.

The expected value of $\bar{r}$ is μ, and the variance of $\bar{x}$ is σ^2/n so that the standard deviation of $\bar{x}$ is:

$$\sigma(\bar{x}) = \sigma(x)/\sqrt{n}$$

Thus as n increases, $\bar{x}$ becomes an increasingly good estimate of μ. It can be shown that the expected value of the sample variance is:

$$E(s^2) = [n/(n-1)]\sigma^2$$

Therefore a reasonable estimate of the variance of the parent population is:

$$\sigma^2 = [n/(n-1)]s^2.$$

For large samples, s and σ are approximately equal, and the difference is unlikely to be of practical significance.

4.2   The normal distribution
This is of fundamental importance in our analysis of molecular geometry. It arises from at least the following considerations.

(a) Some experimental measurements, especially X-ray photon counting for large counts, are normally distributed.
(b) Many observations measure a peak, and the tops of these are often approximately Gaussian. Errors in locating the peak will be distributed normally.
(c) The Central Limit Theorem states that for any parent probability function, the probability function for $\bar{x}$ obtained by sampling is approximately normal with

standard deviation $\sigma/\sqrt{n}$ if n is large. In other words, if we conduct may experiments to sample a value $\bar{x}$ obtaining a different $\bar{x}$ each time, then these $\bar{x}$ will be normally distributed.

(d) Molecular vibrations, which act to smear out the electron density, are approximately harmonic; e.g. for a diatomic molecule:

$$E = -k(r - r_0)^2/2.$$

If this energy is distributed according to the Boltzmann distribution the probability of finding this configuration is:

$$P(E) = A \exp(-E/kT)$$

where A is a normalizing factor. Combining these two equations gives a normal distribution for the probability of finding a classic harmonic molecule with internuclear distance r. This argument, correct in the gas phase, does not normally extend to the solid, but seems to be borne out by analysis of low energy deformations in solids.

(e) Whatever the exact form of the probability distributions of molecular geometries, in practice a normal distribution is usually adequate. Since many statistical techniques have been derived for normal distributions, it is convenient to assume this function in the absence of other information. 'All the world believes it firmly, because the mathematicians imagine that it is a fact of observation, and the observers that it is a theorem of mathematics' (quoted by Poincaré).

The normal density function is given by:

$$P(x) = \exp(-(x - \mu)^2)/2\sigma^{2)}/\sqrt{(2\pi\sigma)}$$

and the normal distribution function by:

$$A(x) = \int_{-\infty}^{x} P(t).dt.$$

The functions are usually tabulated for the case where $\mu = 0$ and $\sigma = 1.0$. In some sciences the variable is then transformed to a z-score, where:

$$z = (x - \mu)/\sigma$$

and:

$$P(z) = \exp(-z^2/2)/\sqrt{(2\pi)}.$$

It can be shown that half the area under a normal curve lies between $+0.67\sigma$ and -0.67σ. The quantity 0.67σ is called the probable error.

It is useful to be able to test whether a distribution is normal. This can be done by using the higher moments, but is more conveiently done with graphical methods, especially the normal probability plot (NPP). For n observations, we calculate the z-scores and sort them. From tables we can find the values of a normally distributed variate which divide $P(z)$ into n equal areas. If these two are plotted, a normal distribution will give a straight line, through the origin with slope 1.

Deviations from normality can be very important and are frequently due to varying degrees of systematic experimental error. Clearly, if the same amount of experimental error is present in each observation, then it will alter only the mean distribution and not the other moments about the mean. If, as is common, each experiment has a varying amount of systematic error, the probability distribution for the occurrence of the error (which may well not be normal), will be convoluted with other errors. This can often give rise to a skewed or even bimodal distribution. These types of distribution, therefore, should be carefully looked at in case systematic errors are responsible. (In crystallography, molecular motion is a common source of systematic error occuring in varying amounts from structure to structure.) The converse is not true: if a distribution is normal, this is no guarantee that systematic errors are not present; they may well be distributed in an approximately normal fashion.

A particularly important reason for deviation from normality is the occurrence of a few 'outliers'. These can be detected by most of the graphical methods of displaying data, whilst they are not easily revealed numerically. Any z-score over 3 is unlikely to result from chance, and the experimental basis for it should be carefully examined. If there are valid reasons for removing the outliers, this can be done and the analysis repeated; the automatic removal of outliers is very dangerous.

4.3   Comparison of populations

Frequently a quantity is measured by two different methods or in different environments, and we wish to know whether they are 'the same'. More precisely, do they belong to different parent populations? If we can determine sample distributions for each, these can be compared by normal probability plots. If, however, we are not able to sample the populations but are able to estimate their means and variances, we can still test whether the populations are different. We construct the t-value.

$$t = (x_i - x_j)/\sqrt{(\sigma_i^2 + \sigma_j^2)}$$

which is distributed as chi-square with 1 degree of freedom. Values of the t-test and chi-square are available in standard tables, which allows us to find the probability that the observed t-value arises by chance from two identical parent populations. This test is widely used in comparison of molecular structure.

An extension of this method occurs when there are several formally independent variables which may be assumed to be normally distributed. An example is in the comparison of two structures which have been determined by different methods or in different laboratories and where both have reported (estimated) standard deviations. If there are n structural parameters (e.g. bond lengths, angles, etc) we can calculate the $n\,t_i$. These should be distributed with a mean of 0 and a variance of 1 so that an NPP (of t_i against expectation) should go through the origin with a slope of 1. If the slope is higher, the standard deviations have been underestimated (which is commonly found by the Cambridge data centre when comparing independent determinations of the same structure.) If there are systematic differences between the structures, the plot will not go through the origin. Alternatively, the quantity:

$$\sum_{i}^{n} t_i^2$$

can be compared with values of chi-square for n degrees of freedom to give a numerical estimate of the probability that the two distributions are identical.

4.4 Bivariate data
Up to now we have concentrated on one-dimensional problems. Much more information can be obtained from multivariate data sets, both in terms of the experimental variance of our parameters, and also of the observed distributions of similar parameters.

If we have n observations of two formally independent parameters, x and y, these have a (bivariate) joint probability distribution. The measure of their statistical dependence is given by the covariance:

$$\sigma^2 = \sum_{i}^{n} (x_i - \bar{x})(y_i - \bar{y})/n.$$

If the parameters are expressed as z-scores the expression for two z-variants z_j and z_k (where i represents observations) an be represented as:

$$r_{jk}^2 = \sum_{i}^{n} z_{ij} z_{ik}/n.$$

The quantity r is the correlation coefficient, and r^2 represents the proportion of the variance that can be explained by covariance. For example, if two variables had a correlation coefficient of 0.9, 81% of the variance can be described with one degree of freedom.

Sometimes it is important to get a feel for the main regions in which data points lie. If there are a few outliers they can be visually very misleading, and their effect can be lessened by 'smearing out' the data. Gaussians are placed at the centre of each data point and summed to give a 2-dimensional scalar array, which can then be contoured. If suitable parameters are chosen for the Gaussians and the contours, the main concentrations of data can be highlighted. This technique extends well to 3-dimensional scatterplots and is also a good way of smearing out the effect of superimposed atoms in superimposed molecules.

4.5 Regression
Regression analyses the variance in a variable y due to the dependent variable x, where

$$y_i = Mx_i + C + \epsilon.$$

Least-squares will give M and C for the regression line of y on x. Since this is not the same line as obtained by regressing x on y (unless the residuals are zero), it is not good practice to regress one geometrical parameter against another, unless there is a clear suggestion that one depends on the other. (Principal components will give a better line through the data.) In cases where one parameter, such as a torsion, might be thought of as having intrinsic variance (perhaps due to crystal-packing forces), a bond length could be considered to be dependent on it, and regression would be appropriate.

4.6 Multivariate data

For multivariate systems the notation is simplified by using vectors to represent the parameters. The n observations of m parameters form a data matrix $\mathbf{Z}$, and the variance/covariance is represented by a covariance matrix $\mathbf{R}$. If we scale the m parameters to zero mean (but not necessarily unit variance) representing them as an m-dimensional vector $\mathbf{p}$, the normal distribution is then:

$$P(\mathbf{p}) = N \exp\left(- \mathbf{p}^{\mathrm{T}}\mathbf{D}\mathbf{p}/2\right)$$

where N is a normalizing factor and $\mathbf{D}$ is the dispersion matrix. If there is no covariance, the off-diagonal terms are zero and the diagonal terms are the reciprocals of the corresponding variances; that is, the m parameters are statistically independent.

The inverse of the dispersion matrix is the covariance or (if z-scores are used) the correlation matrix. Each element represents the bivariate correlation between the corresponding parameters so that the matrix is symmetrical. It is also Gramian, that is, semi-positive definite, in that it has no negative eigenvalues (and only has zero ones if there are exact linear relationships between two or more of the parameters.) It is perhaps coincidental, but extremely attractive, that the mathematical representation of the multivariate probability function is isomorphous to the description of the harmonic molecular force-field. A change of geometry can be represented by a multi-dimensional vector $\mathbf{Z}$, and the energy distortion calculated by an expression similar to that for the probability. Again, as remarked earlier, a Boltzmann distribution of energies gives rise to a population of (harmonically) distorted molecules whose geometries obey a multivariate normal probability function!

In the multivariate case variance is seen as arising from two causes: specific variance, corresponding to the diagonal elements of the covariance matrix, and covariance, corresponding to the off-diagonal terms. Specific variance will arise from: random errors, random amounts of systematic error and effects due to unknown causes (or at least not including in the parameters). Covariance is said to explain variance and can either be used as the basis of regression, where one variable is dependent on one or more other formally independent variables, or in factor analysis where a proportion of the variance is explained by a small number of factors (see later). Covariance matrices arise in both the derivation of parameters from experimental data and in the observational analysis of large bodies of molecular structural data. In both cases it is sometimes possible to estimate whether all the specific variance is due to experimental error.

4.7 Least squares

Least squares is important not only for the analysis of data (for example, fitting a variable to a function of others), but also because it provides an estimate of the errors. It is routinely used, in a non-linear manner, in the refinement of crystal structures, and it provides a useful estimate of some of the errors in the experiment.

The theory of multivariate statistics is implicit in the least squares approach. In least squares we minimize the sums of squares of the residuals between a calculated function and the observed values. For an experiment with n observations, m parameters, and a normal equation matrix $\mathbf{A}$, the elements of the covariance matrix can be estimated as:

$$\sigma_{jk} = A_{jk}^{-1} \sum w_i \Delta_i^2 / (n - m)$$

where

$$\Delta_i = y - <y>.$$

In this estimation it is assumed that the residuals Δ are distributed normally, and systematic deviations from this will invalidate the e.s.d's and estimated covariances (e.c) in the matrix. Nonetheless, owing to the central limit theorem and the transformation of parameters, the refined parameters will often show a normal distribution, as observed in normal probability plots. Thus the least squares method is particularly efficient at transforming systematic errors into a normally distributed error function to be added to the effect of (normal) random experimental observations. We stress again that a normal distribution is thus no guarantee of the absence of systematic errors, especially for a multivariate problem as in X-ray analysis. The correlation matrix is more valuable than often realized. Admittedly it is frequently unpublished in X-ray work, but if parameters are correlated, then the cross-terms can seriously affect their comparison with other experiments. Gas-phase workers and others are more conscious of the importance of correlations which are often more serious than in X-ray work).

4.8   Principal components

The correlation matrix $\mathbf{R}$ can be diagonalized to yield m eigenvalues Λ and an $m \times m$ eigenvector matrix $\mathbf{E}$. This process is often referred to as principal component analysis or, in the behavioural sciences, factor analysis (although this term covers more than the principal components method). It is an extremely powerful way of reducing the formal dimensionality of a problem and is robust, especially when the distribution is approximately normal. It we have several parameters and suspect some correlation, then the principal components will show this to its greatest extent. It is also a useful way for analysing variance and the variance associated with each component can be quantified. Finally, because of the similarity of the mathematics to that of normal mode analysis, it is often found that the factors can be interpreted as normal modes and that observed molecular distortions can be described in terms of dynamic processes. The correlation matrix is set up:

$$\mathbf{R} = \mathbf{Z}^{\mathrm{T}} \mathbf{Z} / n$$

and diagonalized to give the eigenvalues Λ, and the eigenvector matrix $\mathbf{E}$.

$$\mathbf{R} = \mathbf{E}^{\mathrm{T}} \lambda \mathbf{E}.$$

These are then scaled to give the principal axes of the distribution (factors)

$$F = \lambda^{1/2}E.$$

so that

$$R = F^TF.$$

The factors are thus simply linear combinations of the original variables, each factor being an m-dimensional vector and all factors being orthogonal. In effect we have rotated the distribution in m-space such that the axes are those of the inertial hyperellipsoid. In favourable cases there may be only a few significant factors (the others being explainable by error) and the dimensionality of our representation is reduced. Principal components are very useful for explaining variance. If we estimate that, say, 10% of the variance in a 50-dimensional problem is due to known errors and that, say, the first 3 factors explain 80% of the variance we can be confident that the data can be described as resulting from 3 main linear relationships. Whether these are due to structural correlation, systematic errors or a combination of both must be decided subjectively.

The components of each observation along the component (factor) axes are called the factor scores, S.

$$S = EZ$$

If they are scaled by the lengths of the axes of the distribution, the scores will represent the relative importance of the individual factors,

$$S' = \lambda^{1/2}EZ$$

The principal component method can be used with completely independent and non-commensurate variables, for example a mixture of coordinates, charge, etc. The individual factors will be vectors whose components are composed of different measures. The dispersion may be very different along different variables, making comparison difficult. When variables are derived from the same experiment but have very different relations to the experiment (for example a torsion and a bond length), the one with smaller dispersion may have an unduly large effect on the principal component analysis. An added problem arises when there is a co-linearity (exact or approximate) between the variables. This can happen when there is a formal equation of constraint (which might be linear), such as the 3 (non-linear) ones relating the torsion angles in a 5-membered ring. Many parameters describing substituent constants, for example, show colinearity. The use of internal coordinates, therefore, for multivariate analysis should be analysed carefully to eliminate constraints and to make sure that the choice does not implicitly bias the conclusions. The torsion angles, which usually account for most of the variance, have a particular problem with the periodicity: changing an angle from $180°$ to $-180°$ will invalidate any analysis. Possibly it would be useful to use $\sin\tau$ and $\cos\tau$ in the analysis.

There is a particular attraction, however, when all the variables are cartesian coordinates. Now all variables have the same measure and can be directly compared. Moreover there are no hidden constraints (except the 6 redundant orientation and translation ones). Also, in a crystallographic experiment, it is the cartesian coordinates for which errors are derived, rather than internal coordinates. It is suggested, therefore, that principal coordinate analysis (and other multivariate techniques) be carried out on the cartesian coordinates of fitted molecules wherever possible, in preference to an arbitrary selection of internal coordinates.

The correlation matrix will often be singular. If the number of cases, n, is less than the number of parameters m, the matrix will be of rank $\leq n$. There will therefore be at least $m\text{-}n$ zero eigenvalues for which the eigenvectors are undefined. However, the remaining eigenvalues and vectors will be meaningful if a suitable diagonalization method (e.g. Householder) is used. In certain cases, either by chance or for symmetrical molecules, two or more eigenvalues will be equal resulting in degenerate eigenvectors. The use of cartesian coordinates always results in at least 6 zero eigenvalues.

It is difficult to say when a principal component is significant. A good test is whether the eigenvector makes physical or chemical sense; in many cases eigenvectors should be very similar to normal modes as the analysis is isomorphic. It is unlikely that more than three eigenvectors can be interpreted in most cases.

4.9 Other multivariate techniques

Any technique of displaying multivariate data is extremely useful. Several packages are available which allow the graphical inspection of 3-dimensional data fields, and with the judicious use of colour and interactive sectioning, about 5 independent variables can probably be scanned at one time.

Other techniques include cluster analysis and multi-dimensional scaling techniques. They should be used with great care, since the method of choice often depends on the type of data distribution. They will not be described in detail, but examples of graphical output will be given.

Both depend on the construction of the distance matrix, $\mathbf{D}$ where D_{ij} is the distance between observations i and j. The simplest method is to use Euclidian distances, when the matrix is the outer product of the data matrices:

$$\mathbf{D} = \mathbf{Z}\mathbf{Z}^{\mathrm{T}}.$$

Cluster analysis looks for low D_{ij}, that is, for points near to each other in m-space, to form a cluster. These clusters are combined with other clusters, and the whole is representable by a tree, or dendrogram. In cases where clusters are well separated, this is a quick and attractive method of scanning the data. If, for example, it is believed that a molecule exists in several distinct conformations, cluster analysis is a good exploratory method. If, however, these conformations have low energy pathways between them, so that a few intermediate points may occur, the algorithms may behave in substantially different ways.

Other dimension-reducing techniques entail non-linear mapping, which is similar to distance geometry. An iterative method is used to produce a $p \times m$ capitals $\mathbf{V}$, where the dimension p is very low (desirably 3 or fewer). If the outer product:

$$\mathbf{D'} = \mathbf{V}^{\mathrm{T}}\mathbf{V}$$

is close to $\mathbf{D}$, then the observational dimensionality of the data is close to p, and a p-dimensional scatterplot describes the data well.

4.10   Time-dependent data

Molecular dynamics and other simulation techniques produce large amounts of output which can be extremely difficult to analyse. Displaying the trajectory graphically through animation is extremely important, but it should be complemented by statistical analysis. Some of the questions that might be asked are:

(a) Is any part of the molecule more flexible than another?
(b) Does the molecule, or part of it, undergo a substantial change in geometry during the run? Is this a sharp transition? Does the molecule revisit the original conformation?
(c) Is a particular conformation formed during the run?
(d) Are there any periodic fluctuations?

Multivariate methods are extremely valuable, and the points on plots can be connected in sequence. It is unlikely that the trajectory can be represented by a very low dimensionality, but there may be very low energy/large amplitude motions that will show up if cartesian coordinates are used.

A very wide range of techniques are available for the analysis of time series (for example in economics, biology, or sociology) and can be used for variables from the trajectory. Again, graphical plots of variables against time are important, especially those obtained from dimension-reducing techniques. Here are three simple numerical techniques:

(a) Lagged variables. A new variable is formed from an existing one at a different time, that is,

$$x't = x(t + \Delta t)$$

$x't$ could then, say, be correlated with xt or with yt.

(b) Autocorrelation. A variable is correlated with its lagged variable and the correlation $r(\Delta t)$ analysed as a function of Δt.
(c) Moving average. A variate xt is replaced by the average of it and its neighbours, often by using a triangular, weighting function. A simple example would be:

$$x't = (x(t - 1) + 2xt + x(t + 1))/4$$

This has the effect of smoothing the trajectory and removing high-frequency variations.

The combination of dimensionality reduction with any of these should be valauble in detecting low-energy motions and whole molecule transitions. Local transitions are probably very difficult to detect automatically without exhaustive analysis of the data.

5.   PROGRAMS AND PACKAGES

A very wide array of statistical techniques and display packages are available, and the user should certainly use them before attempting to write their own programs. Among the statistical packages and libraries are: SPSS, MINITAB, RS/1, SAS,

GENSTAT, IMSL, NAG; and for display: AVS, WAVEFRONT, UNIRAS, SIMPLE-PLOT. The major database packages also include statistics and often graphics. Most of these will require a flat file of data (corresponding to the data matrix), preferably without missing values (which compromise many statistical techniques).

Sometimes, as in molecular dynamics trajectories, preparing the data matrix automatically is straightforward, since this consists of molecules identical in all except coordinates. Often, however, we wish to analyse parts of molecules (for example beta-turns, sugar rings), and the appropriate atoms in each structure must be matched to a desired fragment. In macromolecules this may be possible when using the atom names in a dictionary, but for small molecules a substructure search routine is required, which must match the atoms. This is available for entries on the Cambridge data file through the program GEOSTAT, where a connection table for the fragment can be defined with great flexibility. The coding of the query should be done carefully, as it is possible to match unwanted fragments (for example different chirality or atom hydridization).

The author has developed a package (DEMOCRITOS) for analysis of molecular geometry which combines substructure searching and a wide range of statistical techniques with a powerful interactive or batch command language. It is also possible to search a wide range of file types, including three databanks mentioned. For macromolecules it complements the BIPED/IDITIS approach as questions can be asked about small molecules (for example metal coordination, sugars, substrates). The case studies have all been prepared with DEMOCRITOS, and some typical input is given.

No examples of intermolecular geometry have been included, but several of the references contain studies of hydrogen bonds and other interactions (e.g. Glusker & Murray-Rust). These illustrate the use of the 'smearing' technique to highlight the most favourable approach of atoms.

6.   CASE STUDIES

Four case studies are now presented which show a selection of the techniques available. The first was performed with GEOSTAT, the others using DEMOCRITOS.

6.1   Case study 1: C-F bond lengths
When analysing a univariate distribution, it is valuable to use graphical techniques, and to investigate outliers individually. As an example, we take the question 'What is the average length of a C-F bond?'. There is no precise answer to this question since C-F bonds occur in a very large number of compounds and in different crystallographic environments. Accurate structures are selected from the Cambridge Data File, using the criterion that the R-factor must be less than 0.05, and that there is no atom heavier than Cl (since heavy atoms lower the accuracy of light atom parameters). Nearly 300 examples of C-F bonds are retrieved (Fig. 1a) with a mean of 1.34 Å and a standard deviation of 0.025 A. The histogram gives clues as to why these values should not be accepted automatically — the distribution is slightly skew,

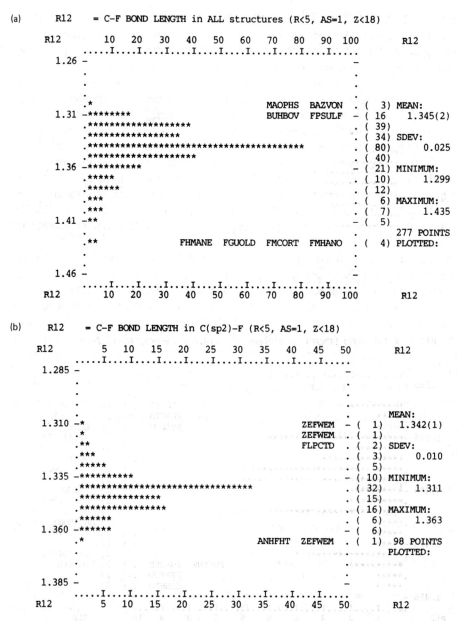

Fig. 1. Univariate statistics on C-F bond lengths in accurate structures from the CCDC file. Histograms (a) to (d) show the progress of the chemical understanding of the underlying populations. Output from GEOSTAT; some diagrams are annotated with the 6-letter Cambridge reference code (REFCODE) (see Table 2) of significant outliers.

(a) All data. The large standard deviation, and the chemical difference between outliers at the two tails (see text) suggest that there are overlapping populations.

(b) Only bonds from Csp^2 to F, selected on chemical criteria in CONNSER. The standard deviation is probably mainly due to experimental error, with some chemical variance.

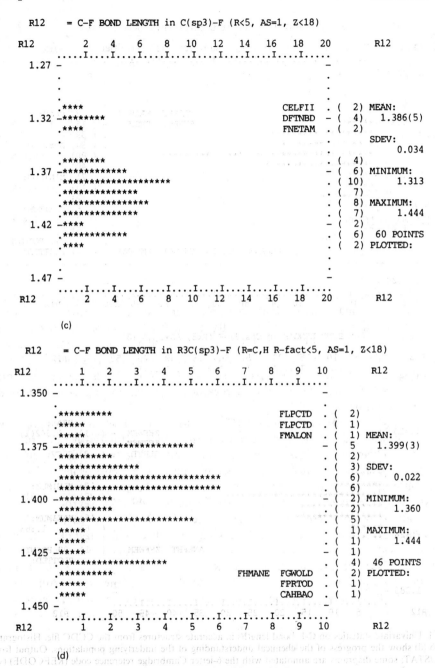

```
  R12     = C-F BOND LENGTH in C(sp3)-F (R<5, AS=1, Z<18)

  R12       2    4    6    8   10   12   14   16   18   20         R12
         ....I....I....I....I....I....I....I....I....I....
  1.27 -                                                    -
          .
          .
          .****                                   CELFII   . (  2) MEAN:
  1.32 -*********                                  DFTNBD   - (  4)   1.386(5)
          .****                                    FNETAM   . (  2)
          .                                                 .      SDEV:
          .                                                 .        0.034
          .********                                         . (  4)
  1.37 -***********                                         - (  6) MINIMUM:
          .******************                               . ( 10)   1.313
          .**************                                   . (  7)
          .****************                                 . (  8) MAXIMUM:
          .**************                                   . (  7)   1.444
  1.42 -****                                                - (  2)
          .************                                     . (  6) 60 POINTS
          .****                                             . (  2) PLOTTED:
          .
          .                                                 .
  1.47 -                                                    -
         ....I....I....I....I....I....I....I....I....I....
  R12       2    4    6    8   10   12   14   16   18   20         R12
```

(c)

```
  R12     = C-F BOND LENGTH in R3C(sp3)-F (R=C,H R-fact<5, AS=1, Z<18)

  R12       1    2    3    4    5    6    7    8    9   10         R12
         ....I....I....I....I....I....I....I....I....I....
 1.350 -                                                    -
          .
          .*********                               FLPCTD   . (  2)
          .*****                                   FLPCTD   . (  1)
          .*****                                   FMALON   . (  1) MEAN:
 1.375 -*************************                            - (  5)   1.399(3)
          .*********                                         . (  2)
          .***************                                   . (  3) SDEV:
          .*****************************                     . (  6)   0.022
          .****************************                      . (  6)
 1.400 -*********                                            - (  2) MINIMUM:
          .**********                                        . (  2)   1.360
          .***********************                           . (  5)
          .*****                                             . (  1) MAXIMUM:
          .*****                                             . (  1)   1.444
 1.425 -*****                                                - (  1)
          .*******************                               . (  4) 46 POINTS
          .**********                      FHMANE  FGWOLD   . (  2) PLOTTED:
          .*****                                   FPRTOD   . (  1)
          .*****                                   CAHBAO   . (  1)
 1.450 -                                                    -
         ....I....I....I....I....I....I....I....I....I....
  R12       1    2    3    4    5    6    7    8    9   10         R12
```

(d)

(c) Bonds from any Csp^3 to F. The very large variance is an indication of overlapping populations.
    (d) Only tertiary alkyl fluorides. The variance is reduced, but not totally explained.

Table 2

GEOSTAT commands to derive Fig. 1. Comments are prefixed by !. The command file will search a data file (in CCDC FDAT format) for all C-F bonds until the end-of-file. Then the histogram will be drawn.

```
FRAG C-F bonds
!       define atoms
AT1 C
AT2 F
!       define bond
BO 1 2
!       define a variable
DEF R12 1 2
ENDFRAGMENT
!       Plot a histogram
HIST R12
```

and there are outliers. The standard deviation (0.025 Å) is also higher than expected, since similar comparisons of functional groups in crystal structures often give an observed s.d. in bond lengths of about 0.007–0.010 Å. Experimental errors would seem to account for only $(0.010/0.025)^2 = 16\%$ of the variance, and a chemical explanation should be sought. When the outliers are inspected, it is found that those with long C-F bond lengths all involve sp^3 carbon atoms, whilst the shortest ones are all to sp^2. Clearly these must be regarded as separate populations, and the analysis should be repeated.

Figure 1b shows the histogram for $100\,C(sp^2)$-F bonds. The standard deviation is now much less, and the mean is probably a useful figure. (In fact there is still some evidence of chemical variation when the compounds in the tails of the distributions are observed, showing that bond lengths are, indeed, a sensitive probe for chemical effects. It might be worth attempting to separate the analysis still further). Figure 1c shows the corresponding plot for $C(sp^3)$-F lengths, which is clearly not normal. Inspection shows that the shortest lengths are all in X-C-F groups where X is an electronegative group such as NO_2. This is a known effect – the effect of withdrawing electrons is to decrease the covalent radius – so the analysis is yet again repeated with only alkyl substituents (that is RR'R"C-F), Fig. 1d. Even here the standard deviation is still high and chemical or crystallographic effects are still present, requiring further analysis to remove. This example shows that even for an apparently homogeneous population, 3 major sub-populations are present, and probably more. Whatever parameter(s) are studied, either uni- or multi-variate, the user should have the ability to inspect the outliers or tails of the distribution quickly.

6.2   Case study 2: ethyl ester conformation
The variation of the precise geometries of ethyl esters, $RC(=O)OCH_2CH_3$, with conformation is explored. This type of analysis would be valuable in adding a new functional group to a forcefield.

The input commands, in DEMOCRITOS language, are given in Table 3, along with the Figures they produce. A query has been prepared (Fig. 2a). A set of accurate structures has been retrieved from the CCDC file, and these are exhaustively searched for fragments (Fig. 2b). (Hydrogen atoms are neglected in the subsequent analysis as they are often poorly located in X-ray structures.) The search is limited; 150 fragments are found and superimposed (Fig. 3) and examined in the spreadsheet. A cluster diagram (Fig. 4) shows two major clusters, attributable to different conformations. A principal components analysis on the fitted cartesians confirms this. Of the 12 non-zero eigenvalues,

Table 3

DEMOCRITOS commands to generate all the data and figures for case study 2. (The graphical commands, for example to open windows, have been omitted). The commands can be issued from batch, interactively, or through a graphical interface. The query, and the associated variable definitions (corresponding to AT, BO and DEF Table 2), are read in from the files ester.geo and ester.cal.

```
!DEMO
!        Conformations of ethyl esters with R < 7
!        All characteristics after ! are comments and can be ignored
FRAGMENT NAMES = ester
!        Read the query in from file (ester.geo) (cf.Table 2)
QUERY FORMAT = geo name = ester1 file = \querydir\ester.geo
!        Read in some commands to calculate variables
@\testdir\ester.cal
QUERY END
FRAGMENT END
!        Draw the query (Fig. 2a)
DRAW QUERY LABEL
!        This sets up the file to read structures from (in this
!        case CCDC FDAT (concatenated). The file is not actually
!        read until the LOOP instruction is issued.
TARGET FORMAT = ccdc file = \datadir\ester.dat
!        This loops through the structures on the target file,
!        until it gets to the end or until 1000 hits have been
!        found. Every entry is exhaustively searched for ethyl
!        esters.
LOOP HITS = 1000
!        Draw the last molecule read in (Fig. 2b)
DRAW TARGET
!        Use cartesian coordinates for analysis
STATISTICS COORDINATES
!        Spreadsheet (Fig. 3)
SPREADSHEET
!        Cluster analysis (Fig. 4)
CLUSTER METHOD = 1
!        Principal components on cartesians; save scores
```

(contd)

Table 3 (*contd*)

```
FACTOR NFACTOR = 2 ADD__SCORES
!       Plot factor scores (Fig. 5)
SCATTERGRAM  #FACT1 #FACT2
!       Change back to internal coordinates and user variables
STATISTICS USER
!       Sort on tor0, and tabulate just the top 10 and bottom 10.
SORT VARIABLE = tor0
TABLES TOP = 10 BOTTOM = 10
!       Histograms and normal probability plots (Figs. 6 a-d)
HISTOGRAM tor1 LIMIT = 0,180
NORMAL__PROBAB tor1
HISTOGRAM o2c3                  !Note no LIMIT given
NORMAL__PROBAB o2c3
!       Scatterplot (note continuation lines with "--")
!       regresses tor1 against o2c3, plots line and gives
!       statistics (Fig. 7)
SCATTERGRAM tor1 LIMIT = 60,180 o2c3 LIMIT = 1.41,1.56 --
        OPTION REGRESSION
!       END DEMO
```

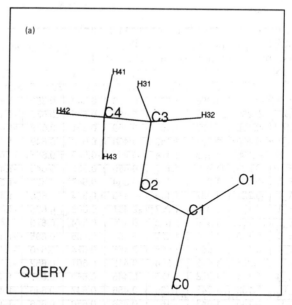

Fig. 2. Accurate structures from CCDC containing ethyl esters.

(a) Query used and the numbering. Atoms C3 and C4 were required to have hydrogen substituents but these were not used in the analysis.

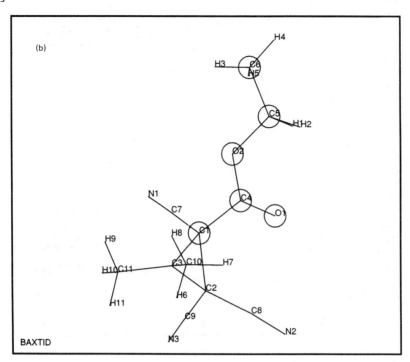

Fig. 2. (b) A typical matched fragment (circled atoms), showing arbitrary atom numbering.

	XC0	YC0	ZC0	XC1	YC1	ZC1	XO1	YO1
ACNPTH10_1	-0.140	1.966	1.087	-0.460	0.548	0.658	-1.453	-0.045
ACNPTH10_2	-0.261	1.930	1.115	-0.403	0.536	0.557	-1.417	-0.087
AECLPA10_1	-0.152	1.937	1.193	-0.459	0.591	0.628	-1.425	-0.060
AEMPYC_1	-0.130	1.901	1.159	-0.458	0.599	0.649	-1.423	-0.072
ALANRE_1	-0.138	1.973	1.134	-0.456	0.549	0.656	-1.442	-0.066
BAGGOF_1	-0.123	1.936	1.177	-0.465	0.587	0.643	-1.437	-0.068
BAKCOF_1	-0.304	1.902	1.179	-0.384	0.546	0.538	-1.398	-0.099
BAKRUA_1	-0.221	1.987	1.116	-0.415	0.524	0.608	-1.433	-0.090
BANYOE_1	-0.156	1.940	1.207	-0.451	0.605	0.635	-1.407	-0.076
BANYOE_2	-0.156	1.959	1.098	-0.455	0.574	0.670	-1.453	-0.060
BANYOE_3	-0.156	1.940	1.207	-0.451	0.605	0.635	-1.407	-0.076
BANYOE_4	-0.156	1.959	1.098	-0.455	0.574	0.670	-1.453	-0.060
BAPYAS_1	-0.225	1.943	1.204	-0.418	0.601	0.652	-1.385	-0.018
BAWPAQ_1	-0.144	1.928	1.175	-0.445	0.569	0.637	-1.424	-0.044
BAXTID_1	-0.132	1.948	1.130	-0.456	0.547	0.645	-1.442	-0.057
BAXTOJ_1	-0.136	1.943	1.161	-0.456	0.556	0.636	-1.420	-0.064
BEBDAN_1	-0.148	1.950	1.129	-0.459	0.552	0.646	-1.442	-0.047
BEBDAN_2	-0.100	1.950	1.184	-0.491	0.571	0.626	-1.447	-0.055
BEBDAN_3	-0.153	1.934	1.150	-0.442	0.560	0.650	-1.425	-0.044
BEBFET_1	-0.302	1.871	1.198	-0.388	0.557	0.543	-1.398	-0.089

Fig. 3. A part of the table (spreadsheet) of the fitted cartesian coordinates of 143 ethyl ester
fragments (numbering as in Fig 2b).

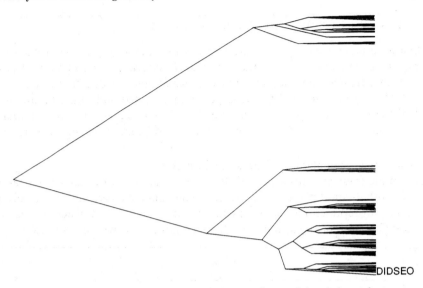

Fig. 4. Preliminary cluster analysis of the cartesian coordinates of the ethyl ester fragments.

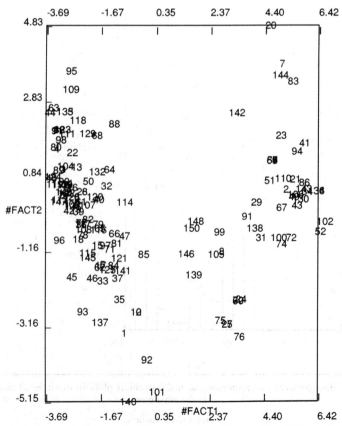

Fig. 5. Principal component analysis of the cartesian coordinates of the ethyl ester fragments. The axes are in Å, as the diagram represents a projection from $(3 \times 6 - 6) = 12$-dimensional cartesian space. Numbers are the serial numbers of the entries (e.g. 1 = ACNPTHI10__1).

11.8, 2.8, 1.1, 0.8, 0.5, 0.5, 0.2, 0.1, 0.1, 0.1, 0.0, 0.0,

the first accounts for 65% of the variance and the second for another 15%, so that the plot (Fig. 5) shows 80% of the variance. Histograms (Fig. 6) show 2 typical internal coordinates and that the two conformations are due to rotation about O2-C3. The variance in r(O2-C3) is larger than expected and might be due to the effect of the O2-C3 torsion. A scatterplot (Fig. 7) and regression shows marginally significant effect ($r = -0.36$), but there is clearly still some unexplained variance.

6.3   Case study 3: exploratory Ramachandran plot

Sixty peptide fragments from the CCDC file were analysed by Ramachandran plot (Fig. 8). (Both d- and l-peptides are present). The data have been smeared to produce a contour plot representing the main concentrations of points. Cluster analyses (Fig. 9) with different algorithms show that the technique must be used with care.

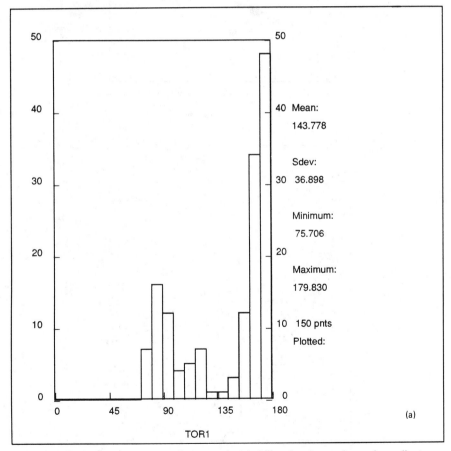

Fig. 6. Histograms and corresponding normal probability plots for two internal coordinates in the ethyl esters.

(a) O2-C3 torsion.

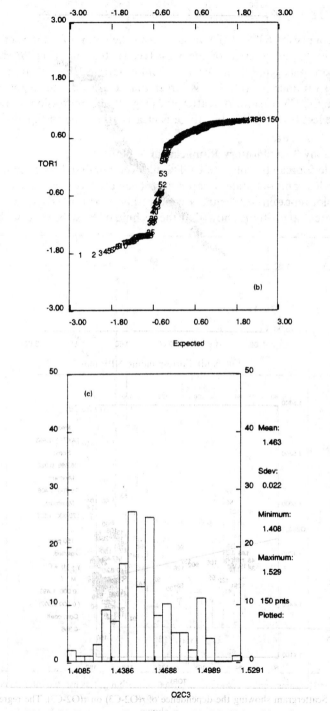

Fig. 6. (b) Corresponding NPP plot. (c) O2-C3 bond length.

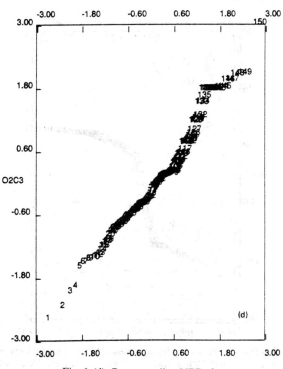

Fig. 6. (d) Corresponding NPP plot.

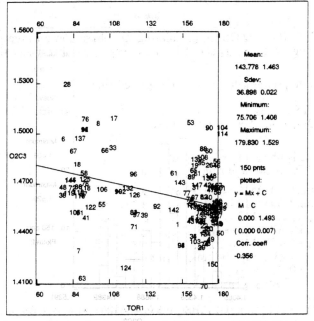

Fig. 7. Scattergram showing the dependence of r(O2-C3) on τ(O2-C3). The regression line
is shown.

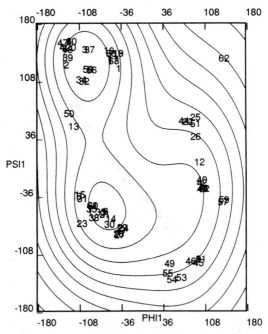

Fig. 8. Exploratory Ramachandran plot for a selection of d- and l-peptides from the CCDC. The distribution of points has been 'smeared out' with point-centred Gaussians, and then contoured.

Table 4

Macro from DEMOCRITOS for calculating the phase and average puckering of a 5-membered ring. Note that this can be used very generally for any ring.

```
!pseudo
!       Calculate pseudorotation in 5-membered ring
!
!       INPUTS
!       at1,at2,at3,at4,at5 are atom names
!OUTPUTS:
!       PHASE is phase of pseudorotation
!       AVPUCK is average ring torsion angle
TORSION junk1 ATOMS = \at1\,\at2\,\at3\,\at4\
TORSION junk2 ATOMS = \at5\,\at1\,\at2\,\at3\
TORSION junk3 ATOMS = \at4\,\at5\,\at1\,\at2\
TORSION junk4 ATOMS = \at3\,\at4\,\at5\,\at1\
TORSION junk5 ATOMS = \at2\,\at3\,\at4\,\at5\
LET junkx = (junk3 + junk5)-(junk2 + junk4)
LET junky = (3.077*junk1)
LET \phase\ = ATAN (junkx,junky)
LET \avpuck\ =
   (ABS(junk1) + ABS(junk2) + ABS(junk3) + ABS(junk4) + ABS(junk5))/5.
!end of pseudo
```

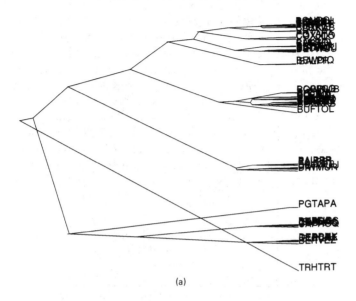

(a)

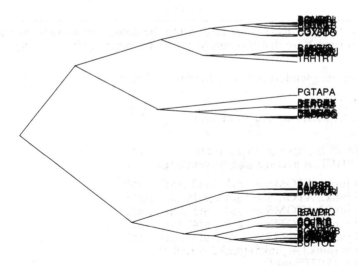

(b)

Fig. 9. Cluster analysis on the cartesian coordinates of the peptides in 8.

(a) Single linkage algorithm.
(b) Group average algorithm.

6.4   Case study 4: molecular dynamics of a peptide

Ninety three frames from a dynamics run on an 11-mer peptide (Fig. 10) *in vacuo* with the program GROMOS are analysed with DEMOCRITOS. The frames have been superimposed and the cartesian coordinates are compared by non-linear mapping (Fig. 11). The effective dimensionality of the trajectory is probably quite high, so that the plot is a poor approximation, but there is clearly no evidence of major periodicity or large-scale transitions. Two side chain torsion angles are subjected to time series analysis (Fig. 12). The moving average shows that the fluctuations are quite small and the conformation does not change markedly. The pseudorotation of Proline 2 is calculated (DEMOCRITOS allows macros and that for pseudorotation is given in Table 4). In this case (Fig. 13) there is a clear shift of phase angle at the start of the trajectory and the ring explores a quite different area of conformational space.

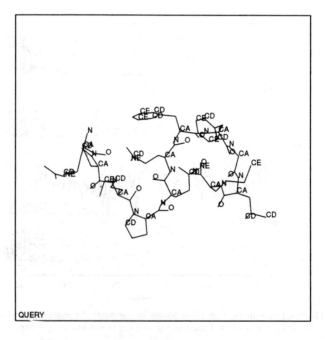

Fig. 10. Analysis of dynamics run on Substance-P. The initial configuration of the peptide.
Only some atoms are labelled, for clarity.

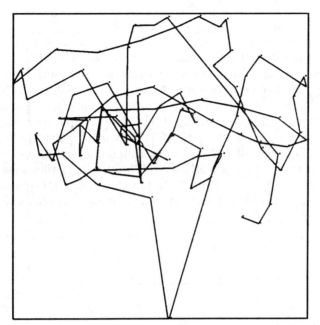

Fig. 11. The trajectory of 93 steps of the dynamic run. The cartesian coordinates of each 'frame' have been fitted by least squares and projected by non-linear mapping into two dimensions.

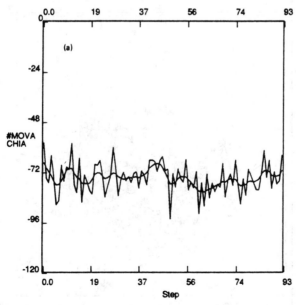

Fig. 12. Time series analysis of torsion angles in the Met side chain. On top of the raw torsion angle is plotted the moving average (a window of ± 3 frames).

(a) χ_2.

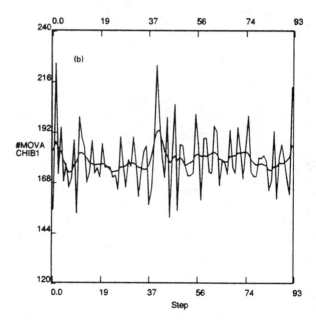

Fig. 12. (b) χ_3.

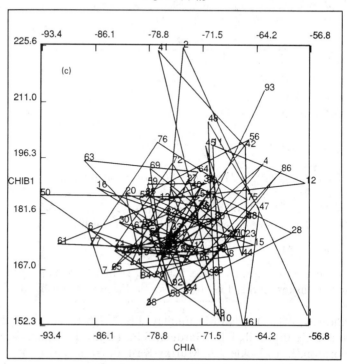

Fig. 12. (c) Sequential variation of χ_3 and χ_2.

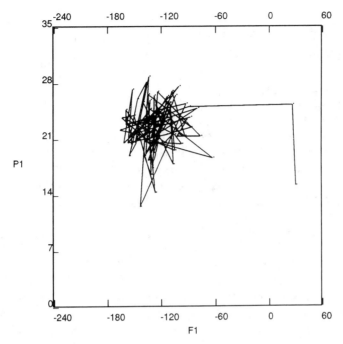

Fig. 13. Variation is pseudorotation parameters (F1 = phase, P1 = pucker) during the trajectory. The start of the trajectory is at (30, 15).

REFERENCES

General

Bernal, J.D. *Science in history*, Third Edition. P.943 Hawthorn Books, Inc. New York, NY

Dunitz, J.D. (1979) *X-ray analysis and the structure of organic molecules*, Cornell Univ. Press

Griffin, J. & Duax, W.L. (1982) *Molecular Structure and Biological Activity*, Elsevier

Horn, A.S. & De Ranter C.J. (1984) *X-ray crystallography and drug action* Oxford Univ. Press

Pauling, L. (1960) *The nature of the chemical bond* (3rd Edition), Cornell Univ. Press

Databases

Abola, E.E., Bernstein, F.C., & ,Koetzle, T.F., (1985). in *The role of data in scientific progress* (ed. Glusker, P.S.), 139–144 Elsevier Science Publishers B.V. North-Holland

Akrigg, D., Bleasby, A.J., Dix, N.I.M., Findlay, J.B.C., North, A.C.T., Parry-Smith, D., Wootton, J.C., Blundell, T.L., Gardner, S.P., Hayes, F., Islam, S., Sternberg, M.J.E., Thornton, J.M., Tickle, I.J., Murray-Rust, P. *Nature*, 335, 745–746, (1988)

Allen, F.H., Bergerhoff, G. & Sievers, R. *Crystallographic Databases*. Data Commission of the International Union of Crystallography, Chester, U.K.

Bergerhoff, G. (1988) Principles of databases for chemistry (Chapter 18) in *Crystallographic Computing* 4, p290–302, ed. Isaacs N.W. and Taylor M.R., Oxford University Press

Analyses of molecular geometry
Allen, F.H. (1980) *Acta Cryst.*, B36, 81–96; (1981)
Allen, F.H. & Kirby, A.J. (1984) *J.A.C.S.* **106**, 6197
Britton, D. & Dunitz, J.D. (1980) *Helv. Chim. Acta*, **63**, 1068
Chandrasekhar, K: & Burgi, H.-B. (1983) *Acta Cryst.* **B40**, 387
Domenicano, A., Murray-Rust, P. & Vaciago, A. (1983) *Acta. Cryst.* **B39**, 457
Huml, K. & Hummel, W. Multivariate analysis of data (Chapter 19) in *Crystallographic Computing* **4**, 303–322, ed. Isaacs N.W. and Taylor M.R., Oxford University Press (1988)
Jeffrey, G.A. & Sundarlingham, M. (1981) *Adv. Carbohydrate Chem. Biochem.*, **38**, 176
Murray-Rust, P. & Bland R. (1978) *Acta Cryst.* B34, 2527
Murray-Rust, P. & Motherwell, W.D.S. (1978) *Acta Cryst.*, **B34**, 2518–2526
Murray-Rust, P. & Glusker, J.P.J. (1984) *J. Amer. Chem. Soc.*, **106**, 1018
Murray-Rust, P. & Motherwell, W.D.S. (1978) *Acta Cryst.*, **B34**, 2537–2546
Murray-Rust, P. & Motherwell, W.D.S. (1979) *J. Amer. Chem. Soc.*, **101**, 4374
Murray-Rust, P. & Raftery, J.E. (1985) *J. Mol. Graph.*, **3**, 60
Norskov-Lauritsen, L. & Burgi, H.-B. (1985) *J. Comput. Chem.* **6**, 216
Rosenfield, R.E., Parthasarathy, R. & Dunitz, J.D. (1977) *J. Amer. Chem. Soc.*, **99**, 4860
Sheldrick, B. & Akrigg, D. (1980) *Acta Cryst.* **B36**, 1615
Taylor, R. & Kennard, O. (1982) *J. Mol. Struct.*, **78**, 1
Taylor, R. & Kennard, O. (1982) *J. Amer. Chem. Soc.*, **104**, 5063
Thomas, N.W. & Desiraju, G.R. (1984) *Chem. Phys. Lett.* **110**, 99
Vedani, A. & Dunitz, J.D. (1985) *J. Amer. Chem. Soc.*, **107**, 7653

4

The representation of molecular structure on a computer graphics system

Ian Tickle
Department of Crystallography, Birkbeck College, Malet Street,
London WC1E 7HX

1. INTRODUCTION: WHAT IS REQUIRED OF A MOLECULAR GRAPHICS SYSTEM?

1.1 Price/performance considerations

Molecules, notwithstanding the traditional chemist's schematic two-dimensional (2D) representation of point atoms connected by lines signifying chemical bonds, are, with very few exceptions, three-dimensional (3D) objects; in addition no molecule is ever static. Thus a picture of a molecule, even if produced on a graph plotter as a stereo pair, is at best merely a snapshot of the real-life situation. The visualization of molecules and their properties on a flat computer graphics display screen therefore poses particular problems for the software designer.

Most other major applications of computer graphics technology, such as computer-aided design (CAD), have had to deal mainly with 2D images, and so have not, on the whole, had to cope with the extra complexity of 3D. For this reason, and also because the high cost increment in going from 2D to 3D, hardware and software suppliers have been until quite recently slow to offer low-cost systems capable of the effective display of molecular structure in all its aspects.

For example, 3D graphics standards are only just now being properly established, even though the corresponding 2D standards have been in place for a considerable time. This has placed an extra burden on the programmer: software developed on one system could not readily be transferred to a different manufacture's hardware, or even to a different model from the same manufacturer.

To quote another example of this kind of problem: the equipment required to produce acceptable stereo images of molecules on a graphics display is regarded by many users of such systems as absolutely essential, and yet, because it is not required by most other applications, it is consequently available from only a very few specialist suppliers at relatively high cost.

The aim is to produce a graphical model that is a 'kinaesthetic' representation, in other words the graphical model has at least the same capacity for movement and modification as one would expect a real model, made of metal or plastics, to have.

It is certainly possible, with some ingenuity, to write programs capable of producing passable 3D representations of molecules on low-cost systems such as personal computers (PCs). However, if real-time motion is desired, such programs are invariably limited to molecules made up of a relatively small number of atoms (say, not more than 100); more complex molecules require much more sophisticated and expensive hardware and software.

Even if one is fortunate to have access to such a high-performance system, it is important to be aware that it has its own limitations. The upper limit on the number of lines that can be displayed whilst still achieving the illusion of smooth 3D motion will be very high (typically 10 000–100 000 per frame at the time of writing, although the rapid march of technology will undoubtedly soon render obsolete these and other performance figures that I quote).

But even these limits can be a serious obstacle in some applications, such as the display of molecular surfaces. Futhermore, if it is desired to use a filled polygon representation instead of a line drawing, then to maintain smooth motion, one must accept a dramatic reduction in the size of molecule that can be displayed, typically by a factor of 100, so again in this case the limit is of the order of a few hundred atoms. Of course one can display a static picture of many thousands of atoms, but then it is usually hard to justify the acquisition of a high-performance system on the basis of producing static pictures alone.

For a thorough review of the various ways of representing molecules on a graphics display, see Plastock & Kalley (1986).

1.2 Programming considerations

The novice programmer can therefore learn some of the software techniques required for molecular graphics by using only a PC and suitable software, even though the program can only be tested with small-molecule data. It is strongly emphasized, however, that if the aim is to develop software for a high-performance system, then the issue of software portability across the different systems has to be considered.

Most PC graphics software provides little more than the ability to draw points and lines of specified colours on the screen; other capabilities are usually also provided, such as the production of graphs and charts, but these are hardly useful for drawing molecules. 3D geometric transformations, such as perspective, scaling, rotation, and translation of the line end-points, which are required to achieve the illusion of smooth motion in 3D, must be coded in the high-level language in use on the PC (such as FORTRAN or C), and interactive data-entry devices are usually limited to the keyboard and a mouse or trackball.

In contrast, a high-performance system will provide a much greater range of useful primitive objects, such as character strings, multiple lines and polygons; there will be a wider choice of attributes, such as line texture, hue, colour saturation, brightness, etc.; there will be the means to specify hierarchies of objects, so that the one-to-one correspondence between the conceptual model and the program structure is clear and much less prone to programming blunders; and most importantly there will be routines for performing all the required 3D transformations by using matrix and vector arithmetic in special-purpose hardware.

The high data throughput is achieved by the use of multiple processors in either pipeline or parallel architecture to transform the graphical data. In addition there will be a wider range of interactive data-entry devices, and the display itself will be of higher resolution and quality than a normal PC colour monitor, and with the option of stereo imaging.

Typical examples of such high-performance graphics systems that are commonly in use for macromolecular graphical display and modelling are the Evans & Sutherland PS300 and ESV series, and the Silicon Graphics Iris 4D series.

An important issue that is relevant here is program modularity. Two main phases of any well-constructed graphics program can always be readily distinguished, namely model generation and model display. First, the generation of the graphical model employs primitives, attributes, and transformations formed into a hierarchical structure; and second, the display of the model involves traversing this structure and produces the illusion of motion by updating the transformations.

Lack of care in organizing the program logic is likely to have a much greater impact on program efficiency on a high-performance system than on a PC. Consequently it is very important to employ correct programming techniques at the outset.

The generation phase need be performed only once for each model, but the display phase has to be repeated with different values of the transformations at least 10 times per second (compare the 16 frames/second used in cinematography) for the brain to perceive smooth motion. Therefore, for maximum efficiency and to avoid unnecessary repetition, it is important to separate carefully the components of the program which fall into the two phases. This is precisely the purpose of program modularity; to keep conceptually distinct parts of the program in separate modules. In fact if this separation is done properly, the display phase need have no knowledge of what objects it is actually displaying; it need only know the transformations that are to be performed.

It is the author's experience that most programmers new to graphics programming have much more difficulty with the display phase than with the generation phase. In the limited space available, it is not possible to cover all aspects in the same detail, therefore this chapter will concentrate mainly on these aspects of model display which programmers find most difficult to grasp.

2. COMPUTER GRAPHICS SYSTEMS: DESCRIPTIVE BACKGROUND

2.1 Architecture of a representative high-performance interactive graphics system

Although it is of course unnecessary for the programmer to have an intimate knowledge of the hardware, it is nevertheless critical that he/she is at least aware of the principal data paths through the system at a schematic level. This is because the need for many of the software concepts to be introduced later, such as display lists, is not readily apparent without a basic knowledge of the machine's 'architecture'. This section therefore brings together these concepts with the associated pieces of hardware; the main flow of data is normally in a unidirectional fashion from beginning (Applications model) to end (Display unit).

For further information on the concepts introduced in the section, consult Foley & van Dam (1982).

2.1.1 Applications model (AM)
This is just the raw data, normally atomic coordinates in Ångstrom units, for one or several molecules, together with labelling information, and application-dependent data such as atomic type, radius, charge, etc. The coordinate system of the AM is usually termed 'world space'; it is sometimes made up of several objects, each with their own local coordinate system, termed 'object space'.

2.1.2 Graphics processor unit (GPU)
This is usually a relatively slow general-purpose computer which runs the graphics program to process the applications model into a form suitable for the display processor, to which it is attached by a high-speed interface. This computer is also responsible for processing information from interactive data-entry devices used for communication between the human operator and the program, and sending the information in appropriate format to the graphics processor. The GPU should not be used for applying transformations to the coordinates; this is the responsibility of the Matrix Arithmetic Processor, which is specially designed for this purpose (see below).

2.1.3 Structured display list (SDL)
This is a representation generated by the GPU by using graphical primitives, attributes, and transformations, of all or part of the AM, usually in high-speed access memory in the graphics system, which is used as a base level from which all interactive transformations are made.

The SDL is effectively a program, and associated data, that loops continuously in the DPU, and asynchronously with the control program running in the GPU.

2.1.4 Display processor unit (DPU)
This is the main processor of the graphics system, responsible for managing the SDL; it cycles through the SDL, interpreting the information as either graphics primitive, attribute, or transformation, and directing it to the next stage. In some systems, the interactive data-entry devices are connected to the DPU instead of, or in addition to, the GPU.

2.1.5 Matrix arithmetic processor(s) (MAP)
This is one, or more often several, special purpose processors, responsible for performing concatenation of transformations and for applying the result to the

graphics primitives coming from the DPU. The transformations can be classified as 'modelling', which alter the relative translational and/or rotational positions of different segments of the graphical model in world space; and 'viewing'. The latter can be considered either as translating/rotating the model in its entirety, or equivalently, since all motion is relative, as moving the observer's viewing position in the opposite direction. The resultant coordinate system, which is in the same units as the world coordinates, is termed 'viewing space'.

Viewing transformations also include the 'windowing' operation, which converts 'viewing coordinates' into a convenient intermediate coordinate system, termed 'normalized viewing coordinates'. Other viewing transformations are the perspective transformation (or other type of projection), and the stereoscopic transformation, which prepares left- and right-eye views for a suitable stereo viewing system.

Note that although the modelling and viewing transformations are conceptually distinct, the hardware makes no such distinction, and all these transformations are performed in an identical manner by using the MAP. For the mathematics behind these transformations, refer to section 3, 'Mathematical background'.

2.1.6   Clipping processor(s) (CP)

This is one or more special purpose processors whose sole function is to clip the transformed primitives, whose positions are now expressed in normalized viewing coordinates, so that only those wholly or partly inside a 3D viewing volume, or 'window' in viewing space, will appear in a designated rectangle, or 'viewport' in screen space, on the screen.

The window is bounded by 3 pairs of clipping planes; however, this will not necessarily have the shape of a rectangular box. If perspective has been applied it will be the volume visible through a rectangular aperture, that is a basal section of a rectangular pyramid, or 'frustum', with the imaginary apex of the pyramid at the eye position. In addition to the 'left', 'right', 'bottom' and 'top' clipping planes bounding the window, clipping is usually also performed at the 'hither' and 'yon' planes, because temporary removal of both close and distant parts of the model often aids comprehension.

Clipping is inherently a numerically intensive operation, and therefore a separate processor is often assigned to each of the six clipping planes.

2.1.7   Viewport mapping processor (VP)

This just scales (or maps) the clipped 3D window to the actual screen viewport size. The viewport may be the whole screen, or just part of it; in fact several viewports can occupy the same screen. It is convenient to think of the viewport as being 3-dimensional, with the third dimension being brightness. The mapping is then 3D to 3D, with no information lost, since the transformed z coordinate is mapped to a brightness scale to produce the 'depth-cueing' effect. The resulting impression on the screen is of a 3D view being observed through a real (2D) window.

The MAP, CP, and VP are often connected in pipeline fashion, for maximum throughput.

2.1.8   *Rasterisation processor(s) (RP)*

These rasterize the primitives, in other words they determine which pixels on the screen need to be illuminated to make up the final picture. In addition, anti-aliasing (smoothing out of pixel steps) is often performed at this stage. The RP's can work in parallel fashion, each one taking care of a particular portion of the screen, although this is not done directly, but rather through the frame buffer.

2.1.9   *Frame buffer (FB)*

This is memory in which the picture is stored temporarily before display. This is required because the television monitor must operate at 50 or 60 frames per second to avoid unpleasant flickering effects, whereas the graphics processors can only send information about the changing parts of the picture, and even then only at a lower rate (typically at least 10 frames/sec). The frame buffer memory can be thought of as consisting of a number of planes, each plane consisting of one bit (binary digit) for every pixel in the display. The number of planes available determines the amount of information that can be stored for each pixel. This information can be colour, brightness, height, visibility, etc., depending on the way it is interpreted by the lookup table.

One further refinement is possible; the frame buffer can be double buffered, that is, divided into two halves containing an equal number of planes. Then, the data coming from the RP can be directed to one half whilst the other half is actually displayed. This avoids the problem where the displayed picture consists of parts of successive frames and there is an obvious 'join' where they do not quite match up.

2.1.10   *Colour lookup table (LUT)*

This is used because there are many more different colours that the TV monitor is capable of displaying that can be stored in the frame buffer memory, unless this is very large. The values of the numbers in the frame buffer can be simply regarded as addresses in the LUT, from which the actual colour, in its red, green, and blue components, is actually obtained. This also gives the programmer the ability of changing the colours very rapidly by simply changing the contents of the LUT, although this is probably of limited usefulness in molecular graphics applications.

2.1.11   *Display unit (DU)*

This is the television monitor and associated amplifying and scanning electronics, which continuously scans the frame buffer, using the LUT to determine the final pixel colours. For optimum picture quality, a high-resolution monitor (typically at least 1280×1024 pixels) with fast anti-aliasing is essential.

2.2   Characteristics of interactive data-entry devices

This section summarizes the characteristics of the interactive data-entry devices in common use with graphics systems.

The 'analogue' characteristic indicates that the device functions by measuring some electrical property such as voltage and returns its magnitude, which must then be passed through an analogue-to-digital converter to the computer; a 'digital' device works typically by counting pulses and returning the count directly to the computer. 'Detente' indicates that the device can return values only in a finite range; conversely, 'no detente' indicates that in principle the device can return an infinite range of values; however, the computer itself can work only with finite values and will therefore impose its own limits.

A 'string' device returns one or more characters; a 'choice' device indicates selection between two or more options; a 'valuator' returns a single value; 'a pick' device indicates selection of an items on the screen; a 'stroke' device is able to draw continuous lines; and a 'locator' returns two or three values simultaneously, thus locating a position in 2D or less commonly 3D.

Devices and functions

Keyboard	string, locator (crude !)
Switches/buttons	choice
Control knobs	analogue, detente, valuator
Control dials	digital, no detente, valuator
Light pen	pick
2D joystick	analogue, detente, pick, locator
3D joystick	analogue, detente, locator
Trackball	digital, no detente, locator
Touch-sensitive screen	digital, detente, pick, locator
Mouse	digital, no detente, pick, stroke, locator
Data tablet with pen or puck	digital, detente, pick, stroke, locator

2.3   3D perception techniques
Various techniques, usually in combination, are employed to enhance the desired 3D effect on the flat display screen. These can be classified as mono- and stereo-scopic, according to whether one or two views are presented to the user's vision, in the latter case corresponding to the views from the positions of the observer's left and right eyes.

2.3.1   Monoscopic techniques
(a) *Depth-cueing with hither and yon clipping* This can be a very effective 3D visual cue, even though brightness variation is rarely a 3D cue in the real world.
(b) *Perspective* This is the effect that distant objects appear smaller than near ones, and parallel straight lines appear to converge to a point on the horizon (except lines parallel to the plane of projection). By itself, perspective is usually not very effective; this is because visual perception employs perspective to judge the distances of familiar objects of approximately known sizes; for example the height of a nearby person can be compared with that of a distant tree to estimate the distance of the tree, but to do this one must have a rough idea of the typical heights of both people and trees. The problem is that the visual system probably does not regard molecules as familiar objects of known size, and therefore has difficulty in forming a 3D impression without further visual cues.

(c) *Motion parallax* This is related to perspective and is the effect observed from a moving vehicle where near objects appear to move in the opposite direction of travel faster than more distant ones. The eye position used to calculate the perspective transformation has to be moved sideways or up/down to achieve this effect, but it is much more effective than perspective alone. This is probably because the human visual system uses motion parallax as a strong visual cue; small but unconscious sideways movements of the head induce the effect.

(d) *Hidden-primitive removal* This is simply obscuration of part of the view by another closer part. By itself, this does not give sufficient visual cue; however, if it is not done consistently, the visual system will receive opposing cues, and confusion will result.

(e) *Real-time rotation* The visual system easily recognizes rotation, either with periodic reversals 'rocking', or continuously in the same direction 'rolling', as a rigid-body motion, and therefore associates it with an object having extent in 3D. However, without other cues (depth, parallax, hidden-primitive), confusion between front and back of the object being viewed can result; the rotation then appears to occur in the wrong direction.

2.3.2 Stereoscopic techniques

The aim here is to present each eye separately with the view it would expect to get; it is very important that neither eye sees any part of the view intended for the other one, and it is precisely in this aspect that many designs fail. A number of devices are available commercially, and they fall into two classes, space and time division. In the former the screen is divided into two halves and displays the two views, which are routed to the corresponding eyes by means of mirrors and/or polaroids. In the latter, the display alternately shows the two views; the left eye is by some means prevented from seeing the right-eye view, and vice versa, and the alternation is sufficiently rapid that the persistence of vision effect eliminates most or all of any flickering produced. These devices employ a mechanical lorgnette or piezoelectric or liquid crystal, in each case more-or-less precisely synchronized with the display alternation.

3   MOLECULAR GRAPHICS: MATHEMATICAL BACKGROUND

3.1   Three-dimensional geometrical operations in matrix/vector notation

In the equations that follow the vector $\mathbf{x}$, with components (x, y, z) is transformed into the vector $\mathbf{x}'$, with components (x', y', z'), by the operation described. In each case the output $\mathbf{x}'$ from one transformation may be the input $\mathbf{x}$ to another.

3.1.1   Translation

$$\mathbf{x}' = \mathbf{x} + \mathbf{t}$$

The translation operation moves an object while preserving its orientation; see

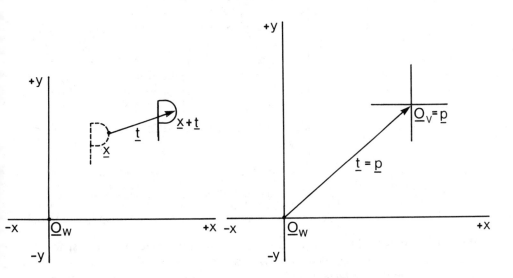

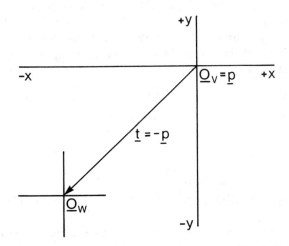

Fig. 1. (a) Translation modelling transformation: object (P) is translated by $\underline{t}$ from $\underline{x}$ to $\underline{x} + \underline{t}$. O_w is the origin of world space.

(b) Translation viewing transformation: viewing space origin $\underline{O}_v$ is translated to point $\underline{p}$.

(c) World space is translated by $-\underline{p}$ so that point $\underline{p}$ moves to $\underline{O}_v$; this is exactly equivalent to (b).

Fig. 1(a). This is used, for example, to translate the origin of viewing space, together with the observer who is fixed in that space, initially to the position **p** of a chosen

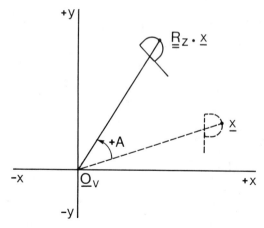

Fig. 2. Rotation modelling transformation: object (P) is rotated around the z axis ($+z$ out of paper) through angle A in viewing space.

atom, or perhaps to the molecular centroid (mean coordinate), in world space. This could equally well be regarded as moving world space and the objects in it by the same amount in the opposite direction ($\mathbf{t} = -\mathbf{p}$), so that the chosen atom or centroid moves to the origin of viewing space, but the former description is in keeping with the concept of keeping the 'world' fixed and having the observer change his viewpoint; see Figs. 1(b) and (c).

Further interactive translations can be made to change the point in the molecule that is at the origin of viewing space. This is necessary because rotations occur about this origin (see next section).

3.1.2   *Rotation*

$$\mathbf{x}' = \mathbf{R} \cdot \mathbf{x}$$

for example

$$\mathbf{R}_z(A) = \begin{bmatrix} \cos A & -\sin A & 0 \\ \sin A & \cos A & 0 \\ 0 & 0 & 1 \end{bmatrix}$$

The rotation operation moves an object around an axis passing through the origin of viewing space, in this example through an angle $+A$ about the coordinate z axis. The positive sense is defined as that producing an anticlockwise rotation when looking from the positive side of the axis towards the origin; see Fig. 2.

Similarly for rotations about the x and y coordinate axes:

$$\mathbf{R}_x(A) = \begin{bmatrix} 1 & 0 & 0 \\ 0 & \cos A & -\sin A \\ 0 & \sin A & \cos A \end{bmatrix}$$

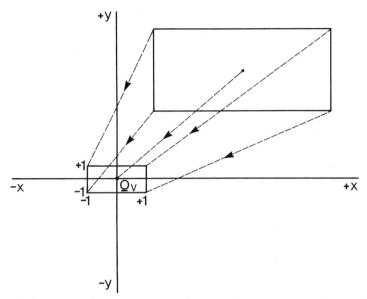

Fig. 3. Windowing transformation: rectangular box in viewing space is mapped to normalized viewing space; unit vectors in this space are indicated by −1 and +1.

$$\mathbf{R}_y(A) = \begin{bmatrix} \cos A & 0 & \sin A \\ 0 & 1 & 0 \\ -\sin A & 0 & \cos A \end{bmatrix}$$

In principle an object can be rotated about any arbitrary axis, but any general rotation can be expressed as a product of three (or more) rotations about the base vectors, and for most purposes it is more convenient to use these rotations.

3.1.3 Scaling

$$\mathbf{x}' = \mathbf{S} \cdot \mathbf{x}$$

$$\mathbf{S} = \begin{bmatrix} S_x & 0 & 0 \\ 0 & S_y & 0 \\ 0 & 0 & S_z \end{bmatrix}$$

Scaling a model of a physical system is usually meaningless; the system exists with the magnitudes Nature has pre-ordained, and therefore scaling is not generally used as a modelling transformation. However, the scaling operation is used as a viewing transformation in place of the windowing operation in the case where no translation is required; see next section.

3.1.4 Windowing

$$x' = \frac{2 \cdot (x - x(\text{min}))}{x(\text{max}) - x(\text{min})} - 1$$

with similar equations for y' and z'.

Substituting $x = x(\text{min})$ and $x = x(\text{max})$, the transformed coordinates are $x' = -1$ and $x' = +1$ respectively. Thus the viewing space coordinates inside the window bounded by the planes $x = x(\text{min})$ and $x = x(\text{max})$ are linearly normalized to the range -1 to $+1$, and similarly for the y and z coordinates.

The positions of the clipping planes, $x(\text{min})$, $x(\text{max})$, $y(\text{min})$, $y(\text{max})$, $z(\text{min})$ and $z(\text{max})$, are in viewing coordinates. They can be given so that the molecule is totally enclosed within the window, or alternatively a smaller volume can be specified, for example to select and magnify a particular region of interest.

The windowing operation can also be written as:

$$\mathbf{x'} = \mathbf{S} \cdot \mathbf{x} + \mathbf{t}$$

demonstrating its relationship to the translation and scaling operations. This effectively centres and scales the molecule by mapping from viewing to normalized viewing coordinates; see Fig. 3.

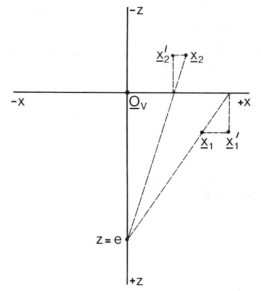

Fig. 4. Perspective transformation: points $\underline{x}_1$ and $\underline{x}_2$ are mapped to $\underline{x}'_1$ and $\underline{x}'_2$ by projecting through the eye position at $(0, 0, e)$ onto the $z = 0$ plane and then shifting back by the original z coordinate. This shows only the x and z coordinates of the points; the y coordinate is transformed in an equivalent way to x.

Usually, the molecule will have already been centred by use of the translation, so then only scaling will be required. In that case, the centre of rotation at the origin of viewing space should be at the centre of the window, so that $x(\text{min}) = -x(\text{max})$, and similarly for y and z. The windowing transformation then becomes just:

$$x' = x/x(\text{max}) \quad \text{and similarly for } y \text{ and } z.$$

The world and viewing coordinate systems are by convention right-handed, that is, holding the thumb and first and second fingers of the right hand at right angles to each other, they point in the positive x, y, and z directions respectively. In some older hardware and texts a left-handed coordinate system is used for both world and viewing space; the directions of the positive x and y axes of viewing space are the same, namely toward the right edge of the screen and upwards respectively, but the positive z axis is into the screen away from the observer, instead of toward the observer as in the right-handed system. This can easily be compensated by applying a scaling transformation with $S_x = S_y = 1, S_z = -1$ immediately before the windowing transformation.

3.1.5   *Perspective*

$$x' = \frac{x}{1 - z/e} \qquad y' = \frac{y}{1 - z/e}$$

$$z' = z$$

This performs a projection on to the $z = 0$ plane through the eye position at $(0, 0, e)$, in normalized viewing coordinates; see Fig 4. It should be mentioned that this is not the only way to specify the perspective projection; other authors differ both on the position of the projection plane and the position of the eye.

Typically, $e = 4$, but if the eye position is moved to infinity so that the factor $1/e$ becomes zero, then this becomes an identity operation, and the result is an orthographic projection, that is perpendicular projection onto the plane of the screen. Normally, in orthographic and perspective projection the z coordinate is lost; in this case we need to keep it as depth-cueing information.

3.1.6   *Stereo*
The usual way to do this is to apply a rotation of + 3 degs for the left-eye view and − 3 for the right-eye. However, a better and simpler way is to do shear operations of the same magnitude:

$$x' = x + 0.05iz \qquad i = +1 \text{ (left)}, -1 \text{ (right)}$$

$$y' = y$$

$$z' = z$$

The factor 0.05 is just 3 degs in radians (roughly). The reason why this is better is that the rotations move wedges of the window in opposite directions thus destroying the stereo effect at the places where it is most noticeable, at the front of the window; see Fig. 5(a). The shear operation also moves wedges out of the clipping planes, but these are at the sides where it is less noticeable; see Fig. 5(b).

3.1.7   *Clipping*
Primitives are not passed on unless:

$$-1 \leq x \leq +1$$

$$-1 \leq y \leq +1$$

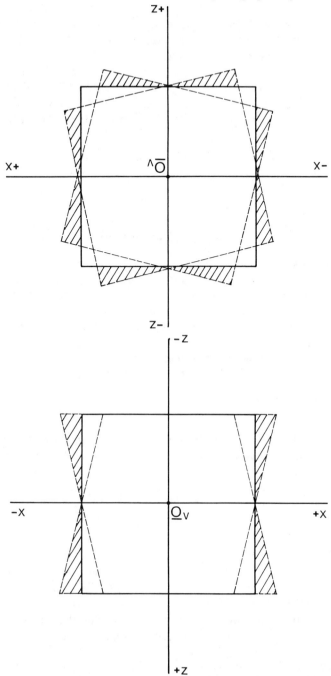

Fig. 5. (a) Stereo transformation using small rotations (the magnitude of the rotation is exaggerated for clarity). The shaded areas would be clipped.
(b) As (a) but using shear transformations; the clipped regions are now not as intrusive.

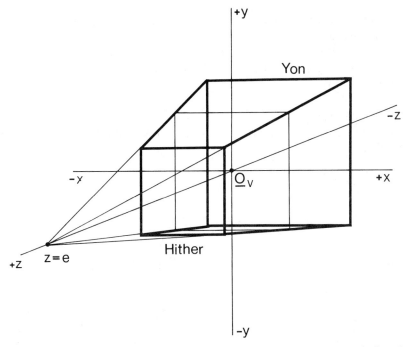

Fig. 6. Perspective projection showing frustum of vision; the six clipping planes are indicated by heavy lines, and the hither and yon planes are labelled.

$$-1 \leq z \leq +1$$

in normalized viewing coordinates. The main reason for working in this intermediate coordinate system is that it is not necessary to pass the positions and orientations of the clipping planes in world or viewing coordinates to the CPs, thus greatly simplifying the clipping arithmetic.

For the perspective projection, the 6 clipping planes enclose a basal section of a square pyramid (frustum) whose vertex lies at the eye position (Fig. 6). For the orthographic projection this becomes a rectangular box (rectangular parallelepiped), or in the case that the window sides are of equal length, a cube. Primitives lying completely outside the clipping planes are not drawn; those lying partially inside are clipped.

3.1.8   Window-to-viewpoint mapping

$$x' = \frac{(x'(\text{max}) - x'(\text{min})) \cdot (x + 1)}{2} + x'(\text{min})$$

with similar equations for y' and z'.

$x'(\text{min})$, $x'(\text{max})$, $y'(\text{min})$, $y'(\text{max})$, $z'(\text{min})$, and $z'(\text{max})$ are the viewport boundaries in screen coordinates, that is, pixels with the origin at the lower left corner of the screen; x' is positive toward the right edge of the screen, y' is positive upward, and the z coordinate is mapped to a brightness scale, using the LUT. This is similar to the windowing operation, except that here the transformation is from normalized viewing coordinates to the final screen coordinates.

A point to note here is that the ratio of the height of the viewport to its width, termed the 'aspect ratio', must be the same as that of the window, otherwise distortion of the picture will occur.

3.2   Coordinate spaces

This just summarizes the coordinate spaces introduced here, with their inter-relationships.

Object coordinates.

$\downarrow$ Place object(s) in world space.

World coordinates

$\downarrow$ View world space in the observer's frame.

Viewing coordinates

$\downarrow$ Scaling and perspective projection.

Normalized viewing coordinates

$\downarrow$ Clip and map to screen viewport.

Screen coordinates.

3.3   Implementation of transformations, using a 4 × 4 matrix (homogeneous coordinates)

A homogeneous coordinate vector has the form: (x, y, z, w). This has the property that multiplying all 4 coordinates by a constant does not change the position of the point defined, for example $(2x, 2y, 2z, 2w)$ is the same point. This is useful when the matrix processor can work only with integers with limited word size. For example, with 16 bits an integer can have values only in the range -32768 to $+32767$, and a problem arises if numbers outside this range have to be represented. The solution is to decrease w. Thus the point (32767, 32767, 32767, 16383) is the same as the point (65534, 65534, 65534, 32766) although the latter cannot be directly represented.

The drawback is that if w is halved, it can still be represented only by an integer, and therefore the rounding errors in the actual x, y, and z coordinates (not the homogeneous ones) double. As z becomes smaller, the actual coordinates are rounded even more coarsely. Thus homogenous coordinates represent a trade-off between range and precision. Most current matrix processors have floating-point capability, so the problem of limited range does not arise in practice, and rounding errors are considerably reduced.

The conventional 3×3 matrix can be used only for rotations, scaling, and stereo; a homogeneous transformation matrix can incorporate translations, windowing, and perspective as well, and is therefore used for all the transformations previously described except clipping and window-to-viewpoint mapping.

In all the matrices that follow, missing elements are zero; also it is assumed that floating-point arithmetic is available, so the w scaling factor is normally unity.

Translation:
$$\begin{bmatrix} 1 & t & x & x+t \\ & 1 & u & . \; y & = & y+u \\ & & 1 \; v & z & = & z+v \\ & & & 1 & 1 & 1 \end{bmatrix}$$

Rotation $[\mathbf{x}' = \mathbf{R}.x]$:
$$\begin{bmatrix} . & . & . & x & x' \\ . & \mathbf{R} & . & . \; y & = & y' \\ . & . & . & z & z' \\ & & 1 & 1 & 1 \end{bmatrix}$$

Scaling:
$$\begin{bmatrix} S_x & & x & S_x.x \\ & S_y & y & = & S_y.y \\ & & S_z & , \; z & S_z.z \\ & & 1 & 1 & 1 \end{bmatrix}$$

Windowing:
$$\begin{bmatrix} 2/A & & -a/A \\ & 2/B & -b/B \\ & & 2/C & -c/C \\ & & & 1 \end{bmatrix} \begin{bmatrix} x \\ y \\ z \\ 1 \end{bmatrix} = \begin{bmatrix} (2x-a)/A \\ (2y-b)/B \\ (2z-c)/C \\ 1 \end{bmatrix}$$

with $A = x(\max) - x(\min)$, $B = y(\max) - y(\min)$, $C = z(\max) - z(\min)$,
$a = x(\max) + x(\min)$, $b = y(\max) + y(\min)$, $c = z(\max) + z(\min)$.

Stereo:
$$\begin{bmatrix} 1 & 0.05i \\ & 1 \\ & & 1 \\ & & & 1 \end{bmatrix} . \begin{bmatrix} x \\ y \\ z \\ 1 \end{bmatrix} = \begin{bmatrix} x + 0.05iz \\ y \\ z \\ 1 \end{bmatrix}$$

$i = +1$ for left eye,   0 for mono, -1 for right-eye.

Perspective with optional stereo:
$$\begin{bmatrix} 1 & 0.05i \\ & 1 \\ & & 1 & -1/e \\ & & -1/e & 1 \end{bmatrix}$$

The stereo transformation is here conveniently incorporated into the perspective matrix, while still allowing the mono option. The windowing and perspective transformations are also usually combined (as 'perspective-window'), but it is easier to understand what is happening if they are written out separately.

The homogeneous perspective matrix above does not give exactly the same result as was given in section 3.1.5. x' and y' are the same, but z' is different:

$$z' = \frac{z - 1/e}{1 - z/e}$$

The reason is that it is impossible to get exactly the desired transformation even with homogeneous coordinates. However, the z' values obtained at the clipping planes (-1 and $+1$) are the same as before, although the value obtained for $z = 0$ is different ($z' = -1/e$). This means that the z' coordinate is non-linear; this is unimportant since this will be mapped to brightness and the eye is unable to detect the difference.

A point concerning the order of matrix multiplication must be made here. Conventionally in matrix algebra, matrices pre-multiply column vectors (that is, matrix on the left), and the result is a column vector; this is the convention adopted throughout this chapter. However, in some texts the matrices post-multiply the vectors (that is, matrix on the right). Consequently the matrices and vectors are all transposed, so that the vectors are all row vectors. The crucial point is that in such a situation all matrices will be printed as the transpose of those shown above.

3.4   Associativity and commutativity of matrix multiplication

3.4.1   Associativity of transformations
The associativity law of matrix multiplication asserts that the result is the same regardless of the way in which a string of matrices are multiplied, provided that the matrices are kept in the same order.
For example:

$$\mathbf{P} \cdot (\mathbf{W} \cdot (\mathbf{R} \cdot (\mathbf{T} \cdot \mathbf{x}))) = (((\mathbf{P} \cdot \mathbf{W}) \cdot \mathbf{R}) \cdot \mathbf{T}) \cdot \mathbf{x}$$

The beauty of this is that instead of multiplying each matrix separately onto the coordinate vectors, all the matrices can be multiplied together first and then the single result matrix multiplied onto the coordinates. This is the importance of the homogeneous matrices; using only 3×3 matrices it is not possible to specify all transformations as matrices, and therefore the above association would not be possible. Since there are normally only a few matrices but possibly thousands of coordinate vectors, this represents a considerable improvement in efficiency.

A typical transformation sequence might therefore be:

$$\mathbf{x}' = \mathbf{V} \cdot [\text{clip}] \cdot (\mathbf{P} \cdot \mathbf{W} \cdot \mathbf{R} \cdot \mathbf{T}) \cdot \mathbf{x}$$

Here, $\mathbf{V}$, $\mathbf{P}$, $\mathbf{W}$, $\mathbf{R}$, $\mathbf{T}$ stand for viewport, perspective, windowing, rotation, and translation transformations.

A crucial point to note here is that the transformation is always applied to the original coordinate vectors; the transformed coordinates are displayed and then discarded. This procedure implies that the matrix product represents the accumulation of all previous operations, which is then multiplied onto the original coordinates, rather than what one might think of as being more natural, namely that the matrix product represents only the changes and the coordinates are continually updated.

Although the second method has the apparent advantage that only one set of coordinates need be maintained in memory, whereas the first requires both the original and current sets, there are actually three reasons for not doing it in the second way. The original coordinates usually need to be kept anyway, in case the user wishes to go back to the initial view; the transformed coordinates can be maintained at lower precision than the original ones; and even if they are maintained at the same precision, rounding errors would gradually accumulate, as a consequence of the continuous cycling round the display loop. It is also true that rounding errors will build up as the matrices are accumulated; however, since the correct form of each matrix is known, rounding errors can be detected and eliminated by a suitable renormalization procedure (see section 4.8).

3.4.2 Commutativity of transformations
The commutativity law of matrix multiplication asserts that, except in special cases, reversing the order of multiplication of two matrices produces a different result. It is useful to know what are the special cases, that is where the matrices 'commute', as then an unnecessary matrix multiplication can be avoided.

$R(p)$ commutes with $R(q)$ only if $p = q$ or $p = -q$.

Rotations about the same axis (or its negative) commute.

$R(p)$ commutes with $t(q)$ only if $p = q$ or $p = -q$.

The same holds for rotations about an axis and translations parallel to the same axis.

$t(p)$ commutes with $t(q)$ for all p, q.

All translations commute, regardless of direction.

Other transformations (for example anisotropic scale, windowing, perspective) are generally non-commutative.

3.5 Bond torsion
Frequently, it is necessary to rotate the whole or part of a molecule around one or more chemical bonds, since torsion about single bonds is usually the lowest energy path for deformation of the molecule. In section 3.1 it was mentioned that rotation about an arbitary axis can be expressed in terms of 3 or more rotations about the base vectors of the coordinate system. Somewhat paradoxically, it is much simpler to express an arbitrary axis rotation in terms of 5 base vector rotations instead of 3.

As before, before applying a rotation in world space it is necessary to shift the object so that a point p on the rotation axis, namely one of the atoms connected by the bond of interest, is at the origin of viewing space. After the rotations are done, the object will be shifted back so that the same point returns to its original position.

One procedure for doing the rotation, though this is not by any means the only way, is to move the object so that the second atom lies on the $+z$ axis; this is done in two steps. Then the object is actually rotated (through angle A below) about z axis, now coincident with the bond. Care must be taken to define the positive sense of rotation about the bond; the usual convention is to consider the nearer atom (at $+z$) as the moving one when looking from a point on the $+z$ side, so that positive is an anticlockwise rotation of this atom. Alternatively, and equivalently, a positive rotation can be defined as a clockwise rotation of the further atom. Finally, the first two rotations are reversed to bring the bond back along its original direction.

The two rotations which bring the bond along the $+z$ axis consist of a rotation about z through an angle $-C$ to bring the bond into the xz plane (in the $+x$ hemisphere), and a rotation about y through an angle $-B$; see Fig. 7. In terms of the direction cosines $(1, m, n)$ (unit vector) of the bond, the angles C and B are given by:

$$C = \tan^{-1}(m/1) \quad \text{and} \quad B = \tan^{-1}((1^2 + m^2)^{1/2}/n)$$

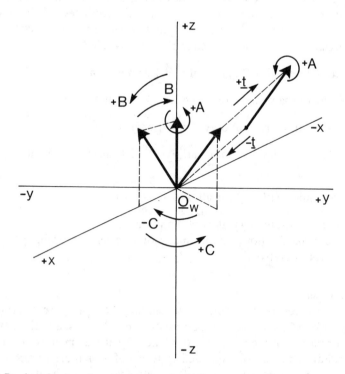

Fig. 7. Bond torsion transformations; these should be followed in the order: $-t$, $-C$, $-B$, $+A$, $+B$, $+C$, $+t$.

Sequence of transformations to produce bond torsion

    Translate $-\mathbf{p}$

    Rotate $\mathbf{R}_z(-C)$

    Rotate $\mathbf{R}_y(-B)$

    Rotate $\mathbf{R}_z(A)$

    Rotate $\mathbf{R}_y(B)$

    Rotate $\mathbf{R}_z(C)$

    Translate $\mathbf{p}$

Some graphics systems can calculate, in one step, an arbitrary axis rotation matrix, which replaces the five rotations above. However, because of the association of matrix transformations, this represents a difference in programming convenience, not execution speed.

Rotation matrix for rotation angle A *about unit vector* (l, m, n):

$$
\begin{bmatrix}
l^2.(1-\cos A)+\cos A & l.m.(1-\cos A)+n.\sin A & l.n.(1-\cos A)-m.\sin A \\
l.m.(1-\cos A)-n.\sin A & m^2.(1-\cos A)+\cos A & m.n.(1-\cos A)+l.\sin A \\
l.n.(1-\cos A)+m.\sin A & m.n.(1-\cos A)-l.\sin A & n^2.(1-\cos A)+\cos A
\end{bmatrix}
$$

4. SOFTWARE CONCEPTS IN COMPUTER GRAPHICS

4.1 Graphics primitives

Graphics primitives are the graphics programmer's model-building components. They are entities predefined by the source of the graphics software library, so that the programmer is freed from concerns about the mechanics of turning a primitive into the collection of illuminated pixels on the screen. An entity is regarded as primitive if it can be produced by a single call to the library, no matter how complex it is.

The programmer need only be concerned about the parameters required to define the geometrical properties (position, length, direction) of the primitive in object or world space. Of course, if the software library does not provide certain primitives, then the programmer's only recourse is to define the missing primitives in terms of simpler ones; for example curves and surfaces can be defined as sets of connected short line segments and polygons respectively.

Typical set of primitives

    Dot

    Line

    Rectangle

    Character   (text symbol with origin in lower left corner.)

    Marker   (centred symbol)

    Polyline   (set of connected lines)

Polygon   (triangle, hexagon, etc.)
Text   (string of characters)
Polymarker   (set of markers)
Circle
Arc
Sphere
Curve
Fill area
Surface

As an example of the construction of a graphical model from primitives at the simplest possible level, a molecule could be represented as a set of dot primitives at the atomic positions, although by itself this representation would be rather uninformative; such a dot representation does, however, have a use in providing targets for picks (see section 4.5). At the next level, lines and polylines are used to represent bonds, and text is used to label some or all of the atoms; and at a higher level, surfaces are used to represent properties such as spatial extent, electric potential, etc.

4.2   Graphics attributes

The appearance of a primitive on the screen is modified by specifying attributes; in addition, a segment, that is, a set of rigidly associated primitives, can have additional attributes.

Primitive attributes
brightness	character font	fill
thickness	character size	pattern
blink	character rotation	texture
dash	string rotation	reflectivity
colour hue		transparency
colour saturation		

Segment attributes:
pick identifier	light source direction(s)
detectability	light source intensity(s)
visibility	light source colour(s)
highlighting	
level of detail	

4.3   Hidden line and surface suppression

There are three methods:

4.3.1   Colour blending

The easiest method is to ignore the problem! However, this is sensible only for transparent surface displays and for line displays, which are inherently transparent. On average, half the line crossings will be back-to-front, and this can be very confusing in complex line drawings, particularly if anti-aliasing is in effect, as this broadens the lines and increases the intersection areas. One solution is to add the values into the frame buffer, rather than just overwriting. This has the effect that the line crossing appears in a different colour, for example red and green add to give yellow, complementary colours add to give white; this highlighting effect can be useful when superposing two or molecules to investigate their similarities.

4.3.2   z-buffering
This is the most general method, but unfortunately also the most time consuming. The algorithm is very simple but effective. Part of the frame buffer is allocated to store the screen z coordinates of every pixel in the viewport (the screen z axis is perpendicular to the screen with the positive direction toward the viewer). Then the picture is generated in the usual way, but every time the colour of a new pixel is calculated its z coordinate is compared with that already in the buffer. If greater, the new colour overwrites the old one; if less, nothing is done. The result is that the pixel colours correspond to the part of the picture nearest the viewer, while those further away are hidden.

4.3.3   Back-facing polygon suppression
This method is used for filled polygon displays. If the polygons are always sent to the SDL with the vertices going round the same way when viewed from outside the object, say clockwise, then if after transformation the vertices still go round clockwise, the polygon must be front-facing; if the vertices go round anticlockwise, the polygon must be back-facing and can be suppressed. This will not work if one object hides another, and z-buffering is then the only solution. Because z-buffering is relatively slow, back-facing polygon suppression can still be used as a first stage of processing.

4.4   Data-entry device interaction
There are two alternative methods for getting information from the data-entry devices into the applications program running in the GPU.

4.4.1   Program polls device
Polling requires the program to initiate the requests for device information from the device controllers. This is inefficient because it cannot know whether the device has new information since the last time it was polled.

4.4.2   Device interrupts program
Each device interrupts the program only when it has new information available (for example dial moved or button pressed). Device information is automatically taken from the device controllers and is placed in an 'event queue', a portion of main memory reserved for this purpose. The program then need only test for a non-empty queue, and then obtain the device information from the queue. This method is therefore much more efficient than polling, though because it is a two-stage process, it is rather more complicated to program.

Regardless of the method used to obtain device information, whether polling or interrupting, new transformation matrices need be calculated only for device data that have changed since the last pass through the display loop, since clearly it is inefficient to repeat calculations when the result is already available.

4.5   Pick testing

The procedure for testing for a 'pick', that is selection of a displayed primitive or segment, is performed by making use of the windowing and clipping operations described in sections 3.1.4 and 3.1.7, as follows:

(1) Set up a square 'pick window' of specified (x, y) dimensions centred on the current cursor position.
(2) On receiving the pick signal from the user, temporarily (1 frame) blank the display.
(3) Save the current windowing transformation on the matrix stack.
(4) Change the windowing transformation to the 'pick window', so that clipping is now performed at the pick window x and y boundaries and the current hither and yon planes (and pick window would map to the screen viewport if the display were enabled).
(5) For a single frame only, define as the display object only the primitives or segments needed for picking. For example, if an atom is to be picked, this would be the set of dot primitives at the atomic positions; if a bond is to be picked, it would be the line drawing of the molecule.
(6) Return the address of the first primitive, or the pick identifier of the first segment to pass the clipping processors.
(7) Finally, disable picking, restore the original windowing transformation, restore the original display object, and re-enable the display.

Having identified exactly what has been picked, further appropriate action can be taken, such as retrieving the coordinates and label of the picked atom.

4.6   Example of structured display list

This uses a model of a car as an example because the object and its transformations are similar and easier to imagine than a molecule; however, the principle is the same.

In this example, a number of new concepts are introduced. 'Push' and 'pop' refer to copying and restoring the matrix that is currently being used to transform coordinates (the 'current transformation matrix' or CTM) on the matrix stack. This is an area of memory reserved in the MAP for this purpose where matrices are moved in and out on a 'last in, first out' (LIFO) basis.

To start, an identity (or unit) matrix must be pushed onto the empty stack to become the initial CTM. Then whenever a new matrix is generated, it is concatenated with the CTM, that is, in the column vector convention the CTM premultiplies the new matrix. The result matrix becomes the new CTM. When a coordinate transformation is required (indicated by "Draw ..."), the CTM premultiplies the coordinate column vectors. Thus the matrices appear in the program, reading from top to bottom, in the same order as in the matrix concatenation, reading from left to right, which, however, is the reverse of the order in which they are effectively applied to the coordinates.

In this way a well-defined hierarchical structure is set up (the levels of this hierarchy are indicated by indenting in the example). As well as push/pop, structure is defined by 'instancing', which is simply another name for 'subroutine' or 'procedure' in high-level languages. This makes a copy of an object by using a different transformation from that originally defined, without having to define the object all over again.

At the end of the display loop (line 'Go to View'), all transformation matrices, except the identity, have been 'popped' (that is, discarded), so that new values of these matrices can be generated for the next pass through the loop (starting at line 'View: ...'). It is assumed here and in the following examples that some means (typically a menu pick) is provided for causing an exit from the display list (via the line: 'End: ...').

Begin: Push identify transformation matrix onto stack
            Concatenate perspective-window transformation

View: Concatenate viewing rotation transformation

Origin: Concatenate viewing translation transformation
            Push current transformation matrix (CTM) onto stack

Move: Translate car (x, y)

Steer: Rotate car (z)
                  [Draw car body in world space]
                Push CTM
                    Translate for front axle $(+ y)$
                    Instance Axle
                Pop CTM
                Push CTM
                    Translate for rear axle $(- y)$
                    Instance Axle
                Pop CTM
              Pop CTM
              Go to View

End: Pop CTM
            Exit

Axle: Instance Wheel
                    Push CTM
                        Reflect for other wheel $(- x)$
                        Instance Wheel
                    Pop CTM
                    Return

Wheel: Push CTM
                        Translate for wheel $(+ x)$
                        Rotate wheel (y)
                            [Draw wheel in object space]

> Pop CTM
> Return

End of SDL

To change the view, the SDL is poked with the appropriate transformation matrices at the addresses labelled View and Origin (the perspective-windowing transformation is not changed in this example). To move the car, the transformation matrices at the addresses labelled Move, Steer, and Spin are changed. Other unlabelled transformations merely define the relationship of one part of the object to another (such as separation between wheels) and are therefore never changed.

4.7   Another simple SDL example

In the previous example, the details of the viewing transformations were rather glossed over, since the intention was to concentrate on the modelling transformations. However, this is not so straightforward to program as it might at first appear, and indeed none of the textbooks on computer graphics that I have consulted acknowledge even the existence of a problem! Novices to graphics programming consequently often experience particular difficulty in this area.

This and the following two sections therefore deal with this problem, and also the related one of manipulating two or more independently movable objects simultaneously. In this example the problem is reduced to its bare essentials; only rotations are used, and only one object is displayed. Note that, for simplicity, it is assumed that the valuators return values directly in units of the angles (degrees or radians); in practice it would probably be necessary to scale the values to give a sensible rotation rate.

The following algorithm is taken from a well-known program as it was originally supplied, and which shall remain nameless because it illustrates how not to do it!

Begin: Push identity transformation matrix onto stack
        Concatenate perspective-window transformation

Loop: Read valuator 1 into rotation angle (1) about x axis
        Read valuator 2 into rotation angle (2) about y axis
        Read valuator 3 into rotation angle (3) about z axis
        Push CTM
            From angle (1) calculate x axis rotation matrix
            Concatenate x axis rotation matrix
            From angle (2) calculate y axis rotation matrix
            Concatenate y axis rotation matrix
            From angle (3) calculate z axis rotation matrix
            Concatenate z axis rotation matrix
                [Draw object]
        Pop CTM
        Go to Loop

End: Pop CTM
      Exit

The intention here was presumably for the valuators 1, 2, and 3 to control rotations of the object about the x, y, and z axes of viewing space. Why doesn't it work? The answer is simple: rotation matrices for different axes do not commute. The program always applies rotation matrices to the object in the order z, y, x, but the user might well want to turn the dials in a different order, say x, y, then x again. How can this be programmed without knowing in advance what the user is going to do (which is obviously impossible)?

The solution is to use increments of the angles, instead of the total angles of rotation, as follows:

Begin: Push identity transformation matrix onto stack
         Concatenate perspective-window transformation
         Read valuator 1 into rotation angle (1) and about x axis
         Read valuator 2 into rotation angle (2) about y axis
         Read valuator 3 into rotation angle (3) about z axis
         Set accumulated rotation matrix $\mathbf{R}_o$ = unit matrix

Loop: Wait for non-empty event queue
         Push CTM

Next: Get next event queue entry
             For valuator (I) entry, get value
             Set angle increment = value − angle (I)
             Set angle (I) = value
             From angle increment, calculate incremental rotation
                 matrix $\mathbf{R}_v$ about axis (I)
             Set CTM = $\mathbf{R}_v$
             Concatenate $\mathbf{R}_o$, so that CTM = $\mathbf{R}_v . \mathbf{R}_o$
             Store CTM into $\mathbf{R}_o$
             If event queue not empty, go to Next
         Pop CTM
         Push CTM
             Concatenate accumulated rotation matrix
                 [Draw object]
         Pop CTM
         Go to Loop

End: Pop CTM
        Exit

This algorithm concatenates the angle increments coming from the valuators into a single accumulated matrix. When using valuators, these angle increments will be about the same axis most of the time, so that the efficiency of this program could be much improved by checking for a change of axis and only then doing the matrix concatenation. When using a locator, such as a trackball, to generate angle increments, this is less likely to be the case, so there may not be much room for improvement. Build-up of rounding errors is then likely to occur much more rapidly, and periodic renormalizations of the accumulated matrix may be required (see next section).

The important feature here is that in order to obtain rotations about the viewing space axes, the new incremental rotation matrix has to be premultiplied onto the current accumulated rotation matrix, whereas the stack only allows premultiplication of the CTM onto the new matrix. This means that the accumulated matrix cannot be kept on the stack, but must be retrieved from and stored back in temporary storage, as shown above.

This is still a considerably simplified example of an SDL. In practice the display loop will be executed partly in the GPU and partly in the DPU; how the split is actually done will depend on the functionality of the DPU. For example, if the valuators are connected to the GPU, then it will be responsible for calculating the rotation matrices and storing them at the appropriate places in the SDL.

4.8   Matrix renormalization

A procedure for renormalizing a rotation matrix, after build-up of rounding errors due to repeated matrix concatenation, is described here. The basic idea is that errors in the rotation matrix will be manifested by apparent distortions of a rigid object, for example the distances between atoms will not remain constant. The distance squared between two transformed points x'_1 and x'_2 is:

$$d^2 = (\tilde{x}_2' - \tilde{x}_1') . M . (x'_2 - x'_1)$$

where ~ indicates transpose (in this case column to row vector) and M is the 'metric tensor' for the space. In cartesian space, that is where the base vectors are orthonormal, the metric tensor is just a unit matrix, and the equation above is just Pythagoras' theorem. In this case, if the rotation matrix R transforms the original cartesian coordinate vector x to the new vector x' (so that $x' = R . x$), then this implies that the product $R . \tilde{R}$ is also a unit matrix, or that the inverse of R is the same as its transpose. This also follows from the fact that the base vectors of the rotated cartesian space, which are the columns of the rotation matrix, must also be orthonormal.

If a distorted space is now assumed, $x' = R' . x$, where R' is the rotation matrix containing rounding errors, then the deviation of the product $R' . \tilde{R}'$ from a unit matrix is a measure of the distortion. R' can be expressed as a rotation followed by a distortion, $R' = D . R$, where $D = E . S . \tilde{E}$. Here, S is a diagonal matrix identical to the scaling matrix in section 3.1.3, but it now represents distortions along three principal axes. These principal axes of distortion are transformed to and from the coordinate axes by the rotation matrix E and its inverse (which, as previously demonstrated, is the same as the transpose). The columns of E and the diagonal components of S are respectively the eigenvectors and eigenvalues of D. Therefore:

$$R' . \tilde{R}' = E . S . \tilde{E} . R . \tilde{R} . E . \tilde{S} . \tilde{E}$$
$$= E . S^2 . \tilde{E}$$

so that E and S are respectively the eigenvectors and the square root of the eigenvalues of $R' . \tilde{R}'$. Hence, knowing E and S, D can be calculated, and therefore $R = D^{-1} . R'$.

4.9 Multiple object manipulation

For full manipulatory functionality, view translations and individual object rotations and translations have to be added to the display loop of section 4.7. Limitations on space prohibit a description of the complete algorithm here, but provided that the principle is understood, namely that the matrix concatenations are performed in the same order that the matrices are generated by the user, and that this is not necessarily the order implied by naive use of the matrix stack, then much of the confusion experienced by novices in this area should evaporate.

There is one further point worth making: normally the user defines only the magnitudes of the rotations and translations to be performed, but the programmer is still responsible for ensuring that these are applied in a consistent and natural way. Unless there are particular reasons for doing otherwise, rotations and translations should occur with respect to the viewing space axes (which coincide with the screen spaces axes), since the user is by definition fixed in viewing space. If they are applied in world space, or indeed in any other arbitrary space, the user has to imagine being projected into a rotating frame of reference, a concept which does not come naturally to the majority of users.

Further, the question of the 'natural' origin of rotations arises. For the view as a whole, this should be the viewing space origin, as otherwise the centre of attention will move as view rotations are performed. Independently movable objects should, however, rotate about their own local origins, so that their rotation remains uncoupled from their translation.

The following table summarizes how these requirements can be realized in practice. Here subscript n refers to object number, or display list segment, n. Object o refers to world space; there may or may not be an actual object fixed in world space.

	Operation:			
	$R_o =$	$t_o =$	$R_n =$	$t_n =$
R_v:	$R_v . R_o$	$R_v . t_o$	$R_v . R_n$	$R_v . t_n$
Increment: t_v:	—	$t_v + t_o$	—	$t_v + t_n$
R_s:	—	—	$R_s . R_n$	—
t_s:	—	—	—	$t_s + t_n$

R_o and t_o are the current accumulated rotation matrix and translation vector for world space, or equivalently the current viewing transformation.

R_n and t_n are the accumulated rotation matrix and translation vector for object number n.

R_v and t_v are the incremental rotation and translation applied simultaneously to all objects in world space, in order to change the viewing transformation.

R_s and t_s are the incremental rotation and translation applied only to object number n.

Row 1, column 1 of the table shows $R_o = R_v . R_o$, which was the concatenation performed in the previous example (section 4.7). The remaining entries in row 1 show how the other matrices and vectors are to be concatenated when the view rotation is altered. In particular, R_v concatenates all translations, t_o becomes $R_v . t_o$ and t_n becomes $R_v . t_n$, whereas in row 3, R_s does not affect t_n. This achieves the desired effect of rotation of the view about the viewing space origin, whereas individual object rotations occur about object origins.

4.10   Typical program structure

What follows is an outline description of the structure of a representative molecular graphics program. It is built up from several levels of user interaction; the higher the level, the more critical is the response time; thus input and processing of text, which are slow, are placed at the lower levels, whereas visual interaction requires fast response times and occurs at the highest level.

(a) 0th level user interface – invoke program from operating system.
(b) Initialize counters, flags, constants, etc.
(c) 1st level user interface – input of text, for example filenames, or invoke Database Query Language processor to select, label, and/or colour substructures.
(d) Get coordinate data, compute initial centre and scale to fit the picture on the screen, and create structured display list (SDL) in graphics memory. Specifically:

Open segment.
Generate window-to-viewport and perspective-window-stereo
transformations.
Generate initial rotation and translation transformations, saving
pointers to display list.
Generate picture with graphics attributes and primitives.
Close segment.

(e) Begin display loop.
(f) Display segments. That is,
Despatch SDL to DPU for application of current transformation, clipping, viewport mapping, rasterization, and storage in frame buffer for display.
(g) 2nd level user interface – interaction via screen menu picks with options to return to any previous stage, or initiate serial or concurrent task, for example analysis or modification of the model, generation of backdrop, or hard copy dump.
(h) 3rd level user interface – get interactive device inputs for changed rotation/translation/scaling/clipping parameters. Update display list matrices at relevant places, using saved pointers.
(i) Repeat from (e) until exit signalled.

REFERENCES

Newman, W.M. & Sproull, R.F. (1979) *Principles of interactive computer graphics*, McGraw-Hill, 2nd ed.

Foley, J.D. & van Dam, A. (1982) *Fundamentals of interactive computer graphics*, Addison-Wesley.

Plastock, R.A. & Kalley, G. (1986) *Theory and problems of computer graphics* Schaum's Outline Series in Computers, McGraw-Hill

Harrington, S. (1987) *Computer graphics: a programming approach*, McGraw-Hill, 2nd ed.

Hubbard, R.E. (1989) *Computer-aided molecular design*, ed. Richards, W.G., IBC Technical Services

5

Potential energy functions

Sarah L. Price[1] and Julia M. Goodfellow[2]
[1]Department of Chemistry, University College, Gower Street, London WC1H 0AJ.
[2]Department of Crystallography, Birkbeck College, Malet Street,
London WC1E 7HX

1. INTRODUCTION

The potential energy of intramolecular and intermolecular interactions is an important concept in computer modelling. Such energy functions are used with a variety of mathematical techniques such as optimization (called molecular mechanics or minimization), Monte Carlo simulation, and molecular dynamics algorithms. The basic concept is that, given a molecular structure (that is, cartesian coordinates for all the atoms), we can calculate the energy of interaction between all atoms within the molecule (intramolecular), and this will have low values for the conformations which occur in nature. We can also use these functions to calculate the intermolecular energy between two molecules such as a drug molecule interacting with proteins or DNA. The total potential energy is assumed to be a function of the number and type of chemical species within the molecule and the distance between all pairs of atoms. To calculate the potential energy, it is divided into a number of terms which correspond to physical effects such as electrostatic interactions, dispersion and repulsion energies, bond distance, and bond angle distortion.

In principle, we can calculate the intermolecular and intramolecular forces from quantum mechanics, since it is assumed that distant parts of a molecule, such as distant residues in a protein, interact in the same way whether in the same or different molecules. The potential energy of the interaction arises from the forces between all nuclei and electrons within a molecule. The behaviour of a molecule can then be described by the Schrödinger equation. The concept of a potential energy surface requires that we assume that the nuclei are at rest and that we calculate the distribution of electrons in the field of the nuclei (the Born–Oppenheimer approximation). This calculation is then repeated for different assumed bond lengths and angles to give the potential energy surface. However, an exact solution to this equation is possible for only a few simple cases.

Although modern quantum mechanics provides approximate solutions to the Schrödinger equation for systems of up to 50 atoms (and this limit is rapidly increasing), this is not sufficient for the study of proteins and oligonucleotides consisting of many thousands of atoms. Even if we could undertake one approximate quantum mechanical calculation on one protein, it is not feasible to consider repeating this calculation for the large number of conformations which would be necessary in order to realistically characterize its potential energy surface. Therefore, computer modelling of macromolecules often entails the use of empirical potentials (rather than pure *ab initio* potentials) which can be derived from the quantum mechanics of small fragments combined with experimental data (Lifson 1981). Moreover, these models entail the calculation of the interactions between atoms rather than electrons.

2   INTRAMOLECULAR POTENTIALS

2.1   Bonded interactions

The geometry of a molecule is defined by the covalent bond lengths and bond angles as well as the torsion angles around each bond (see chapter 2 on geometry). Thus, the main components of the intramolecular potential involve an evaluation of the deformation energy due to strained covalent bonds, angles, and torsion angles. To evaluate these, it is necessary to define the perfect case and the penalty function when the bond is distorted.

Although the potential energy due to the deformation of a diatomic model was due to Morse, it is usual to describe bond stretching by a simpler model in which each covalent bond acts as a stiff spring, although the Morse function would give a more realistic representation. Thus, the energy of bond deformation becomes

$$E_{bond} = K_b(b - b_o)^2$$

where K_b is the spring constant defining the strength of the interaction and b_o is the perfect bond distance for a given two atoms. K_b is usually determined by spectroscopy while b_o comes from X-ray diffraction studies on small molecule crystals. For a whole molecule, it is necessary to sum such interactions over all pairs of bonded atoms.

Bending energy (deformation of bond angles) is treated in a similar manner. Thus,

$$E_{angle} = K_\theta(\theta - \theta_o)^2$$

where K_θ again represents the strength of the bending motion and θ_o the equilibrium bond angle. Both the bond and angle terms tend to be fairly rigid and therefore have a large force constant. Thus, for example, C–C single bonds tend to be very similar in length in different structures, and the bond angle depends primarily on the number of atoms which are connected to the central atom, for example, four bonded atoms tend to have tetrahedral angles.

Most macromolecules fold into three-dimensional conformations which are determined by conformation or torsion angles. These are defined as rotation around a given bond, such as the C–C bond in ethane, and are far more flexible than bond distance or bond angle terms, and so a wider range of torsion angles are observed. Thus the energy changes involved in rotation are relatively small and the spring constant is weak. They also tend to be periodic in nature with the exact periodicity depending on the number of atoms attached to the two atoms defining the bond about which rotation can take place. For example, the ethane torsion has three equivalent minima so the energy, E_{tor}, has three-fold periodicity. In general,

$$E_{tor} = E_\varphi [1 + \cos (n\varphi - \delta)]$$

where K_φ is the force constant, n the periodicity, and δ a reference angle at which the potential is a maximum.

It may be necessary to define improper torsion angles such as those involved in minimizing out-of-plane bending by an atom bonding to three other atoms. Sometimes improper torsion angles, involving non-bonded distances, are used as a mathematical tool to keep a conjugated group planar.

A few potential functions contain cross-terms which take account of correlations between the lengths of two adjacent bonds or a bond length and a bond angle term. Such correlations exist, and these cross-terms have been found essential for the analysis of vibrational spectra, but they are usually neglected. However, recent studies indicate that these terms might be important in the correct evaluation of molecular energy and geometry (Hagler *et al.* 1989).

2.2   Non-bonded interactions

Usually, three terms are included under the umbrella of non-bonded interactions. These are the electrostatic, dispersion, and repulsion energies which occur between non-bonded atoms within a molecule or between molecules.

2.2.1   *Electrostatic*

The rearrangement of electrons on the formation of a molecule results in an electrostatic field around the molecule which is generally represented by assigning atoms a negative or positive charge. These partial atomic charges can be calculated directly from quantum mechanical calculations on molecular fragments. Electrostatic interactions between atoms can be expressed mathematically by Coulomb's law such that

$$E_{elec} = q_i q_j / 4\pi\epsilon_0 \epsilon R_{ij}$$

where q_i and q_j are the partial atomic charges on atoms i and j, R_{ij} is the distance between these atoms, ϵ_0 is the permitivity of free space, and ϵ is the relative dielectric constant. Sometimes the dielectric constant, ϵ, is made proportional to the distance between the atoms (or given a constant value greater than the vacuum value of unit) in order to mimic the effective environment within the essentially apolar interior of a protein surrounded by polar solvent. The summation is taken between all atoms if an intermolecular energy is required, or between all atoms greater than three or four bonds away within a molecule.

2.2.2   *Repulsion and dispersion energy*

Even between inert gas atoms, there are repulsive forces at short range and attractive forces which cause the gas to condense at low temperatures. Although each atom may be neutral, the electron cloud may be distorted such that there is an instantaenous dipole induced in one molecule. Neighbouring molecules feel the field generated by this instantaneous dipole resulting in an instantaneous dipole within the second molecule. This attractive force goes as R_{ij}^{-6} where R_{ij} is the distance between atoms i and j. It is a purely quantum mechanical effect arising from the correlation in motions between electrons. The coefficient, C_{ij}, has been shown to depend on the polarizabilities of the atoms. Thus,

$$E_{\text{disp}} = -C_{ij}/R_{ij}^6.$$

There is also a repulsive term, E_{rep}, between two atoms when they become so close that their electron clouds overlap. It increases so steeply as the separation between atoms decreases that it is often called a repulsive wall. It is often modelled as a term depending on the inverse twelfth power of distance. Such a functional form rises very steeply as required and can be calculated quickly if R^{-6} is already known from the calculation of the dispersion term. However, it is known that an exponential form is more accurate, but this has the disadvantage of requiring two coefficients for each atom pair rather than the one coefficient required by the R^{-12} paramaterization. For these reasons, non-bonded interactions in macromolecules are usually represented by the simpler R^{-12} form. Some studies have shown that R^{-9} is as good if not better for biological molecules.

Thus,

$$E_{\text{rep}} + E_{\text{disp}} = A_{ij}/R_{ij}^{-12} - C_{ij}/R_{ij}^{-6}$$

where A and C are the coefficients for the repulsive and attractive terms for each pair of atoms. It is more informative to describe these interactions in terms of the depth, ϵ, and position, σ, as formulated by Lennard Jones. Thus,

$$E_{\text{LJ}} = 4\epsilon[(\sigma/R_{ij})^{12} - (\sigma/R_{ij})^6].$$

However, this equation is deceptively simple as we require a pair of coefficients (either ϵ and σ or A and C) for each combination of pairs of atoms. Often a combination rule is used to derive the coefficients for unlike pairs of atoms based on empirically derived values for the interaction between like atoms such as

$$A_{ij} = (A_{ii}A_{jj})^{1/2}$$

and

$$C_{ij} = (C_{ii}C_{jj})^{1/2}$$

2.3   HYDROGEN BONDS

The three-dimensional structures of biological macromolecules are stabilized by the presence of hydrogen bonds between secondary structural elements in proteins and between the bases in DNA. They occur when a polar hydrogen atom interacts with an atom which has a partial negative charge. They are thought of as predominantly electrostatic in nature and have been treated as such by the Lifson/Hagler school who have used non-bonded parameters with the same R^{-1}, R^{-12}, R^{-6} terms as in the forms described above. Others have introduced a r^{-10} and r^{-12} specific hydrogen bond term between the hydrogen atom and hydrogen bond acceptor in order to get empirically acceptable predictions of hydrogen bond lengths.

2.4 Solvent

Many simulations of macromolecules were initially carried out *in vacuo* but with dielectric constants not equal to unity to mimic solvent effects. However, the increase in the power of modern computers has lead to the inclusion of implicit solvent (water molecules and counter-ions) around protein and DNA. There are many models for water (Finney *et al.* 1986), and this has been a major area of interest in itself because of the problems of finding a model which can represent the anomalous properties of water in solid, liquid, and gas phases. The currently most common models are the SPC model (Berendsen *et al.* 1981) and the TIP3P and TIP4P models (Jorgensen *et al.* 1983). In these relatively simple models, water is represented by three charges centred on the two hydrogen atoms and at a point either centred on the oxygen atom positions (SPC and TIP4P) or on the bisector between the hydrogen atoms about 0.15 Å from the oxygen (TIP4P). There is also a non-bonded interaction which depends on the distance between the oxygen atoms. As many macromolecules are naturally hydrated, it is clearly important to get the correct balance between water–water and water–solute interactions in any calculation.

3 FORCE-FIELDS

There are a number of complete sets of potential energy parameters which describe the interactions between, for example, all atoms in a protein or nucleotide. These have their roots in the pioneering work of Scheraga and colleagues (Momany *et al.* 1974, 1975) and Lifson/Hagler and co-workers (Lifson *et al.* 1979). Some of the most recent traditional parameterizations for proteins, the OPLS models, are described in Jorgensen & Tirado–Rives (1988). Details of individual force-fields used by the software packages CHARMM and AMBER can be found in Brooks *et al.* (1983), Weiner *et al.* (1984, 1986). Improved potential energy functions for nucleics acids have also been described by Nilsson & Karplus (1986).

3.1 Comparisons

There have been relatively few comparisons of the molecular force-fields used to represent macromolecules. Hall & Pavitt (1984) tested a number of such force-fields when applied to the energy minimization of three cyclic hexapeptides. They concluded that the most effective potential was that of Kollman and co-workers (Weiner *et al.* 1984) 'not withstanding its use of "united atoms" for CH, CH_2, and CH_3 groups'. Since then, Weiner et al. (1986) have published all atom representations. Hall & Pavitt also found that force-fields in which hydrogens bonded to electronegative atoms are not specified explicitly, are less accurate.

A more recent study that used the AMBER, CHARMM, and ECEPP force-fields concluded that their predictions for the low-energy conformations of (Asn-Ala-Asn-Pro)$_9$ were significantly different (Roterman, Gibson & Scheraga 1989) and, indeed, none even gave predictions of the phi–psi energy dependence of the alanine dipeptide which were completely compatible with experimental results (Roterman *et al.* 1989).

The effect of different potential energy functions on the location of solvent hydrogen bonding sites has been tested by Vovelle & Goodfellow (1986). They found that the model chosen to represent the water molecule had a large effect on which potential hydrogen bonding sites were in fact at an energy minimum. However, the choice of partial electronic charges and repulsion and dispersion coefficients for the solute atoms affected the magnitude of the interaction energy and the exact location of the solvent molecules with respect to the solute.

3.2   Critique of current force-fields

In the light of these comparisons, it seems clear that we do not yet have one definitive force-field for biological molecules. To appreciate the likely accuracy of the commonly used force-fields, we should examine the assumptions implicit in the models in the light of what we know about intermolecular forces for smaller systems. (Rigby *et al.* 1986 is a useful introductory text; Maitland *et al.* 1981 gives fuller details).

(1)   The assumption of an effective pair potential

The force-fields all make the pairwise additive approximation, that is, they assume that the interaction energy of a set of molecules is just the sum of the interaction energies between every pair of molecules. Thus, the energy of three molecules, i, j and k is assumed to be $U_{ijk} = U_{ij} + U_{jk} + U_{ik}$. This implies that bringing in a third molecule does not change the interaction between the first two molecules. This is clearly quite a gross approximation, as can be seen by considering an ion close to a readily polarizable atom, such as argon. The electric field of the ion will distort the argon atom, giving rise to the polarization energy from the interaction of the charge with the induced dipole moment. However, if another ion of the same charge is placed symmetrically the other side of the argon atom, there is no electric field at the argon and so no induced dipole. Thus the dipolar polarization energy is zero, not twice that of the argon–ion pair, as would be calculated in the pairwise additive approximation.

Formally, we can define a three-body potential U^3_{ijk} as the difference between the energy of the three molecules and the sum of the pair potentials, and use $U_{ijk} = U_{ij} + U_{jk} + U_{ik} + U^3_{ijk}$ to calculate the energy of the trio of molecules. For four molecules, we would sum over the pair potential, three-body and four-body potentials, and so on. Very little is known about the three, four, or other many-body terms, except in the case of the rare gas atoms, but they are generally assumed to be small in comparison with the uncertainties in the intermolecular pair potential. Certainly, polarization effects from ions are an extreme example of non-additive intermolecular interactions, though it has been estimated that the three-body terms contribute 10% to the lattice energy of argon, and so these effects are not negligible even for non-polar systems.

By making the pairwise additive approximation, and ignoring the existence of the many-body effects, we are hoping that the non-additive effects can be absorbed into the pair potential in some ill-defined averaged way. Thus effective pair potentials which provide an excellent description of the solid and liquid phases of chlorine (Rodger *et al.* 1988, Wheatley & Price 1990) do not predict the properties of the gas well, because the many-body terms which have been absorbed into the model potential do not affect intermolecular interactions in the gas. The assumption that an effective potential can represent the interactions of biological molecules in different environments will be even poorer, as even if the system does not contain any ions, the making and breaking of hydrogen bonds involves significant polarization of the molecular charge distribution.

Some of the standard force-fields are effective in that they are also supposed to have absorbed the effects of the solvent in some averaged way, so that calculations with these potentials which do not explicitly include water molecules in the model, aim to simulate the behaviour of the molecules in water. This is a very crude model for studying a process at the atomic level, where the size of a water molecule is comparable to the dimensions of the molecular fragments being docked, as the presence or not of a water molecule between two molecular fragments that would like to be in van der Waals' contact has more than a minor effect on the interaction!

(2)   The united atom approximation
Some force-fields do not have an interaction site on hydrogen atoms, but assume that the hydrogen atom's effects are represented by the model potential for the bonded heavier atom. This approximation has the considerable advantage of cutting down the number of interaction sites, and thus the computer time required for the calculations, very significantly. Also, there is no need to specify the positions of the hydrogen atoms, which makes it easier to use X-ray molecular structures, where the positions of the hydrogen atoms are often not resolved.

The use of an isotropic untied N atom to represent the electrostatic effects of a NH group is extremely poor, as it is the charge separation along this bond which makes it a hydrogen bond donor. Moreover, Hall & Pavitt (1984) have shown that this is a poor approximation in practice, and thus current force-fields have sites on protons bonded to nitrogen.

A united atom representation of a methyl (CH_2) group can be quite a good approximation, as there is little charge density associated with the hydrogen atoms, and the bond is not particularly polar. Thus, the long-range intermolecular effects of the protons are small enough to be absorbed into a united atom. If a methyl group is freely rotating, the effective shape of its repulsive wall may be adequately represented by a spherical united atom. However, the repulsive effects of united atoms which are not freely rotating, such as CH_2 groups, could be too poorly represented for use in predicting 'van der Waals' packing' of molecules, since a united atom potential cannot predict the crystal structures of the paraffins. The AMBER force-field was updated in 1986 (Weiner *et al.*) to give an all-atom representation.

(3)   Transferability

Force-fields define all the potential parameters (except the charges) according to the atomic types of the atoms involved in the interaction. (This scheme cannot be used for the charges, as it would not always give the correct net charge for the molecule). The definition of the different atomic types varies between the force-fields, though atoms with different atomic numbers, or in different states of hybridization, will generally be defined as different types, with different potential parameters. Other subdivisions have been introduced as and when found empirically necessary. For example, CHARMM has different parameter sets for carbonyl, carboxyl, hydroxy, and water oxygens, whereas AMBER has different types for carbonyl, carboxyl, ether or ester, and alcohol oxygens. In assuming that, for example, all carbonyl carbon atoms have the same potential parameters, we are assuming that they all have the same charge density.

This assumption that atomic charge densities (and therefore associated potential parameters) are transferable between molecules is justified, and is derived from the basic tenets of organic chemistry. Certainly the same functional group behaves in a sufficiently similar way in different molecules to allow organic chemistry to be systematic. However, organic chemistry also shows that the reactivity of a functional group is affected by the nature of the bonded atoms, an observation that is rationalized in terms of short-range inductive effects along the bonds redistributing the charge density between the atoms. The redistribution of charge is often reflected in the model for the electrostatic interactions. However, it is very rare for the definition of atomic types, and thus the other potential parameters, to take full account of the nature of the functional groups bonded to atom. Thus, the accuracy of the force-field will be limited by the extent to which the atoms which are assumed to have the same parameters actually have the same charge density. We would expect the transferability to be good when the atom is bonded to the same functional groups in the molecule of interest as in the model molecules used to parameterize the force-field. However, if the bonded functional groups differ markedly in electronegativity, then the potential parameters will be much less transferable.

(4)   The assumed functional form

The model force-field cannot represent the interactions more accurately than the best fit of the assumed functional form to the actual unknown potential which can be obtained by optimizing the parameters. The functional forms of many terms in the potential are very simple, computationally convenient first approximations to the actual potential. For example, the radial form for the non-bonded interactions is usually a Lennard–Jones 12–6 potential, with two parameters to vary the position and depth of the well as described in a previous section of this chapter. However, we know that the shape of the Lennard–Jones potential is a poor approximation to the actual shape of the intermolecular potential for two rare gas atoms, such as argon. We know from perturbation theory that the long-range form of the dispersion interaction between two atoms can be represented by the infinite series

$$U_{\mathrm{disp}} = -C_6/R^6 - C_8/R^8 - C_{10}/R^{10} - \dots,$$

but the Lennard–Jones form uses only the first term. Similarly, the short-range repulsion between two atoms decays approximately exponentially with separation. However, Lennard–Jones, working before the advent of computers, had to model the repulsive wall by an inverse power potential, in order to have a model that is mathematically tractable. If we compare the Lennard–Jones potential with a modern accurate representation for the intermolecular potential of argon,

$$U(R) = \epsilon \exp[\alpha(1 - r)] \sum_{i=0}^{5} A_i(r - 1)^i + \sum_{j=0}^{2} C_{2j + 6}/(\delta + r)^{2j + 6},$$

where $r = R/\rho$, it is clear that the Lennard–Jones radial form cannot have the flexibility to describe the non-bonded interactions between the atoms exactly.

Another implicit assumption in most of these force-fields is that the non-bonded and electrostatic interactions between the atoms depend only on their separation (the isotropic atom–atom model). This is equivalent to assuming that the molecules interact as if the molecule is composed of spherical atomic charge densities. This is a reasonable zeroth order approximation to the molecular shape, but completely ignores the non-spherical features in the valence electron distribution, such as π or lone pair electron density, which are predicted by theories of chemical bonding. Thus, in principle, we would expect the intermolecular interaction between two atoms in different molecules to depend not only on their separation, but also on the relative orientation on their valence electron density (anisotropic atom–atom potentials).

(5) Reasonable parameterization
The functional form of the force-fields may be very simple, but nevertheless, the number of potential parameters which are required for even a family of molecules with relatively few atomic types is enormous. For example, the CHARMM force-field (Brooks *et al.* 1983) for proteins, nucleic acids, and prosthetic groups, has 29 atomic types, and requires 59 sets of bond stretching parameters. It therefore uses 406 parameters for the non-bonded repulsion and dispersion interactions which are therefore necessarily derived from a set of parameters for each atomic type, using crude combining rules. The sources of the parameters vary between force-fields, though often force-fields have some parameters in common. Some parameters can be fixed independently, for example the minimum energy bond lengths can be derived from crystal structures, or the electrostatic parameters obtained from some form of analysis of *ab initio* wavefunctions for model molecules. However, in all force-fields, there are some parameters which have to be obtained empirically, i.e. by being adjusted until the force-field predicts some property of the molecule in satisfactory agreement with experiment.

The need to obtain a large number of parameters empirically severely limits the confidence that we can place in the results of the simulations. If we attempt to find too many parameters empirically, the fitting problem becomes very ill-defined, so we are nessarily restricted to simple functional forms. Even when, by trial and error, a set of parameters is found which will predict selected sets of experimental data with reasonable accuracy, this does not imply that the force-field can be used with confidence to predict any other property of any molecule which can be constructed from the defined atomic types. The main reason to be careful of placing too much faith in the results of such predictive calculations is that different regions of the force-field are sampled in different simulations, and the force-field may not extrapolate well outside the region sampled in the fitting.

One reason for poor extrapolation is that the assumed functional form is inadequate. For example, crystal structure analysis (Nyburg & Faerman 1985) shows that two chlorine atoms (bonded to carbon) can approach each other 0.4 Å more closely if they are in a head-to-head near-linear arrangement (that is, C–Cl $\cdots$ Cl–C) than side-by-side. Thus, if we assume that the van der Waals radius of chlorine is isotropic and does not vary with direction (as in most force-fields), the value obtained from a crystal structure with a head-to-head intermolecular contact would give a poor prediction of crystal-packing involving side-to-side contacts.

A second, closely related reason, is that the fitting procedure may not be very sensitive to certain potential parameters. For example, the crystal structure used in the fitting may not have any close repulsive contacts of a certain type, and so the values of the repulsive parameters (perhaps implied through combination rules) could give a hopeless prediction of a crystal structure which did have that type of repulsive interaction.

The above illustrations over-simplify the very real problems met in parameterizing force-fields empirically. Certainly the successes of various force-fields often results from a cancellation of errors between the different terms, implying that improving the model for one component, such as the electrostatic terms, could result in a worse overall potential. The best force-field for a given simulation is likely to be the one which has been parameterized for very similar molecules by using experimental data similar to those being simulated. It is salutary to note that the number of quite different sets of isotropic atom–atom intermolecular potentials that have been proposed for small organic molecules (Pertsin & Kitaigorodsky 1987) such as hydrocarbons, as this implies considerable sensitivity to the choice of functional form and parameterization data even for relatively simple systems.

Hence it is not surprising that many of the results of biological simulations are disturbingly sensitive to the choice of force-field, though relatively few comparisons have been made. Thus, although the simulations are valuable in stimulating thought about a process, and any of the current force-fields may be good enough for many purposes (certainly they are all a great improvement on a mechanical space-filling molecular models), the detailed results should be viewed with some caution. It is essential to be able to compare some results with experimental data to give credibillity to the predictions and insights derived from the simulation.

4.   THE WAY FORWARD FOR BIOLOGICAL FORCE-FIELDS: STATE-OF-THE-ART POTENTIALS FOR SMALL MOLECULES

The above critique shows that we need to improve the accuracy of biological force-fields, and that this cannot be done purely empirically. The main problem lies with the non-bonded and electrostatic contributions. We can hope to improve the description of these terms by considering current model intermolecular potentials for smaller molecules. This section describes some recent developments in the description of intermolecular forces which may be incorporated into the next generation of biological force-fields.

There is compelling evidence that the isotropic atom–atom potential model cannot give realistic simulations for all small molecules, as it is incapable of predicting even the observed crystal structure for Cl_2 (Price & Stone 1982) and OCS (Deakin & Walmsley 1989). Indeed, the diverse low-temperature crystal structures of the homonuclear diatomics cannot be accounted for by varying the parameters in an isotropic atom–atom plus point quadrupole model (English & Venables 1974). A solution to this problem is to drop the assumption that the interaction between the atoms depends only on their separation, and introduce anisotropy into the model potential which reflects the anisotropy of the valence charge distribution. By varying both the form and the strength of the anisotropy in the electrostatic and repulsion terms, it is possible to predict a field of stability for all the observed lowest-temperature crystal structures of the homonuclear diatomics (Price 1987), with the parameters correlating with the molecular charge distribution. Thus, it is clearly desirable to introduce anisotropy into the model potentials of larger molecules, but this cannot be done empirically because of the problem of determining sufficient parameters in a form flexible enough to describe the different shapes of the atomic charge distributions. The next sections will outline how this can be done, using the monomer wavefunctions; the reader is referred to recent reviews for the mathematical details (Stone & Price 1988, Price 1988).

4.1   Distributed multipole electrostatic models

A major improvement on the atomic point charge electrostatic model can be obtained by using a set of multipoles (charge, dipole, quadrupole, etc.) on each atomic site to represent the atomic charge distribution. The higher multipole moments represent the electrostatic effects of the non-spherical features in the local charge distribution, such as lone pair or pi electron density. Since if a molecule was a superposition of neutral spherical atomic charge densities, there would be no electrostatic force outside the molecular charge density, and we can ascribe all the electrostatic interactions to the distribution of the valence electrons. Thus the anistropy in the electrostatic model can be very important.

The sets of distributed multipole moments can be obtained by analysing an *ab initio* charge density for the molecule, using some recipe for splitting it up between the atoms. There are several such recipes, though provided that all multipoles up to at least quadrupole are included, the choice of method has little effect on the calculated electrostatic interaction energies (Spackman 1986). The great advantage of this approach is that, in principle, it can be used to calculate electrostatic energies to the accuracy of the *ab initio* wave function, and does not require any empirical assumptions, though the atomic multipole moments obtained from the analysis do correlate well with our chemical pictures of bonding. In principle, the set of multipole moments at each site should be infinite, but in practice the multipole series converges very rapidly after the quadrupolar term, provided that there are sufficient sites in the molecule, such as a site at every atom.

One interesting consequence of the development of distributed multipole electrostatic models is that, since they enable electrostatic energies to be calculated quickly and accurately, it is possible to assess the importance of electrostatic forces in determining molecular interactions. For example, Buckingham & Fowler (1985) showed that the structure of a few dozen diverse van der Waals complexes of small molecules could be predicted by finding the minimum in the electrostatic interaction energy (as calculated by using Stone's distributed multipole analysis (Stone 1983)) subject to the constraint that the molecules did not approach each other more closely than allowed by their van der Waals radii. This result implies that the electrostatic energy generally dominates the orientation dependence of the intermolecular potential for these hydrogen bonded complexes, an observation which has been confirmed by expensive intermolecular perturbation theory calculations of the different components for several systems. The electrostatic term also appears to dominate the interactions between aromatic molecules, such as benzene (Price & Stone 1987), and in small $N-H\cdots O=C$ hydrogen bonded complexes (Mitchell & Price 1989). It will be interesting to see whether electrostatic forces also dominate interactions involving polypeptides, DNA, drug molecules, etc, as is widely believed.

Distributed multipolar models are beginning to be used for biological systems, as the distributed multipoles can be transferred between molecules to build up models for larger molecules. For example, a distributed multipole model for a polypeptide can be built from calculations on dipeptides (Faerman & Price, 1990). As mentioned above, in order that the atomic charge distributions are even approximately the same, it is necessary for at least the neighbouring bonded functional groups to be the same in both molecules, so calculations on quite large model molecules are required. However, advances in computer technology now make it possible to obtain the necessary wave functions for molecules the size of dipeptides quite routinely.

4.2   Polarization and dispersion

Since polarization and dispersion forces, like the electrostatic force, are long range, they can also be described rigorously in terms of the properties of the charge distributions of the isolated molecules. However, distributed polarizability and dispersion models are intrinsically much more complicated than distributed multipole models for the electrostatics, as they describe the changes in the molecule's charge distribution due to the presence of the other molecule. Thus, the electric field from one molecule not only causes the local polarization of an atoms charge density, but also causes charge to move from one atom to another, giving rise to non-local polarizabilities. This results in a rigorous expression (Stone 1985) for the polarization energy involving a sum over all pairs of sites in both molecules; that is, there are contributions which involve four atoms.

The distributed polarizabilities can be derived from the monomer wave function, though the results are very sensitive to the quality of the wave function. A distributed dispersion model can also be derived from the distributed polarizabilities, by the usual integrations. In the special case of linear molecules, the results can be transformed into a pairwise additive sum over the atom and bond centre sites (Stone & Tong 1989). However, the combination of the general non-pairwise additivity of these terms, and the expense of obtaining a sufficiently good wave function to give worthwhile values to the polarizabilities, means that considerably more work is required before these methods can be applied to organic molecules.

4.3   Anisotropy in the repulsion

The non-spherical features in the charge distribution are small compared with the total charge density, and so it is not surprising that the density contour maps of molecules do not show 'rabbits ears' sticking out in the lone pair directions. Hence we would not expect very marked anisotropy in the position of the repulsive wall; nevertheless, since the repulsion energy varies so steeply with separation, a variation of 0.1 Å or less in the position of the repulsive wall can have a major effect on the possible packing of molecules. Certainly the anisotropy in the repulsion around a chlorine atom has a major effect on the crystal-packing of Cl_2 (Price & Stone 1982) and p-dichlorobenzene (Munowitz et al. 1977). Unfortunately, there is no rigorous method of determining the anisotropy of the repulsion from the monomer wavefunction. However, anisotropic repulsive potentials for diatomic molecules as diverse as HF and N_2 have been derived empirically by fitting either to crystal structures or ab initio dimer potential surfaces (Brobjer & Murrell 1983, Price 1986). Recently, the empirical observation that the repulsion energy correlates with the overlap of the undistorted monomer charge densities has been used successfully to derive functional forms and parameters for the atom–atom repulsion for linear molecules (Wheatley & Price 1990). If this method fulfils its initial promise, it could enable the development of anisotropic repulsion potentials for organic molecules.

4.4   The position for small molecules

Despite considerable efforts, we do not have a definitive intermolecular potential for any polyatomic molecule, though this may change within the next few years. A fairly recent paper about an attempt to derive such a definitive potential for nitrogen was entitled 'Towards an intermolecular potential for nitrogen' (Ling & Rigby 1984). Perhaps the most progress has been made with chlorine, where two potentials, one mainly empirical (Rodger et al. 1988), the other based on a synthesis of the distributed multipoles, dispersion and overlap repulsion models (Wheatley & Price, 1990), have been shown to be capable of reproducing several properties of both the solid and liquid state. However, even for this non-polar molecule, the potentials did not transfer successfully to the gas phase since they are effective potentials which have absorbed many body effects into the parameterization.

The representation of the many body forces still remains a major barrier to progress for model potentials for even these very small molecules.

Thus state-of-the-art intermolecular potentials are atom–atom models with complex forms for both the radial and orientation dependence. Thus biological force-fields will be considerably more sophisticated and complex in form before we can reasonably expect them to be accurate over the entire range of the potential surface which could be sampled in realistic simulations. However, much valuable insight has been gained by the current models, and we can expect that computer simulation will be an even more powerful tool as the force-fields become more realistic.

ACKNOWLEDGEMENTS

JMG would like to thank the Wellcome Trust for a research leave fellowship.

REFERENCES

Berendsen, H.J.C., Postma, J.P.M., van Gunsteren, W.F. & Hermans, J. (1981) Interaction models for water in relation to protein hydration in *Intermolecular forces* (ed. Pullman, B.) Reidel, Dordrecht, 331–342.

Buckingham, A.D. & Fowler, P.W. (1985) A model for the geometries of van der Waals complexes, *Canad. J. Chem.* **63**, 2018–2025.

Brobjer, J.T. & Murrell, J.N. (1983) The Intermolecular Potential of HF, *Molec. Phys.*, **50**, 885–899.

Brooks, B.R., Bruccoleri, R.E., Olafson, B.D., States, D.J., Swaminathan, S. & Karplus, M. (1983);, CHARMM: A program for macromolecular energy, minimization and dynamics calculations', *J. Comp. Chem.* **4**, 187–217.

Deakin, A.A. & Walmsley, S.H. (1989) Potential functions and the lattice dynamics of carbonyl sulphide, *Chem. Phys.*, **136**, 105–113.

English, C.A. & Venables, J.A. (1974) The structure of the diatomic molecular solids, *Proc. Roy. Soc. A*, **340**, 57–80.

Faerman, C.H. & Price, S.L. (1990) A transferable distributed multipole model for the electrostatic interactions of peptides and amides, *J. Amer. Chem. Soc.*, **112**, 4915–4926.

Finney, J.L., Quinn, J.E. & Baum, J.O. (1986) The water dimer potential surface, in *Water Science Reviews* **1** (ed. F. Franks), 93–170, CUP, Cambridge.

Hagler, A.T., Maple, J.R., Thacher, T.S., Fitzgerald, G.B. & Dinur, U. (1989) Potential energy functions for organic and biomolecular systems, in *Computer simulation of biomolecular systems. Theoretical and experimental applications* (eds van Gunsteren, W. and Weiner, P.K.) 149–167, Escom, Leiden.

Hall, D. & Pavitt, N. (1984) An appraisal of molecular force fields for the representation of polypeptides, *J. Comp. Chem.* **5**, 441–450.

Hurst, G.J.B., Fowler, P.W., Stone, A.J. & Buckingham, A.D. (1986) Intermolecular forces in van der Waals dimers, *Int. J. Quant. Chem.* **29**, 1223–1239.

Jorgensen, W.L. & Tirado-Rives, J. (1988) The OPLS potential functions for proteins, *J. Am. Chem. Soc.* **100**, 1657–1666.

Jorgensen, W.L., Chandrasekhar, J., Madura, J.D., Impey, R.W. & Klein, M.L. (1983) Comparison of simple potential functions for simulating liquid water, *J. Chem. Phys.* **79**, 926–935.

Lifson, S. (1981) Potential energy functions for structural molecular biology, Nato Advanced Study Institute on *Current methods in structural molecular biology* (D.B. Davies *et al.*)

Lifson, S., Hagler, A.T. & Dauber, P. (1979) Consistent force field studies of intermolecular forces in hydrogen bonded crystals. 1. Carboxylic acids, amides and the C=O..H— hydrogen bonds, *J. Am. Chem. Soc.* **101**, 5111–5121.

Ling, M.S.H. & Rigby, M. (1984) Towards an intermolecular potential for nitrogen, *Molec. Phys.* **51**, 855–882.

Maitland, G.C., Rigby, M., Smith, E.B. & Wakeham, W.A. (1981) *Intermolecular forces their origin and determination*, Oxford University Press.

Momany, F.A., Carruthers, L.M., McGuire, R.F. & Scheraga H.A. (1974), Intermolecular potentials from crystal data. III Determination of empirical potentials and application to the parking configurations and lattice energies in crystals of carboxylic acids, amines and amides', *J. Phys. Chem.* **78**, 1595–1620.

Momany, F.A., McGuire, R.F., Burgess, A.W. & Scheraga, H.A. (1975), Energy parameters in polypeptides. VII Geometric parameters, partial atomic charges, nonbonded interactions, hydrogen bond interactions an intrinsic torsional potential in naturally occuring amino acids, *J. Phys. Chem.* **79**, 2361–2381.

Munowitz, M.G., Wheeler, G.L. & Colson, S.D. (1977) A critical evaluation of isotropic potential functions for chlorine. Calculations on the three phases of *p*-dichlorobenzene at 100K, *Molec. Phys.*, **34**, 1727–1737.

Nilsson, L. & Karplus, M. (1986) Empirical energy functions for energy minimization and dynamics of nucleic acids, *J. Comp. Chem.* **7**, 591–616.

Nyburg, S.C. & Faerman, C.H. (1985) A revision of van der Waals atomic radii for molecular crystals: N, O, F, S, Cl, Se, Br and I bonded to carbon, *Acta Cryst. B* **41**, 274–279.

Pertsin, A.J. & Kitaigorodsky, A.I. (1987) *The atom–atom potential method*, Springer-Verlag, Berlin.

Price, S.L. (1986) The limitations of isotropic site-site potentials to describe a N_2–N_2 intermolecular potential surface, *Molec. Phys.* **58**, 651–654.

Price, S.L. (1987) The structure of the homonuclear diatomic solids revisited – a distorted atom approach to the intermolecular potential, *Molec. Phys.*, **62**, 45–63.

Price, S.L. (1988) Is the isotropic atom–atom model potential adequate? *Molec. Simuln.*, **1**, 135–156.

Price, S.L. & Stone, A.J. (1982) The anisotropy of the Cl_2–Cl_2 pair potential as shown by the crystal structure. Evidence for intermolecular bonding or lone pair effects? *Molec. Phys.*, **47**, 1457–1470.

Price, S.L. & Stone, A.J. (1987). The electrostatic interactions in van der Waals complexes involving aromatic molecules, *J. Chem. Phys.* **86**, 2859–2868.

Rigby, M. Smith, E.B., Wakeham, W.A. & Maitland, G.C. (1986). *The forces between molecules*, Oxford University Press.

Rodger, P.M., Stone, A.J. & Tildesley, D.J. (1988) The intermolecular potential of chlorine: a three phase study, *Molec. Phys.* **63**, 173–188.

Spackman, M.A. (1986) A simple quantitative model of hydrogen bonding, *J. Chem. Phys.*, **85**, 6587–6601.

Roterman, I.K., Gibson, K.D. & Scheraga, H.A. (1989) A comparison of the CHARMM, AMBER and ECEPP potentials for peptides. I. Conformational predictions for the tandemly repeated peptide (Asn–Ala–Asn–Pro)$_9$, *J. Biomolec. Struc. & Dyn.*, **7**, 391–420.

Roterman, I.K., Lambert, M.H., Gibson, K.D. & Scheraga, H.A. (1989) A comparison of the CHARMM, AMBER and ECEPP potentials for peptides. II phi–psi maps for N-Acetyl Alanine N′-Methyl Amide: Comparisons, contrasts and simple experimental tests, *J. Biomolec. Struc. & Dyn.*, **7**, 421–454.

Stone, A.J. (1985) Distributed polarisabilities, *Molec. Phys,.*, **56**, 1065–1082.

Stone, A.J. & Alderton, M. (1985) Distributed multipole analysis. Methods and applications, *Molec. Phys.* **56**, 1047–1064.

Stone, A.J. & Price, S.L. (1988) Some new ideas in the theory of intermolecular forces: Anisotropic atom–atom potentials, *J. Phys. Chem.* **92**, 3325–3335.

Stone, A.J. & Tong, C.S. (1989) Local and non-local dispersion models, *Chemical Phys.* **137**, 121–135.

Vovelle, F. & Goodfellow, J.M. (1986) The effect of different force fields on the probable hydration sites of urea, in *Biomolecular stereodynamics III* (ed Sarma R.H. & Sarma M.H.) Adenine Press, NY 251–276.

Weiner, S.J., Kollman, P.A., Case, D.A., Chandra Singh, U. Ghio, C., Alagona, G., Profeta, S. & Weiner, P. (1984). A new force field for molecular mechanical simulation of nucleic acids and proteins, *J. Am. Chem. Soc.* **106**, 765–784.

Weiner, S.J., Kollman, P.A., Nguyen, D.T. & Case, D.A. (1986), An all atom force field for simulations of proteins and nucleic acids, *J. Comp. Chem.* **7**, 230–252.

Wheatley, R.J. & Price, S.L. (1990) An overlap model for estimating the anisotropy of repulsion, *Molec. Phys.* **69**, 507–533.

Wheatley, R.J. & Price, S.L. (1990) A systematic intermolecular potential for chlorine, *Molec. Phys.* **71**, 1381–1404.

6

Biomolecular mechanics

A.M. Hemmings

1. INTRODUCTION

Techniques employing potential energy functions (PEFs) are commonly used to probe the complex interrelationships between the structure, dynamics, and function of biological macromolecules. The objectives of such theoretical methods encompass a gamut of applications ranging from the calculation of small corrections to experimental results, such as X-ray crystallographic bond length measurements, through to the prediction of molecular properties which elude direct measurement. For small molecules, methods such as these are collected under the general umbrella term of molecular mechanics, and have often been described in the literature (Boyd & Lipkowitz 1982, Bukert & Allinger 1982, White *et al.* 1989). The application of techniques of this kind to large molecules of biological interest requires consideration of questions not only of scale (that is, number of interaction centres) but also of the form of the potential function to be used. For these reasons we choose to separate terms, and for our present purposes we shall refer to the alternative expression *biomolecular mechanics*.

It is perhaps a combination of the conceptual simplicity of molecular mechanics techniques and their speed and ease of implementation in computer programs which has led to their extensive use in computer modelling of biological molecules. To perform a calculation we need only a (one hopes differentiatable) potential energy function to provide an analytical representation of the molecular potential energy surface (PES) for the molecule or molecule(s) of interest and a set of coordinates to describe the relative positions of the interaction centres. The simplest of all the methods entails straightforward calculation of potential energy for specific conformations of macromolecules (representative points on the molecular PES) with or without explicit representation of the solvent phase and counter-ions. When this is coupled with the various methods of non-linear optimization we arrive at the technique of energy minimization. Here we seek to relax the molecular conformation by locating a molecular conformation corresponding to the point of minimum energy on the PES. Only a local minimum (that closest to the starting conformation) is usually found, although modifications to the basic algorithms can provide alternative solutions (Hemmings *et al.* 1992).

Knowledge of the potential energy surface in the Born–Oppenheimer approximation in principle allows us to calculate many useful properties of a biomolecular system (Hudson 1974). However, the large number of degrees of freedom in a typical biological macromolecule precludes adequate sampling of phase space and thus calculation of accurate molecular properties. If structural information only is required, then, so long as the PEF chosen can provide a *reasonable* representation of the gross features of the ground state PES in the vicinity of the time- and space-averaged solution, the major features of the structure will be returned. In this context we may choose to draw analogies with X-ray structural analysis and discuss the *resolution* we require of the PES. In so doing we can conveniently sub-classify the various popular applications of potential energy functions in the field of biomolecular mechanics.

Low resolution of structural detail may conceivably involve only information concerning morphology. Thus, we need not include terms in our PEF which contribute to the fine detail of the PES. This has several advantages. Firstly, computation times will be faster owing to the simplicity of the model, and, secondly, the radius of convergence of optimization methods will be increased. Investigations of this type include that of the packing of domains in model-built protein structures (Najmudin 1990), the packing of secondary structural elements (Chou *et al.* 1985) and simplified approaches to the general protein folding problem (Levitt 1983). Especially in the case of the latter, however, without additional information (for example, distance restraints from 2D NMR measurements) biomolecular mechanics alone is insufficient to tackle the problem.

Medium resolution analyses require correspondingly more detail in the PES to be successful, implying greater complexity in the PEF. More important here are the *relative* energies of alternative minima, as these will be important in determining conformer probabilities. Work of this type typically necessitates investigations of local protein structure, such as loop conformation (Fine *et al.* 1986, Bruccoleri *et al.* 1988), investigations of relative binding affinities of similar ligands to the same receptor (Blaney *et al.* 1982, Wipff *et al.* 1983), and energy minimization in protein model-building protocols (Hemmings 1987, Najmudin 1990). Increased complexity of the PES here leads to a reduced radius of convergence for standard non-linear optimisation techniques. This, in turn, provides the impetus for the surge in interest in optimization methods based on simulated annealing (Kirkpatrick *et al.* 1983).

Theoretical calculations of the structures of enzyme-substrate complexes are examples of high resolution analyses. Here, accurate potential energy functions are an absolute necessity, carefully parameterized by using *appropriate* experimental information, that is, that which will provide detailed information to determine the shape of the PES in the region of interest (for example, vibrational frequencies) and the relative depth of the minima (for example, quantum mechanical calculations). The requirements on the PEF are exacting, as the energy differences required approach the practical limit of the resolution available of the force-field. Specialized functional forms (Stone & Alderton 1985) may be necessary, and, more often than not, hybrid quantum-mechanical/biomolecular mechanical models devised to take into account important non-classical effects (Rullmann *et al.* 1989, Arad *et al.* 1990).

   In this chapter we shall review the field of energy calculations on biological macromolecules, using potential energy functions. To do this we must first briefly discuss the basics of univariate and multivariate optimization methods, as these form the basis of energy minimization algorithms.

2. OPTIMIZATION METHODS

The vast majority of optmizations performed in the field of computational biomole-cular mechanics, using analytical potential energy functions, can be described as unconstrained minimizations of multivariate non-linear objective functions. Excellent discussions of optimization theory are available in the literature (Bunday 1985, Scales 1985). Generally speaking, all optimization methods of this type are iterative, and, if at the start of the kth-iteration the current estimate of the minimum of the function is denoted by $\mathbf{x}_k$, the new estimate, $\mathbf{x}_{k+1}$, will be obtained from

$$\mathbf{x}_{k+1} = \mathbf{x}_k + \alpha_k \, \mathbf{p}_k \tag{1}$$

where $\mathbf{p}_k$ is a suitable search direction and α_k is a scalar usually obtained by linear search. In this process, a search must be made along the direction of the vector $\mathbf{p}_k$ in an attempt to find a new point $\mathbf{x}_{k+1}$ that represents a minimum in this direction or that gives a desired reduction in function value.

2.1 Univariate optimization
The fundamental problem here is the univariate minimization of the function $F(\mathbf{x}_k + \alpha \mathbf{p}_x)$ with respect to α. Univariate minimization methods can be divided into two classes. The function comparison methods such as golden section search (Scales 1985) rely on function evaluations for various values of α only. Polynomial interpolation methods use function and first derivative information to fit quadratic or cubic polynomial functions to the energy surface along the search vector and predict α as the minimum of the interpolating function.

2.2 Multivariate optimization
Several methods are available for solving an unconstrained minimization problem. These can be classified into two broad categories known as the direct search methods and gradient methods. The direct search methods require only objective function evaluations, and do not use the partial derivatives of the function in finding the minimum, hence they are often called the non-gradient methods. Examples include the simplex method (Nelder & Mead 1965) and pattern search (Hooke & Jeeves 1961). They are most suitable for problems involving a relatively small number of

variables and are, in general, less efficient than the gradient methods. The latter methods, as their name implies, require, in addition to evaluations of the function, the evaluation of first and possibly higher order derivatives of the objective function.

As the form of potential energy functions are such that it is relatively inexpensive to calculate partial first derivatives with respect to the coordinate variables, the gradient methods are overwhelmingly favoured for optimization purposes. In this section we look at the most commonly used multivariate optimization methods for macromolecular energy minimization. Methods such as Newton's method and the various variable metric quasi-Newton methods will not be covered here. The interested reader is referred to the excellent monograph by Scales (1985) for full details.

2.2.1   The method of steepest descents

To appreciate the explicit form of the search direction as used by the steepest descent optimization method let us firstly consider the Taylor expansion of F_{k+1} in terms of F_k and $\mathbf{g}_k$ as $\alpha_k \to 0$:

$$F_{k+1} = F(\mathbf{x}_k + \alpha_k \mathbf{p}_k) \approx F_k + \alpha_k \mathbf{g}_k^{\mathrm{T}} \mathbf{p}_k. \tag{2}$$

If $F_{k+1} < F_k$, as is desired for a minimization of the objective function, then $\mathbf{g}_k^{\mathrm{T}} \mathbf{p}_k < 0$. Rewriting equation (2) we have

$$F_{k+1} - F_k \approx \alpha_k \|\mathbf{g}_k\| . \|\mathbf{p}_k\| \cos\theta, \tag{3}$$

where θ can be regarded as the angle between the two vectors $\mathbf{p}_k$ and $\mathbf{g}_k$. To maximize the decrease in the function over the iteration we should attempt to minimize $\cos\theta$. This occurs when $\theta = \pi$ and thus, for a sufficiently small value of α_k, the greatest reduction in function value is obtained for the search direction

$$\mathbf{p}_k = -\mathbf{g}_k. \tag{4}$$

The negative gradient direction is called the steepest descent direction and its use in the iteration gives rise to the method of steepest descents (SD). This is perhaps the best-known multivariate optimization method, and it has a long history: the use of the negative of the gradient vector as a search direction for function minimization was first made by Cauchy in 1847 (Cauchy 1847). With exact linear search the SD

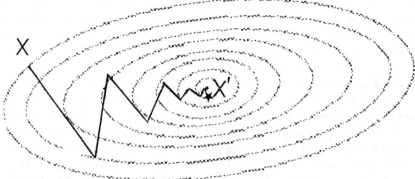

Fig. 1. The progress of the steepest descent method on a hypothetical contoured quadratic function.

method can be shown to be linearly convergent. However, the convergence properties are poor as successive search directions are necessarily orthogonal. Fig. 1 shows the progress of an optimization on a typical quadratic function generating a sequence of points following a characteristic zigzag path from **x** towards the minimum, **x'**.

2.2.2   The conjugate gradient method

The convergence characteristics of the SD method can be greatly improved by its conversion to a conjugate gradient (CG) method as methods of this type possess the desirable property of quadratic termination. Thus, if such an algorithm is used to minimize a quadratic function, F, displaying a positive definite Hessian matrix, **G**, by making a sequence of exact linear searches along each of the vectors $\mathbf{p}_k$ in turn, and these vectors are mutually conjugate with respect to **G**, then the exact minimum of the function, F^*, will be found in at most n searches, where n is the number of independent variables. Since any general function can be reasonably well approximated by a quadratic function in the vicinity of a minimum, then it would be expected that a CG method would find this solution in a finite number of iterations.

The problems then becomes one of generating a series of mutually conjugate search vectors $\mathbf{p}_k$ which, when used with exact linear searches according to equation (1), will minimize a quadratic function with a positive definite Hessian matrix. In general, we can express the search direction for the kth iteration, $\mathbf{p}_k$, as a linear combination of $-\mathbf{g}_k$ and $\mathbf{p}_{k-1}$ by

$$\mathbf{p}_k = -\mathbf{g}_k + \beta_k \mathbf{p}_{k-1} \tag{5}$$

where the value of β_k must be found so as to make $\mathbf{p}_k$ conjugate to $\mathbf{p}_{k-1}$. There are various possible choices for β_k, of which a commonly used variant is that due to Fletcher & Reeves (1964)

$$\beta_k = \frac{\mathbf{g}_k^T \mathbf{g}_k}{\mathbf{g}_{k-1}^T \mathbf{g}_{k-1}} \tag{6}$$

The proof that the search direction $\mathbf{p}_k$ generated by equation (5) will automatically be conjugate to all previous search directions is straightforward (see Scales 1985), and will not be repeated here. When applied to non-quadratic functions, such as is the case for application to the problem of optimizing against macromolecular potential energy functions, the exact minimum will not normally be obtained in a finite number of steps. The problem then becomes one of choosing the search vector once n iterations have been carried out (Powell 1977). Practical experience has shown that the simple strategy of resetting the search vector to the steepest descent direction is acceptable, and this is the most frequently adopted method in practical applications of the conjugate gradient scheme.

Conjugate gradient methods, being of first-derivative type, remove the necessity for calculation of second derivatives of the objective function while retaining quadratic convergence properties. Their major attraction, particularly in application to problems with many independent variables, lies in their meagre computer storage requirements. Only $3n$-vectors of storage are required for the Fletcher–Reeves method; all other gradient methods of comparable efficiency require the storage of an $n \times n$ matrix or its lower triangle. This factor is obviously of paramount importance when attempting to energy minimize macromolecular systems typically consisting of > 1000 atoms and thus > 3000 degrees of freedom.

2.3   Transition state optimization

The ability to move systematically on a molecular potential energy surface from one stable molecular geometry to another through one or more saddle points (transition states) is obviously a highly desirable objective. A facile pathway linking two stable geometries or linking reactant(s) to specific product(s) is synonymous with stating that the interconversion process may occur with a reasonable probability. In this section a brief introduction to transition state optimization algorithms is given. Transition state optimization is of primary importance in the directed perturbation conformational analysis method (DPCA) (Hemmings *et al.* 1992) discussed later in this chapter.

2.3.1   *Constrained Newton–Raphson optimization*

The idea of progressing uphill from one minimum, then downhill toward another, was the basis of the early gentlest ascent method for locating transition states proposed by Crippen and Scheraga (Crippen & Scheraga 1971). In this application a short step is taken along the lowest normal mode direction followed by energy minimization in the subspace orthogonal to it, leading to an iterative sequence moving away from the initial minimum along a low-energy pathway. The disadvantage of this method is that it is time-consuming (a complete energy minimization for each iteration), and that it will not, in fact, locate a transition state but will simply indicate when such a point has been passed.

Cerjan & Miller (1981) proposed a walking algorithm using derivative information that does not require subspace optimizations via a modified NR algorithm in which constraints on the usual step length are applied by means of a Lagrange multiplier. Modifications to this algorithm were later suggested to ensure stability of search (Simons *et al.* 1983), including a 'trust radius' inside which a local quadratic approximation to the potential is sufficiently accurate for the NR algorithm to succeed.

The basic form of the algorithm is as follows. Let us begin with the form of the ordinary Newton update given by

$$\alpha . \mathbf{p}_k = -\mathbf{G}^{-1}.\mathbf{g}_k. \tag{7}$$

Leaving aside the difficulties in calculating and inverting the Hessian matrix ($\mathbf{G}$), there are two problems with the NR method for use in locating transition states. Firstly, the step length (that is, the norm of $\mathbf{x}$) may be so large that the truncation of the Taylor series expansion is no longer sufficiently accurate. Secondly, if the Hessian matrix is positive definite, as it will be near a minimum, then the NR step will move toward the minimum rather than away from it as desired. Both of these problems can be ameliorated by constraining the step length to some predetermined value, δ; this is most easily implemented by means of a Lagrange multiplier. Consider the Lagrangian function

$$L(x,\lambda) = V(\mathbf{x} + \mathbf{x_o}) + \frac{\lambda}{2}(\Delta^2 - x^\mathrm{T}x). \tag{8}$$

Setting $\partial L/\partial \mathbf{x} = 0$ determines the stationary points of the function on the boundary determined by Δ and leads to

$$\mathbf{x} = (\lambda\mathbf{I} - \mathbf{G})^{-1}\mathbf{g} \tag{9}$$

$$\Delta^2 = \mathbf{g}^\mathrm{T}(\lambda\mathbf{I} - \mathbf{G})^{-2}\mathbf{g} \tag{10}$$

where I is the matrix. Equation (10) may be solved for λ given Δ, and then equation (9) solved for the step, $\mathbf{x}$. Performing the unitary transformation to a basis which diagonalizes G leads to expressions which may be used to rationalize the consequences of the possible solutions for λ from equation (10). Letting the eigenvalues and eigenvectors of $\mathbf{G}$ be denoted by b_i and v_i gives the equivalent relationships

$$\mathbf{x} = \Sigma_i(\lambda - b_i)^{-1}(v_i.g).v_i \tag{11}$$

$$\Delta^2 = \Sigma_i(\lambda - b_i)^{-2}(v_i.g)^2. \tag{12}$$

Thus, the new potential energy to second order is

$$V^* = V(\mathbf{x_o}) + \Sigma_i(\lambda - b_i)^2(v_i.g)^{\ 2}(\lambda - \frac{b_i}{2}). \tag{13}$$

If a solution to equation (13) exists such that $b_1 < \lambda < b_2$ (assuming $b_i < b_{i+1}$), then the step $\mathbf{x}$ will have the characteristic that it will be directed along the gradient, or uphill, in the v_i direction, and will oppose the gradient along all other eigenvector directions. If, furthermore, λ is chosen so that $\frac{1}{2}b_1 < \lambda < \frac{1}{2}b_2$, then equation (13) shows that the contribution to the expected energy change will be negative along all directions except for that along v_i.

The basis of the method is that, starting from a minimum energy conformation possessing a Hessian with all positive eigenvalues, a step of fixed length is taken that proceeds uphill along the current softest eigenvector while simultaneously decreasing the energy of the system along all other directions. As one nears a transition state, the lowest eigenvalue will become negative and the characteristic of the normal NR technique to converge to the closest stationary point can be exploited (λ set to zero). To explore the local structure of the PES along modes corresponding to eigensolutions other than the lowest one (stiff mode walks), a coordinate scaling along the required eigenvector can be performed to scale the corresponding eigenvalue to become the lowest in the system. As one approaches a transition state the desired direction generally becomes the lowest mode of the system and the scaling becomes redundant. To implement this idea there must be some mechanism for keeping track of the chosen eigendirection. At each step then, the direction of search is generally taken to be that of the current eigenvector with the largest projection on the previous search direction (Simons et al. 1983). Modifications for its use with many-variable systems have also been published (Nguyen & Case 1985).

3. RESTRAINED REFINEMENT OF MACROMOLECULAR STRUCTURE

The process of macromolecular structure determination by X-ray crystallography entails the extraction of detailed atomic positional and thermal parameters from available experimental data in the form of structure factor amplitudes (and occasionally MIR phases) (see Blundell & Johnson 1978). Unfortunately, however, it is invariably found to be the case that the refinement of structural models is crucially hindered by problems arising from the relatively small excess of experimental observations over model parameters. This is particularly pertinent for protein structure refinement where the resolution of the diffraction data is limited for several reasons (Blundell & Johnson 1978) and is generally much lower than that routinely available for small molecules. In consequence it has become customary to use least squares refinement methods which simultaneously derive a molecular model to fit both the diffraction data and additional observations associated with known molecular stereochemical features. The stereochemical observations restrain the model to be compatible with prior knowledge regarding the distributions structural coordinates about ideal values. Commonly, restraints will be included related to bonding distances, planarity of groups of atoms, chirality at asymmetric centres, non-bonded atomic contacts, torsion angles, non-crystallographic symmetry, and thermal parameters.

Many of these restraints can be implemented by means of observational functions which are equivalent to the forms found in typical potential energy functions as used in biomolecular mechanics. This suggests a close correspondence between the two techniques, but what happens when energy minimization alone is used to refine a protein structure? Simple energy minimization of refined protein structures has been performed (Gelin & Karplus 1975, Ooi et al. 1978, Yoshioki et al. 1983) and noted for a propensity to increase the crystallographic residual (R-factor) in all but a few cases in which it showed only a moderate decrease (Levitt 1974, Ferro et al. 1980). This is symptomatic of a major, acknowledged shortcoming of energy minimization as applied to refined protein structures, which is that since it is formulated in terms of a single, unique conformation it is, as such, inherently unsuited to the job of description of poorly ordered systems such as solvent phases or disordered polypeptide structure. However, when combined in a consistent fashion with refinement against diffraction data, extremely useful refinement methods can result. Naturally, the question of the relationship between X-ray and energy refinement arises in this context, and the problem of their relative weighting in a combined restrained X-ray refinement scheme has been discussed (Moss 1980).

Several major restrained structure factor least squares refinement programs for macromolecules are now available, falling into two major categories. These differ not so much by the form of the potential energy function used to augment the experimental observations (as all programs use very similar functional forms), but more by the optimization method employed. The programs of the first type are exemplified by RESTRAIN (Haneef et al. 1985). This program uses the Gauss–Newton theory of function optimization to solve the system of least squares normal equations, and it has been used in the refinement of a large number of important biological macromolecules including that of the HIV-1 proteinase (Lapatto et al. 1989), a target for the development of drugs to combat AIDS. The X-PLOR program of Brünger *et al.* (1987) is of the second type, and it can perform a simulated annealing optimization by generating molecular dynamics trajectories at elevated system temperatures on an effective energy surface resulting from a combination of experimental and restraint potentials. With the advent of widely accessible supercomputing resources refinement it is inevitable that procedures of this type will become increasingly popular.

4.　ENERGY MINIMIZATION AND PROTEIN STRUCTURE

A common application of biomolecular mechanical energy minimization is in the geometrical and stereochemical optimization of protein models constructed by means of one (or a combination) of several modelling procedures. These include homology modelling (discussed in the following section), distance geometry-based methods (Ripka 1986), and protein folding simultations (Levitt 1983). In this context, the role of energy minimization has been reduced to that of stereochemical regularisation and optimization of side-chain packing for models usually found to display poor geometry. These are undoubtedly important tasks to be performed, but the competence of the method even in this regard must be questioned when so many of the parameters from the force-field can be, and are, altered by researchers in an *ad hoc* manner.

There have been sporadic attempts to delineate the effects of energy minimization on protein structure both in terms of the isolated protein (with implicit models for solvation) and with the inclusion of the intermolecular degrees of freedom resulting from explicit representation of solvent molecules (Ferro 1979). Further investigations have focused on the effects of crystal environment (Gelin & Karplus 1979), inclusion of counter-ions (Singh *et al.* 1985), and spatial constraints (Bruccoleri & Karplus 1986). A comparison of several different potential energy functions has been made for small, crystalline, cyclic peptides (Hall & Pavitt 1984). However, analyses of molecules such as these may be considered to be of limited practical relevance to parallel calculations on proteins as they are too small to display extensive secondary structure and because the large number of intermolecular contacts often results in different crystal and solution structures (Tonelli & Brewster 1972). The results of crystal-packing calculations on the flexible small molecule, Leu-enkephalin, serve to emphasize the importance of these observations (Glasser & Scheraga 1988).

Whitlow & Teeter (1986), using the high resolution structure of the small hydrophobic protein, crambin, performed over 70 minimizations changing various force field parameters in a comprehensive assessment of the effects of energy minimization on protein structure. The focus of the calculations was to discover the parameterization of a basic potential function (choice of van der Waals' radii, effective dielectric constant, etc.) and the nature of the model used (inclusion of intermolecular contacts, inclusion of crystal solvent, etc.) to accurately reproduce the geometry of a protein in a crystalline environment. Given that both static and dynamic disorder contribute to the spatial and temporal average structure refined in an X-ray analysis, the objective of the calculations was thus to parameterize an *average* molecular PEF designed solely for energy minimization. Such a PEF would therefore not necessarily be of use in, say, a molecular dynamics simulation, as the corresponding PES is non-realistic, including as it does time-averaged and space-averaged information together with implicit inclusion of entropic effects such as hydrophobic forces.

What then were their conclusions? Perhaps, unsurprisingly, the optimal conditions found were similar to those long since adopted by other users of the technique. For example, inclusion of explicit solvent in the molecular model by means of a Monte Carlo-generated water bath resulted in closer correspondence for the surface of the protein than otherwise. This is in agreement with EM calculations on the aspartic proteinase, endothiapepsin, both *in vacuo* and including solvent molecules at sites revealed by X-ray crystallography (Hemmings 1987). Nevertheless, the absence from the protein PEFs of terms necessary to model effects such as hydrophobicity will not be revealed by calculations of this type. This is, in itself, an area deserving continuing close consideration.

5.   PREDICTION OF LOCAL PROTEIN CONFORMATION

Before moving on to address the use of biomolecular mechanics in the derivation of protein models by schemes using sequence homology or distance restrains from, usually, 2D-NMR data, let us briefly turn our attention to a potentially much simpler problem, that of the prediction of small regions of protein conformation where most of the structure is known.

This situation commonly arises in the process of protein structure solution by X-ray crystallography, usually because of disorder, although biomolecular mechanics is not often used in such situations. In other situations one is interested to predict the structure of a mutant protein that differs from that of a previously determined one by the substitution of a single amino acid. In other cases, particularly in the modelling of protein structures by homology, the problem is to determine the conformation of short regions of polypeptide chain assuming an appropriate model for the remainder of the structure. The best known example of this can be found in the modelling of the antibody hypervariable loop conformations in the immunoglobulins (Bruccoleri *et al.* 1988).

These problems are basically similar and in theory readily solved if two assumptions can be made. Firstly, one must have access to a method to map the conformational PES of the parent molecule, and, secondly, one must assume that the resultant change in the PES is small and is localized in the site of the mutation. Then, assuming that a method is available to screen the plausible conformations generated from energetic criteria for the most probable of the set, a prediction of local polypeptide conformation can be made.

Various algorithms have been proposed and used to predict local protein structure. Shih *et al.* (1985) used the concept of localized structural perturbation to model a site-directed mutant of lysozyme. Loop-closure algorithms have received attention from several groups and have been used in prediction. The most successful of these, the CONGEN procedure of Bruccoleri & Karplus (1987), has been used to successfully predict antibody complementarity-determining regions (CDR). Similar algorithms have been published by Snow & Amzel (1986) and Moult & James (1986).

6. MODELLING OF PROTEIN STRUCTURE

The three-dimensional structures of proteins that have been solved by X-ray crystallography show that they form families in which homologous amino acid sequences possess highly similar folding patterns. Well-known examples of such families include the globins, immunoglobulins, cytochromes, and the serine and aspartic proteinases. Indeed, the three-dimensional structures of proteins have been observed to evolve more slowly than amino acid sequence, and a strong structural relationship can be seen to persist even when the homology of the sequences falls at the lower limit of detectability when using current sequence alignment methods (Doolittle 1986). The discovery of these familial relationships and the relative ease with which primary structural information can be obtained has led to attempts to model protein tertiary structure from primary sequence comparisons and the structures of their known homologues. This forms the basis of the method of homology modelling.

Browne *et al.* (1969) were the first to adopt this scheme in their construction of a model of α-lactalbumin from the crystallographic structure of lysozyme. This was soon followed by a structural model for the α-lytic proteinase from that of the serine proteinase, elastase (McLachlan & Shotton 1971). Many further examples can be found in the literature, including models for human insulin-like growth factor based on bovine insulin (Blundell *et al.* 1978) and for β-crystallins based on bovine γ-crystallin (Inana *et al.* 1983). A comparison of two proposed models for *Streptomyces griseus* trypsin with the experimentally determined structure has led to an evaluation of the nature and magnitude of the errors likely in comparative model building (Read *et al.* 1983). The model for immunoglobulin D1.3 constructed by Chothia and co-workers (1986) was also compared with the cystal structure. However, such estimates are perhaps less appropriate for models constructed by using the more rigorous model building techniques developed in recent years, particularly those developed by Blundell and co-workers (Blundell *et al.* 1988).

Nevertheless, given the complexity of protein architecture, the inherent subjectivity of aspects of the model building process even in highly experienced hands can result in models which display physically unrealistic close steric contacts between atoms. It has therefore become customary in model building exercises to employ energy minimization procedures to optimize amino acid packing and to remove these unrealistic atom–atom contacts from the final model. Warme *et al.* (1974) were the first to use such a procedure on their model for α-lactalbulin based on the crystal structure for lysozyme. Greer, too, has constructed models for haptoglobin, mammalian serine proteinases, and thrombin from those of chymotrypsin, trypsin, and elastase by comparative model building followed by energy minimization (Greer 1980, 1981).

Novotny *et al.* (1984), recognizing a general reluctance to rigorously assess the correctness or otherwise of model built protein structures, constructed, energy minimized, and analysed patently incorrect models for mouse myeloma immunoglobu-lin light chain variable domain and hemerythrin. These proteins have the same number of amino acids but very different native structures and sequences. The aims of this study were to test the two principal assumptions of protein modelling, namely that only homologous side chains can be modelled onto a known protein backbone, and that empirical potential energy functions can be used to gauge the correctness of the models. The results were to show that even under the extreme test conditions, detailed and careful analysis was required to distinguish between the correct and grossly misfolded structures, and that the absence of close non-bonded contacts, while necessary, was not a sufficient condition for the validity of a model built protein structure (see also Novotny 1988). Thus, while the salient features of an *in vacuo* PES can be reproduced by a simple PEF, hydrophobic and solvent-mediated effects are modelled poorly or just not modelled at all in calculations of this type.

6.1   Modelling the aspartic proteinases

Renin is an aspartic proteinase intimately involved in the humoral regulation of blood pressure. Its sole detectable action is the cleavage of the N-terminal decapeptide of its endogenous plasma glycoprotein substrate to produce angiotensin I. This in turn is proteolytically processed by angiotensin converting enzyme (ACE) to form the potent pressor octapeptide, angiotensin II. The fine specificity of renin makes it, in contrast to the proteolytically promiscuous ACE, a good candidate for rational antihypertensive design. For many years no atomic structure of renin was available from X-ray crystallography despite determined effort. However, while structures of the native enzyme and of its complexes with inhibitors refined from high resolution X-ray data are obviously desirable, much useful information on the molecular basis of enzyme–substrate and enzyme–ligand interaction and specificity of renin can be obtained from inspection of models constructed with reference to the previously derived three-dimensional structures of homologous enzymes. For this reason a model of the tertiary structure for human renin was proposed on the basis of comparative model building (Sibanda *et al.* 1984, Sibanda 1986), using as templates the known 3-dimensional structures of other aspartic proteinases, particularly that of endothiapepsin. The model was completed by the use of extensive conjugate gradient energy minimization, using a Cray 1S supercomputer and a standard protein PEF (Hemmings *et al.* 1985, Hemmings 1987). Ramachandran plots of the (φ, ψ)-torsion angles for the initial and energy minimized human renin models are presented in Fig. 2. The distribution of (φ, ψ)-pairs in the final model is more reminiscent of the distributions found for high-resolution protein structures than the initial. Another indicator of correctness, the number and geometry of intramolecular hydrogen bonds, is summarized for the models in Table 1. Here, results for initial and an intermediate human renin model are compared with those from an energy minimized model for endothiapepsin. It would be expected that two homologous enzymes of approximately the same size would share similar hydrogen bonding statistics. Energy minimization is seen to have begun the process of optimization of hydrogen bond geometries.

For an enzyme of fungal origin such as endothiapepsin to serve as a good model for a mammalian enzyme such as human renin, it is at least necessary that amino acid changes in the major elements of secondary structure leading to large changes in local density are compensated by appropriate adjacent residue changes in order to preserve good packing and hydrogen bonding capacity. A good example of such

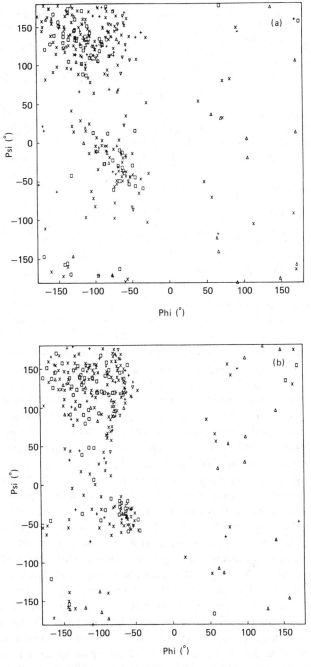

Fig. 2. Ramachandran plots of the initial (a) and energy minimized (b) human renin models.
Δ, glycine; ∇, proline; □, β-branched amino acids; +, aromatic; ×, remainder.

Table 1.   The geometry of intramolecular hydrogen bonds in the initial (init.) and energy minimized (final) models of human renin. Statistics for an energy minimized crystal structure of endothiapepsin (EPR122F) are presented for comparison

Model	Category[a]	Number	Mean (σ)			Correlation coefficient[b]
			l(H-A)/Å	θ(D-H-A)/°	θ(H-A-AA)/°	
Human	main-main	142	2.03 (0.25)	154 (13)	141 (19)	−0.27
renin	main-side	30	2.00 (0.32)	146 (14)	120 (23)	−0.19
(Init.)	side-side	2	2.02 (0.00)	133 (16)	120 (14)	*
Human	main-main	155	2.02 (0.15)	151 (18)	134 (20)	−0.43
renin	main-side	69	2.03 (0.12)	150 (12)	123 (22)	−0.18
(Final)	side-side	15	2.06 (0.24)	151 (13)	126 (20)	−0.34
	main-main	183	1.97 (0.12)	150 (12)	134 (19)	−0.54
EPR122F	main-side	92	1.98 (0.14)	149 (13)	116 (19)	−0.41
	side-side	34	1.88 (0.17)	157 (15)	122 (21)	−0.68

Hydrogen bond statistics for the original and energy minimized structures of human renin.
Symbols used: D donor
H hydrogen
A acceptor
AA acceptor antecedent
[a] Hydrogen bonds divided into categories by the nature of the interacting atoms, that is, as being found in the main- or side-chain segments of amino acid residues.
[b] Correlation coefficients calculated between the H–A distance and the D–H–A angle.

compensatory changes is found in the strands q_N and r_N of the 6-stranded basal sheet. Here, the substitutions of the aligned and solvent inaccessible residues 153 Ala→Phe, 165 Tyr→Ile, and 155 Leu→Tyr lead to a situation where the side-chain phenolic hydroxyl group of Tyr155 in human renin can be placed in an almost identical position to that of Tyr165 in endothiapepsin (see Fig. 3). However, if simple substitution of the relevant side chains is made to follow the orientation of original side chains, then the requisite packing will not result. In fact, the χ_2-torsion angle of Phe153 in the human renin model must change by 93° (4.3σ for all χ_2-torsion angle changes) on energy minimization to preserve the local amino acid packing. In this way, the total volume for the three residues mentioned above in the energy minimized structures is 512 Å^3 in endothiapepsin and 504 Å^3 in human renin as calculated by the Voronoi procedure (Richards 1974). Thus, it appears that energy minimization can correct errors in side-chain orientation. However, this is possible only where the correct orientation corresponds to the local energy minimum; in other cases molecular dynamics simulated annealing procedures may be of greater usefulness.

7.   THE MULTIPLE MINIMA PROBLEM IN PROTEIN CONFORMATIONAL ANALYSIS

In attempting to locate all of the conformations available to a molecule, and therefore also the conformation of lowest energy, that is, the global minimum, computer programs have been written which can perform systematic scans through dihedral angles in the initial model to map the potential energy of the system as a function

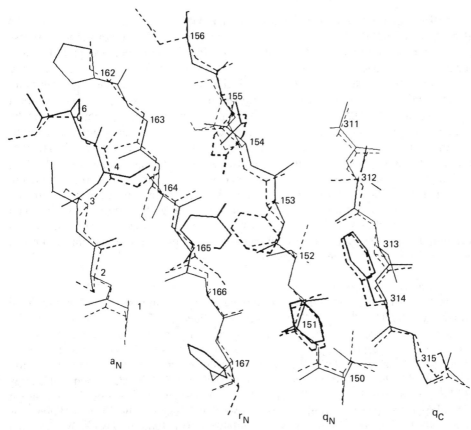

Fig. 3. Accommodation of a substitution between the hydrophobic cores of endothiapepsin and human renin. A least squares superposition of sections of the basal sheet from the relaxed (energy minimized) endothiapepsin (solid line) and human renin (broken line) models.

of conformation. When coupled to an optimization of the system potential energy at each grid point, this rather straightforward approach can give interesting details of the conformational preferences of, for example, amino acid side chains (Gelin & Karplus 1975). It is, however, impossible to provide anything other than a restricted mapping of a small region of the multi-dimensional PES for a macromolecule. Stochastic exploration of energy surfaces by a Monte Carlo-like approach has been demonstrated for small flexible molecules (Saunders 1987). However, given the number of independent variables in typical biomolecular systems, it is obvious that the number of energy minimizations should be kept as low as possible. For this reason, stochastic approaches such as this are of limited appeal. Smart conformational analysis approaches, such as those described in this section, have greater potential for application to recurrent problems in the investigation of polypeptide and protein structure. In section 7.2 a brief survey is made of other approaches aimed at the more difficult task of surmounting the problem of multiple minima in predictions of protein folding.

7.1   Directed perturbation conformational analysis
Bearing in mind that for a molecule any conformational interconversion process must proceed via a transition state on the PES for that molecule, we have the basis for another approach to the multiple minima problem. In this way, given a starting energy minimum conformation, the most efficient way to locate further energy minima in its vicinity is to firstly locate the transition states that separate them. Once a transition state has been found, standard energy minimization techniques can be used to locate the alternative energy minimum. Each new energy minimum point can then serve as a starting point for further transition state searches and thus further minima. This is the basis of the directed perturbation conformational analysis (DPCA) technique (Hemmings *et al.* 1992) as implemented in the Beijing Insulin Group molecular modelling program, BIGMOL. Obviously, if this procedure is repeated *ad infinitum* all possible minima will be located, and the global energy minimum can then be simply chosen by inspection of relative energy. However, the procedure is best applied to the problem of optimizing an initial 'best guess' conformation known to lie in the vicinity of the preferred one.

7.1.1   The DPCA algorithm
Given a starting conformation and having energy minimized it to find a local minimum, the DPCA algorithm proceeds by means of a series of searches for transition states by using initial search directions parallel and antiparallel to the eigenvectors corresponding to the N lowest eigenvalues of the system at this point (thus, a value of $N = 3$ gives a total of 6 search directions). Once a new transition state has been found and added to the transition state (TS) list, subsequent energy minimization from it will lead to an alternative energy minimum conformation (or to an energy minimum found at some previous stage in the search). Each new conformation is added to an energy minimum (EM) list and can serve as a starting point for further transition state searches. In this way a local search of the molecule PES can be made. The algorithm is presented in detail in Hemmings *et al.* (1992).

Having decided on the use of torsion angles as conformational variables as the most efficient representation of internal distortion coordinates, this algorithm requires a potential which can express the energy of the molecule as a function of variables of this type alone. The empirical conformational energy program for polypeptides (ECEPP) developed by Scheraga and co-workers (Momany *et al.* 1975) satisfies this requirement and was incorporated into the program. A user-specified set of independent torsional coordinates are used to describe the essential degrees of freedom of the molecule in question. The selection of these is entirely at the discretion of the user, but will not normally exceed 200 because of problems with convergence. The first and second derivatives of the potential function with respect to the selected independent torsional coordinates are calculated analytically by using efficient formulae (Noguti & Gō1983, Abe *et al.* 1984, Wako & Gō1987) modified to allow for systems consisting of more than one molecule.

7.1.2   Applications of the method
To assess the efficiency of the DPCA method a series of analyses of simple homooligopeptides in conformations representative of short stretches of secondary

structure commonly found in proteins were performed. The molecules chosen for study included the N-acetyl, N'-methylamide derivatives of hexa-L-alanine, hexa-L-valine, and deca-L-alanine. In addition, a simple mono-L-alanine derivative was used in a more exhaustive search of conformational space.

Initial models for these molecules were constructed by using ideal internal coordinate values taken from the ECEPP force-field (Momany *et al.* 1975). These models were, in all cases, built initially with torsion angles in the α_R region of conformation space with $(\varphi, \psi) = (-60°, -40°)$ except for an additional model of the hexa-L-alanine derivative constructed in a generally extended conformation with $(\varphi, \psi) = (-83°, -153°)$. The latter was chosen as a result of the analysis of the PES of the mono-L-alanine derivative. The x_1 side-chain torsion angles of the hexa-L-valine derivative were all set to 180° and all peptide groups set in the trans-planar conformation.

The assignment of molecular degrees of freedom depended on the model, but in each case involved only torsion angles. For the first of the models, N-acetyl,N'-methyl-L-alaninamide, five torsional variables were assigned including the φ and ψ angles. For the remaining models only the main-chain φ and ψ torsion angles for each residue of the hexa-L-alanine derivative (12 variables) and the deca-L-alanine derivative (20 variables) were unconstrained. In the N-acetyl,N'-methyl-hexa-L-valinamide model in addition to the (φ, ψ) degrees of freedom, the χ_1 side-chain torsion angles were unconstrained (18 variables). In each oligopeptide model all peptide torsion angles, ω, were constrained.

The conformational analyses of these models were performed with the BIGMOL program. The ECEPP force-field was used to provide the molecular potential function. The derivatives of the potential were calculated by using a modification of the efficient algorithm of Wako & Gō (1987). Transition state optimizations were carried out by using initial search directions parallel and antiparallel to the eigenvectors corresponding to the three lowest frequency eigensolutions of the Hessian matrix calculated at each minimum energy search start point. Energy minimizations were performed by using a sequence of conjugate gradient (Powell 1977) and quasi-Newton–Raphson (Fletcher 1970) optimization methods to accurately locate each minimum energy point. In the general case, a maximum of 30 energy minima on the PES was requested of the DPCA algorithm.

To assess the efficiency of the DPCA method relative to molecular dynamics approaches to the question of local conformational analysis (MDCA), a simulation of the deca-L-alanine derivative was performed with the AMBER molecular mechanics program (AMBER Version 3.0) (Singh *et al.* 1986). An all-atom force field was used with cartesian coordinates as degrees of freedom. Owing to the small size of the molecule no non-bonded interaction cut-off was employed. A dielectric constant of $\varepsilon = 1$ was used in the calculation of electrostatic interactions. After energy minimization *in vacuo*, using the conjugate gradient method, the molecule was heated from 0 K to 300 K in 50 K steps over a period of 6 psec, using an integration time step of $\delta = 2$ fsec. With the same time step, a further 14 psec of simulation was performed with coordinate sets extracted every 1 psec for energy minimization. All energy minimized coordinate datasets possessed root mean square (rms) values for the elements of the residual first derivative vector of less than 0.01 kcal mol^{-1} Å^{-1} at termination.

7.1.3   Results

Starting from a molecular conformation in the α_R-helical region of (φ, ψ)-space of N-acetyl,N'-methyl-L-alaninamide, the DPCA algorithm was rapidly able to generate a set of 9 energy minimum conformations and details of the transition state conformations that separate them. The efficiency of the search, expressed as the percentage of transition state searches that led to new energy minima, was 80%. The details of these confrmations are presented as Table 2. The geometry of the energy

Table 2.   Energy minimum (EM) points on the potential energy surface of N-acetyl,N'-methyl-L-alaninamide

EM index	Φ	T	ΔE
1	-68	-46	0.0
2	-172	-60	$+4.0$
3	-96	01	-1.4
4	77	-52	$+22.1$
5	-83	153	-2.2
6	44	-71	$+22.8$
7	44	60	$+1.1$
8	-150	84	-1.0
9	60	174	$+5.3$

minimum points agree reasonably well with previous theoretical calculations on this small molecule (Rossky *et al.* 1979, Scarsdale *et al.* 1983). The global energy minimum conformation was found in the $C_{7,eq}$ region at $(\varphi, \psi) = (-83°, 153°)$, lying 2.2 kcal mol^{-1} below the α_R form.

The results of the analyses of the molecular PES local to two markedly different starting conformations of the hexa-L-alanine derivative in the α_R form and the extended form are presented as Fig. 4. The extended form shows greater flexibility, that is, it shows a larger number of low-lying transition state structures which can be readily sampled to locate alternative energy minima well separated from the initial energy minimum conformation. This can be inferred from the distribution of energy barriers to be crossed before locating alternative energy minima (see Fig. 5). In the case of the α_R form, the maximum rms deviation of any conformation from the starting energy minimized conformation is 3.7 Å. For the β form the corresponding maximum rms deviation is 2.3 Å. These deviations are much greater than those found from standard energy minimization or molecular dynamics procedures (Hemmings 1987). The substitution of valyl for alanyl side chains in the α-form to give the hexa-L-valine derivative leads to a considerable stiffening of the helix and to a constriction of the amount of conformational space searched by the DPCA algorithm. The distributions of relative energies for transition state structures and energy minima for this system are presented as Fig. 6. Note that the algorithm is capable of locating alternative energy minima approximately 74 kcal mol^{-1} below that of the energy minimized starting structure.

For the deca-L-alanine derivative the goal to find 30 distinct energy minimum conformations was achieved by the DPCA algorithm after 67 transition state

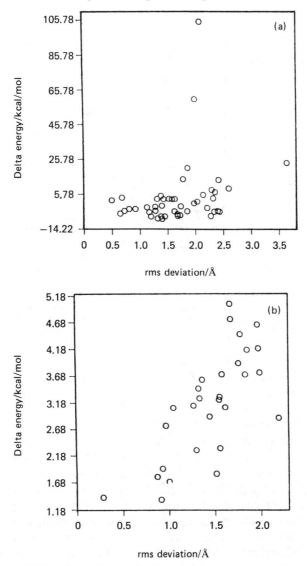

Fig. 4. Plots of difference energy versus rms atomic deviation for energy minimum conformations from the EM stack relative to the energy minimized starting structure for (a) the α-form and (b) the β-form of the hexa-L-alanine derivative.

optimisation searches yielded a total of 32 unique transition states. Fig. 7 shows a sequence of least squares comparisons of molecular conformations representative of points on the molecular PES generated sequentially by the DPCA algorithm. It shows the energy minimum structures of indices 1 and 5 from the EM stack which are separated by the transition state structure of index 4 from the TS stack. Note that while the transition state structure differs only slightly from that of its parent structure (rms deviation 0.4 Å, $\Delta E = +23$ kcal mol^{-1}), the minimum energy structure

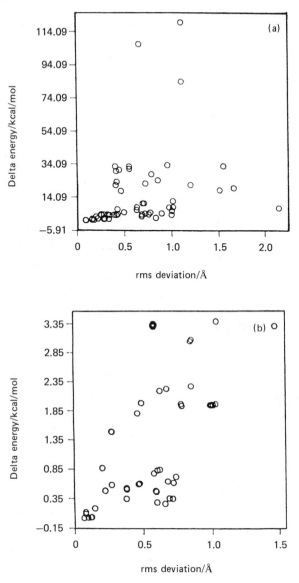

Fig. 5. Plots of difference energy versus rms atomic deviation for transition state structures
from the TS stack relative to their individual parent energy minima (that is, the minimum
from which a transition state is found) for (a) the α-form and (b) the β-form of the hexa-L-
alanine derivative.

located from it shows considerable distortion from the initial. In fact, this alternative
conformation is 8 kcal mol^{-1} lower in energy than that of the parent and shows an
rms devviation of 1.4 Å. We can see that the N-terminus of the helix has begun to
unwind, and this process is continued as further transition states and energy minima
are located (not shown).

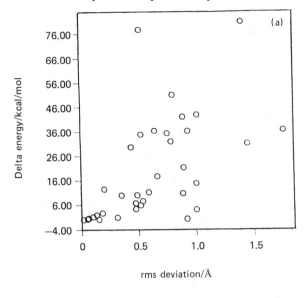

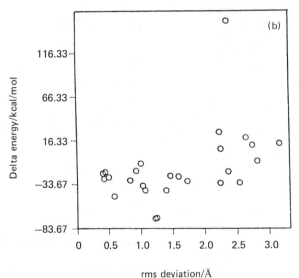

Fig. 6. Plots of difference energy versus rms atomic deviation for (a) transition state structures and (b) energy minimum structures for the α-form of the hexa-L-valine derivative.

Analysis of the fifteen energy minimized conformation sof N-acetyl,N'-methyl-deca-L-alaninamide resulting from the molecular dynamics trajectory were compared with the $t = 0$ psec structure to reveal the range of conformational space available to such a system during a typical molecular dynamics simulation. Of immediate note is that the procedure generates only 4 closely similar conformations for this molecule. These representative conformations, presented in Fig. 8, differ only in the orientation of the blocking N-acetyl and N'-methylamide groups, and no significant distortion

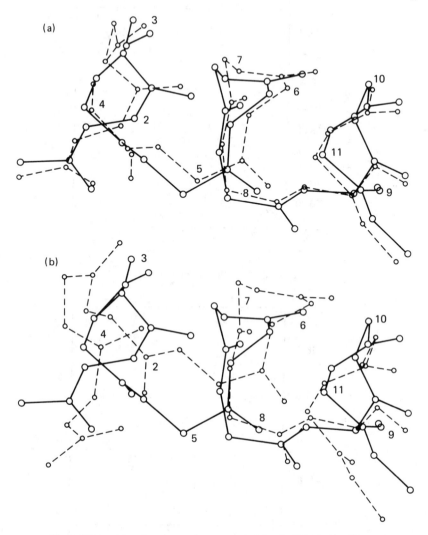

Fig. 7. Comparison of conformations generated by the DPCA algorithm.
(a) A comparison of the initial energy minimized conformation (solid lines) and the fourth conformation from the TS stack (dotted lines) for the deca-L-alanine derivative.
(b) A comparison of the initial energy minimized conformation (solid lines) and the fifth conformation from the EM stack (dotted lines) for the deca-L-alanine derivative. Only main-chain, non-hydrogen atoms displayed.

of the molecular helix was noticed. The all-atom rms deviations for the structures resulting from energy minimization after $t = 6, 9$, and 19 psec of simulation relative to the $t = 0$ psec structure were 0.6, 0.7, and 0.5 Å, respectively. These three structures lay 0.7, 2.0, and 0.3 kcal mol^{-1} below the energy of the initial structure as calculated in the AMBER all-atom force field.

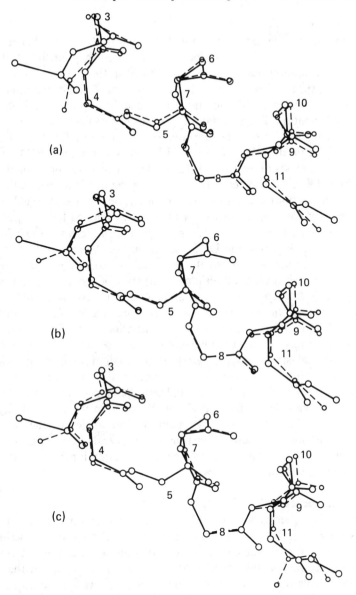

Fig. 8. Results of molecular dynamics simulated annealing of N-acetyl,N'-methyl-deca-L-
alaninamide.
(a) A comparison of the t = 0 psec and energy minimized t = 6 psec conformations;
(b) A comparison of the t = 0 psec and energy minimized t = 9 psec conformations;
(c) A comparison of the t = 0 psec and energy minimized t = 19 psec derivatives.
Only main-chain, non-hydrogen atoms displayed. In each case, the t = 0 psec structure is
shown with solid bonds.

7.1.4   *Discussion*

From the preceding discussion it is evident that the DPCA algorithm can produce from a reasonable starting structure (perhaps generated by modelling techniques) a set of alternative equilibrium structures distributed in the vicinity of the original in conformational space. These energy minima represent conformational substates available to the molecule and should be included in any discussion of preferred molecular conformation. The expectation value for observables such as conformation can then be calculated from the appropriate distribution function. The DPCA algorithm is also efficient. While the total CPU-time spent in the DPCA and MDCA conformational analyses of the deca-L-alanine derivative were approximately similar (DPCA required 4 h, MDCA required 6 h for 20 psec trajectory generation and 4 h for energy minimization), the amount of conformational space searched by the two methods is clearly not. The number of distinct energy minima located and their rms deviations from the initial structure are much greater in the case of DPCA. Thus, it appears from these data that the DPCA algorithm is comparatively more efficient than MDCA for sampling conformational space. It is beyond question that the precise details of the conformations and energetics of the equilibrium structures revealed by the DPCA algorithm may be influenced by the constraint of bond lengths and angles. However, the magnitude of these effects may, in fact, be rather small (Hemmings 1987), and furthermore, each conformation is intended to serve only as a starting point for more exhaustive analysis. For the case of the directed perturbation conformational analysis of a protein system rather than of small oligopeptides, some changes in the details of the calculation will be necessary. Firstly, degrees of freedom will be assigned only to specific torsion angles in the immediate region of interest of the protein. For example, in the case of a modelled loop region, flexibility need be assigned to only the main- and side-chain torsion angles of the loop and to neighbouring parts of the structure. Obviously, the fewer degrees of freedom included in the calculation, the greater the volume of conformational space that can be searched for given computer resources.

7.2   Other approaches

The group lead by Scheraga at Cornell University has been very active in developing algorithms for polypeptide and protein conformational analysis. These algorithms have been used with reasonable success in prediction of the conformations of small biologically active polypeptides (up to 20 amino acids in length). In this section a brief review is made of some of these approaches along with an indication of their applicability to the somewhat larger problems of interest to those working in the field of molecular design.

In the self-consistent electrostatic field (SCEF) procedure (Piela & Scheraga 1987) it is assumed that each residue in the final conformation of a molecule should have optimal electrostatic energy. In practical terms, this condition is fulfilled by deforming the molecule from a trial conformation in such a way that the dipole moment of each residue is optimally aligned in the electrostatic field created by the whole molecule. After each local deformation, an optimization of the potential for the whole molecule is carried out, taking all interactions (not only those being electrostatic in nature) into consideration. This process can be repeated and an optimal conformation found iteratively. When applied to a model of the 19 residue N-acetyl,N'-methyl poly-(L-alanine) amide, a presumed global minimum α-helical conformation was readily located from a distant starting point.

The Metropolis Monte Carlo algorithm can generate a sequence of configurations for a system of particles according to a chosen ensemble by appropriate choice of transition probabilities. However, the search of conformational space for a large molecule using even a classical potential function can be extremely time consuming. Nevertheless, the limiting distribution would allow one to identify the global minimum energy conformation. Li & Scheraga (1987) developed a method to speed the search of conformational space by using a Monte Carlo-type approach augmented by energy minimizations. Firstly, the starting conformation is energy minimized. Then a random change (Δ) is made to a randomly chosen torsion angle in the range $0 < \Delta < 2\pi$, and the energy of this new conformation is also minimized. The Metropolis criterion is used to decide whether to accept or reject the new conformation, thus completing one iteration. This sampling strategy can be modified to sample torsion angles with different frequencies, depending on their type. With this method eighteen randomly generated distinct starting conformations for the polypeptide enkephalin converged to the same global minimum.

These two procedures can be combined and augmented by an *ad hoc* technique to model thermal fluctuation effects to give the so-called electrostatically driven Monte Carlo procedure (Ripoll & Scheraga 1988). Here, the SCEF technique gives a diagnosis based on the current orientations of the dipoles of the protein with respect to the local electric field. This diagnosis can then be used in conjunction with the random sampling technique to generate a further conformation which can be energy minimized and compared with the previous minimum. The Metropolis criterion is then used as before to decide its fate. If the new conformation is rejected it is not discarded but stored for use if the basic algorithm fails to generate any new conformation after a set limited number of perturbations. Then, one of the previously discarded conformations is used as a new starting point. In this way, a rather crude model of perturbation due to thermal effects is included. This method was tested by using again a terminally blocked 19-residue poly-(L-alanine) chain. The presumed global energy minimum conformation of a right-handed α-helix was achieved, starting from both the fully extended and α_L-form.

8. LIGAND BINDING

5.1 Solvation

There is a wealth of X-ray crystallographic and thermodynamic data on the relevance of hydration to the structure, dynamics and function of biomacromolecules (Edsall & McKenzie 1979, 1983). This has provided the impetus for computer modelling investigations of the hydration of proteins and nucleic acids. Such calculations represent a common application of potential energy functions in biomolecular mechanics. We shall not consider here the many applications of solvent-biomolecular PEFs using Monte Carlo (Goodfellow 1987) or molecular dynamics (van Gunsteren *et al.* 1983) simulations techniques, but we shall highlight only a handful of calculations using energy minimization representative of the many in this field. In addition, Warshel and co-workers have noted that the solvent configurational space in the vicinity of a polarizing solute is characterized by the presence of many minima of similar energies and they have constructed several models for the interaction of aqueous solvent with solutes (Warshel 1979, King & Warshel 1989). The interested are referred to the discussions of these models for relevant background material.

A simple algorithm has been developed to investigate the hydrogen bonding of aqueous solvent in the high-resolution 1.2 Å X-ray structure of hexagonal 2Zn-insulin (Hemmings *et al.* 1992b). This system represents a rather unusual case among protein X-ray structures in that more than 95% of the crystal solvent was refined as part of the final molecular model. The objective of the simulation was to generate a series of low-energy solvent configurations using rigid water and protein models and a standard intermolecular potential, that is, a combination of the protein potential of Weiner *et al.* (1986) and the water potential TIP3P (Jorgensen *et al.* 1983). This algorithm seeks to place water hydrogens by building up solvent shells about a solute molecule in much the way that one would assume hydration would occur naturally. This is expected to give best agreement for the solvent sites in the first solvation shell. The results were analysed in terms of closed cages of water molecules solvating the protein as was seen for the high-resolution structure of crambin (Teeter 1984).

Goodfellow and her co-workers have been very active in structural studies of the interactions of solvent molecules with proteins (Goodfellow *et al.* 1989) and DNA (Vovelle & Goodfellow 1989). For example, using a Meiko computing surface they have been able to parallelize the energy minimization program, CARTE, which uses Powell's method (Goodfellow *et al.* 1990) to minimize the energy of interaction between a water molecule and a solute with respect to three eulerian angles defining the solvent orientation. By repeating the calculation for solvent sites distributed on a cubic grid about the solute they can map the response of the water as a function of position and can compare the results with analyses of the distributions of water molecules around high-resolution protein structures (Thanki *et al.* 1988).

8.2 Relative binding energies

Calculations of relative free energies by perturbation or thermodynamic integration methods based on molecular dynamics or Monte Carlo sampling are rapidly becoming the techniques of choice for this type of work (Wong & McCammon 1986, Bartlett & Marlowe 1987). However, careful analyses have shown that there still remains considerable scope for uncertainty in the application of the simulation techniques themselves and the protocols used to effect the mutation. Even with increased computational power these calculations are very costly, and one might reasonably ask in certain cases if more simple computational models may provide a more parsimonious route to an answer, if its only use is to provide an indication as to whether a more rigorous assault on that particular problem is necessary.

When presented with the question as to which of two chemically similar ligands would form the most energetically favourable complex with a receptor of known conformation, one might suppose that a technique such as energy minimization would be appropriate. Indeed, the method has found a certain degree of popularity (DeTar 1980, Wipff et al. 1983, Oatley et al. 1984, Hemmings 1987, Dauber-Osguthorpe et al. 1988). However, leaving aside questions as to the accuracy of the PEF to be used, it has also become evident that this simulation technique itself needs modification if grossly misleading results are not to be obtained. To illustrate this point let us look at an example of the application of straightforward energy minimization to a simple problem so as to demonstrate the limitations of the method. This can then be contrasted with a recent advance in methodology which introduces the flexibility necessary to model more complex cases.

Blaney et al. (1982) simulated the interaction of thyroid hormone analogues with the human plasma protein, thyroxine (T_4) binding prealbumin (TBPA), using molecular mechanics calculations. With starting geometries derived from the high-resolution X-ray structure of prealbumin and difference electron density maps of the prealbumin-thyroxine complex, they were able to qualitatively reproduce the experimentally observed relative free energies of association of the analogues to the binding protein. This particular simulation typifies the rather exacting criteria for successful application of simple energy minimization to the calculation of relative binding affinities. Firstly, TBPA has a very deep and well-defined binding cleft with only small conformational changes in receptor structure on association, and, secondly, there is very limited conformational flexibility in the thyroxine analogue ligands (only four major torsional degrees of freedom). Even so, despite the fact that in this case the criteria were satisfied, a simple model of differential solvation contributions to the free energy of binding based on the energetics of transfer from water to the gas phase of simple model compounds was necessary to produce the correct qualitative ordering of the relative binding affinities. Thus, in addition, the modelling of non-covalent association is made extremely difficult by the absence of an adequate method for dealing with solvent.

The questions as to the influence of energy minimization techniques themselves on the results of a relative binding energy analysis have been addressed. According to Haneef (1990), comparisons of binding energies can be carried out only for similar molecules when calculated in simple ('equivalent') minima. This idea was cleverly demonstrated by performing energy minimization calculations on the binding of trimethoprim to dihydrofolate reductase. In the case where *no* interactions between ligand and receptor were included the method delivered binding energies in the range ± 40 kcal mol^{-1}, even though in these models the ligand did not interact with the enzyme. The inescapable conclusion to be drawn is that variables like the total number of degrees of freedom have a marked effect on the course of numerical minimization algorithms. To alleviate this problem a modified energy minimization method was forwarded, its aim being to simultaneously minimize all molecules contributing to the binding energy difference in the same simulation, guaranteeing convergence in each case to equivalent energy minima. The method was successfully used to calculate the relative binding energies of two avian lysozymes to the monoclonal antibody D1.3.

REFERENCES

Abe, H., Braun, W., & Gō, N. (1984) Rapid calculation of first and second derivatives of conformational energy with respect to dihedral angles for proteins. *Comp. Chem.* **8**, 239–247.

Arad, D., Langridge, R., & Kollman, P.A. (1990) A simulation of the sulphur attack in the catalytic pathway of papain using molecular mechanics and semi-empirical quantum mechanics. *J. Am. Chem. Soc.*, **112**, 491–502.

Bartlett, P.A. & Marlow, C.K. (1987). Evaluation of intrinsic binding energy from a hydrogen bonding group in an enzyme inhibitor. *Science* **235**, 569–571.

Blaney, J.M., Weiner, S.J., Dearing, A., Kollman, P.A., Jorgensen, E.C., Oatley, S.J., Burridge, J.M., & Blake, C.C.F. (1982) Molecular mechanics simulations of protein-ligand interactions: binding of thyroid hormone analogues to prealbumin. *J. Am. Chem. Soc.* **104**, 6424–6434.

Blundell, T.L. & Johnson, L.N. (1976) *Protein crystallography*. Academic Press, London.

Blundell, T.L., Bedarkar, S., Rinderknecht, E., & Humbel, R.E. (1978) Insulin-like growth factor. A model for tertiary structure. *Proc. Natl. Acad. Sci. USA* **75**, 180–184.

Blundell, T.L., Carney, D., Gardner, S., Hayes, F., Howlin, B., Hubbard, T., Overington, J., Singh, D.A., Sibanda, B.L. & Sutcliffe, M. (1988) Knowledge-based protein modelling and design. *Eur. J. Biochem.*, **172**, 513–520.

Boyd, D.B. & Lipkowitz, K.B. (1982) Molecular mechanics. The method and its underlying philosophy. *J. Chem. Ed.* **59**, 269–274.

Browne, W.J., North, A.C.T., Phillips, D.C., Brew, K., Vanaman, T.C. & Hill, R.L. (1969) A possible three-dimensional structure of bovine α-lactalbulin based on that of hen's egg-white lysozyme. *J. Mol. Biol.* **42**, 65–86.

Bruccoleri, R.E. & Karplus, M. (1986) Spatially-constrained minimisation of macro-molecules. *J. Comp. Chem.* **7**, 165–175.

Bruccoleri, R.E. & Karplus, M. (1987) Prediction of the folding of short polypeptide segments by uniform conformational sampling. *Biopolymers*, **26**, 137–168.

Bruccoleri, R.E., Haber, E., & Novotny, J. (1988) Structure of antibody hypervariable loops reproduced by a conformational search algorithm. *Nature*, **335**, 564–568.

Brünger, A.T., Kuriyan, J., & Karplus, M. (1987) Crystallographic R-factor refinement by molecular dynamics. *Science* **235**, 458–460.

Bukert, U. & Allinger, N.L. (1982) *Molecular mechanics*. A.C.S. *Monograph* 177, American Chemical Society, Washington D.C.

Bunday, B.D. (1985) *Basic optimisation methods*. Edward Arnold, London.

Cauchy, A.L. (1847) Methode generale pour la resolution des systemes d'equations simultanees. *C.R. Acad. Sci., Paris*, **25**, 536–538.

Cerjan, C.J. & Miller, W.H. (1981) On finding transition states. *J. Chem. Phys.* **75**, 2800–2806.

Chothia, C., Lesk, A.M., Levitt, M., Amit, A.G., Mariuzza, R.A., Phillips, S.E.V., & Poljak, R.J. (1986). The predicted structure of immunoglobulin D1.3 and its comparison with the crystal structure. *Science* **233**, 755–758.

Chou, K.-C., Némethy, G., Rumsey, S., Tuttle, R.W., & Scheraga, H.A. (1985) Interactions between an α-helix and a β-sheet. *J. Mol. Biol.* **186**, 591–609.

Crippen, G.M. & Scheraga, H.A. (1971) Minimisation of polypeptide energy. XI. The method of gentlest ascent. *Arch. Biochem. Biophys.* **144**, 462–466.

Dauber-Osguthorpe, P., Roberts, V.A., Osguthorpe, D.J., Wolff, J., Genest, M. and Hagler, A.T. (1988) Structure and energetics of ligand binding to proteins: *Escherichia coli* dihydrofolate reductase-trimethoprim, a drug-receptor system. *Proteins* **4**, 31–47.

DeTar, D.F. (1980) Computation of peptide-protein interactions: Catalysis by chymotrypsin. *J. Am. Chem. Soc.* **103**, 107, –110.

Doolittle, R.F. (1986) *Of URFs and ORFs. A primer on how to analyze derived amino acid sequences.* Univ. Science Books, Mill Valley, California.

Edsall, J.T. & McKenzie, H.A. (1979) Water and proteins I. *Adv. Biophys.*, **10**, 137–207.

Edsall, J.T. & McKenzie, H.A. (1983) Water and proteins II. *Adv. Biophys.* **16**, 53–183.

Ferro, D.R. (1979) In: *Report on CECAM workshop: Simulation of enzyme catalysis.* CECAM, Orsay, France. 141–188.

Ferro, D.R., McQueen, J.E. Jr., McCown, J.T., & Hermans, J. (1980) Energy minimisations of rubredoxin. *J. Mol. Biol.* **136**, 1–18.

Fine, R.M., Wang, H., Shenkin, P.S., Yarmush, D.L. & Levinthal, C. (1986) Predicting antibody hypervariable loop conformations. *Proteins*, **1**, 342–362.

Fletcher, R. (1970) A new approach to variable metric algorithms. *Computer J.* **13**, 317–322.

Fletcher, R. & Reeves, C.M. (1964). Function minimisation by conjugate gradients. *Comp. J.* **7**, 149–154.

Gelin, B.R. & Karplus, M. (1975) Sidechain torsional potentials and motion of amino acids in proteins: Bovine pancreatic trypsin inhibitor. *Proc. Natl. Acad. Sci. USA*, **72**, 2002–2006.

Gelin, B.R. & Karplus, M. (1979) Side-chain torsional potentials. *Biochemistry* **18**, 1256–1268.

Glasser, L. & Scheraga, H.A. (1988) Calculations on crystal packing of a flexible molecule, Leu-enkephalin. *J. Mol. Biol.* **199**, 513–524.

Goodfellow, J.M. (1987) Computer simulation of hydration networks around amino acids. *Int. J. Biol. Macromol.* **9**, 273–280.

Goodfellow, J.M., Saqi, M., Thanki, N., Baum, J.O., & Finney, J.L. (1989) Monte Carlo calculations on proteins: hydration and electron transfer processes. In: *Theoretical chemistry and molecular biophysics: a comprehensive survey.* Adenine Press, New York.

Goodfellow, J.M., Jones, D.M., Laskowski, R.A., Moss, D.S., Saqi, M., Thanki, N., & Westlake, R. (1990) Use of parallel processing in the study of protein-ligand binding. *J. Comp. Chem.* **11**, 314–325.

Greer, J. (1980) A model for haptoglobin heavy chain based on structural homology. *Proc. Natl. Acad. Sci. USA* **77**, 3393–3397.

Greer, J. (1981) Comparative model building of the serine proteinases. *J. Mol. Biol.* **153**, 1027–1042.

Hall, D. & Pavitt, N. (1984) An appraisal of molecular force fields for the representation of polypeptides. *J. Comp. Chem.* **5**, 441–450.

Haneef, I., Moss, D.S., Stanford, M.J., & Borkakoti, N. (1985) RESTRAIN: restrained structure-factor least-squares refinement program for macromolecular structures. *Acta Crystalogr.* **A41**, 426–433.

Haneef, M.I.J. (1990) Calculations of ligand binding energies using a robust energy minimisation technique. *J. Mol. Graphics* **8**, 45–51.

Hemmings, A.M. (1987) Towards the rational design of inhibitors of human renin. PhD thesis, University of London.

Hemmings, A.M., Foundling, S.I., Sibanda, B.L., Wood, S.P., Pearl, L.H., & Blundell, T.L. (1985). Energy calculations on aspartic proteinases. *Biochem. Soc. Trans.* **13**, 1036–1041.

Hemmings, A.M., Chang, W.-R., & Liang, D.-C. (1992a) Theoretical approaches to protein structure-function analysis. *Science in China Ser. B.* **35**, 304–318.

Hemmings, A.M., Chang, W.-R., & Liang, D.-C. (1992b) An atomic model for aqueous solvent in the 1.2Å resolution structure of 2Zn insulin. (in preparation).

Hooke, R. & Jeeves, T.A. (1961). Direct search solution of numerical and statitical problems. *J. Assn. Comp. Mach.* **8**, 212–229.

Hudson, B.S. (1974) Intermolecular Forces, Molecular Structure and Molecular Vibrations. In: Chen, S.-H. & Yip, S. eds. *Spectroscopy in biology and chemistry.* Academic Press, New York.

Inana, G., Piatigorsky, J., Norman, B., Slingsby, C. & Blundell, T.L. (1983) Gene and protein structure of a β-crystallin polypeptide in murine lens. *Nature*, **302**, 310–315.

Jorgensen, W.L., Chandrasekhar, J., Madura, J.D., Impey, R.W., & Klein, M.L. (1983) Comparison of simple potential functions for simulating liquid water. *J. Chem. Phys.* **79**, 926–935.

King, G. & Warshel, A. (1989) A surface constrained all-atom solvent model for effective simulations of polar solutions. *J. Chem. Phys.*, **91**, 3647–3661.

Kirkpatrick, S., Gelatt, C.D. Jr., & Vecchi, M.P. (1983). Optimisation by simulated annealing. *Science* **220**, 671–680.

Lapatto, R., Blundell, T.L., Hemmings, A.M., Overington, J., Wilderspin, A., Wood, S., Merson, J.R., Whittle, P.J., Danley, D., Geoghegan, K.F., Hawyrlik, S., Lee, S., Scheld, K., & Hobart, P.M. (1989) X-ray analysis of of HIV-1 proteinase at 2.7Å resolution confirms structural homology among retroviral proteinases. *Nature*, **342**, 299–302.

Levitt, M. (1974) Energy refinement of hen egg-white lysozyme. *J. Mol. Biol.* **82**, 393–420.

Levitt, M. (1983) Protein folding by restrained energy minimisation and molecular dynamics. *J. Mol. Biol.*, **170**, 723–764.

Levitt, M. & Lifson, S. (1969) Refinement of protein conformations using a macromolecular energy minimisation procedure. *J. Mol. Biol.* **46**, 269–279.

Li, Z. & Scheraga, H.A. (1987) Monte Carlo minimisation approach to the multiple minima problem in protein folding. *Proc. Natl. Acad. Sci. USA* **84**, 6611–6615.

McLachlan, A.D. & Shotton, D.M. (1971) Structural similarities between α-lytic proteinase of *Myxobaxter* 495 and elastase. *Nature New Biol.* **229**, 202–205.

Momany, F.A., McGuire, R.F., Burgess, A.W. & Scheraga, H.A. (1975) Energy parameters in polypeptides VII. *J. Phys. Chem.* **79**, 2361–2380.

Moss, D.S. (1980) In: *Refinement of protein structures*. Machin, P.A. & Campbell, J.W., eds. Daresbury Laboratory, Warrington, UK. pp 9–12.

Moult, J. & James, M.N.G. (1986) An algorithm for determining the conformation of polypeptide segments in proteins by systematic search. *Proteins* **1**, 146–163.

Najmudin, S. (1990). X-ray Crystallographic Analysis of the eye lens and related proteins. PhD thesis. Univ. of London. (In preparation).

Nelder, J.A. & Mead, R. (1965) A simplex method for function minimisation. *Comp. J.*, **7**, 308–313.

Nguyen, D.T. & Case, D.A. (1985) On finding stationary states on large-molecule potential energy surfaces. *J. Phys. Chem.* **89**, 4020–4026.

Noguti, T. & Gō, N. (1983) A method of rapid calculation of a second derivative matrix of conformational energy for large molecules. *J. Phys. Soc. Japan*, **52**, 3685–3690.

Novotny, J., Bruccoleri, R., & Karplus, M. (1984). An analysis of incorrectly folded protein models. Implications for structure predictions. *J. Mol. Biol.* **177**, 787–818.

Novotny, J., Rashin, A.A., & Bruccoleri, R.E. (1988) Criteria that discriminate between native proteins and incorrectly folded models. *Proteins*, **4**, 19–30.

Oatley, S.J., Blaney, J.M., Langridge, R., & Kollman, P.A. (1984) Molecular mechanical studies of hormone-protein interactions. *Biopolymers* **23**, 2931–2941.

Ooi, T., Nishikawa, K., Oobatake, M., & Scheraga, H.A. (1978) Flexibility of bovine pancreatic trypsin inhibitor. *Biochim. Biophys. Acta* **536**, 390–405.

Piela, L. & Scheraga, H.A. (1987) On the multiple-minima problem in the conformational analysis of polypeptides. I. Backbone degrees of freedom for a perturbed α-helix. *Biopolymers* **26**, S33–S58.

Powell, M.D.J. (1977) Restart procedures for the conjugate gradient method. *Math. Prog.* **12**, 241–254.

Read, R.J., Brayer, G.D., Jurasek, L., & James, M.N.G. (1984) Critical evaluation of comparative model building of *Streptomyces griseus* trypsin. *Biochemistry*, **23**, 6570–6575.

Richards, F.M. (1974) The interpretation of protein structures. Total volume, group volume distributions and packing density. *J. Mol. Biol.*, **82**, 1–14.

Ripka, W.C. (1986) Computer-assisted model building. *Nature*, **321**, 93–94.

Ripoll, D.R. & Scheraga, H.A. (1988) On the multiple-minima problem in the conformational analysis of polypeptides. *Biopolymers* **27**, 1283–1303.

Rossky, P.J., Karplus, M., & Rahman, A. (1979) A model for the simulation of an aqueous dipeptide solution. *Biopolymers* **18**, 825–854.

Rullmann, J.A.C., Bellido, M.N., & van Duijnen, P.Th. (1989) The active site of papain. An all-atom study of interactions with protein matrix and solvent. *J. Mol. Biol.* **206**, 101–118.

Saunders, M. (1987) Stochastic exploration of molecular mechanics energy surfaces.

Hunting for the global minimum. *J. Am. Chem. Soc.* **109**, 3150–3152.

Scales, L.E. (1985) *Introduction to non-linear optimization*. Macmillan, London.

Scarsdale, J.N., van Alsenoy, C., Klimkowski, V.J., Schäfer, L., & Momany, F.A. (1983) *Ab initio* studies of molecular geometries. 27. Optimised molecular structures of N^{α}-acetyl-N-methylalaninamide. *J. Am. Chem. Soc.* **105**, 3438–3445.

Shih, H.H.-L., Brady, J., & Karplus, M. (1985) Structure of proteins with single-site mutations: A minimum perturbation approach. *Proc. Natl. Acad. Sci. USA* **82**, 1697–1700.

Sibanda, B.L., Blundell, T.L., Hobart, P.M., Fogliano, M., Bindra, J.S., Dominy, B.W., & Chirgwin, J.M. (1984) Computer graphics modelling of human renin. Specificity, catalytic activity and intron-exon junctions. *FEBS Lett.*, **174**, 102–111.

Sibanda, B.L. (1986) Structural studies of mammalian aspartic proteinases, renin and chymosin. PhD thesis, Univ. of London.

Simons, J., Jorgensen, P., Taylor, H., & Ozment, J. (1983) Walking on potential energy surfaces. *J. Chem. Phys.* **87**, 2745–2753.

Singh, U.C., Weiner, S.J. & Kollman, P.A. (1985) Molecular dynamics simulations of d(C-G-C-G-A).d(T.C.G.C.G) with and without 'hydrated' counterions. *Proc. Natl. Acad. Sci. USA*, **82**, 755–759.

Singh, U.C., Weiner, P.K., Caldwell, J.W., & Kollman, P.A. (1986) *AMBER(UCSF) Version* 3.0. Dept. Pharmac. Chem., Univ. California, San Francisco.

Snow, M.E. & Amzel, L.M. (1986) Calculating three-dimensional changes in protein structure due to amino-acid substitutions. *Proteins*, **1**, 267–279.

Stone, A.J. & Alderton, M. (1985) Distributed multipole analysis. Methods and applications. *Mol. Phys.* **56**, 1047–1064.

Teeter, M.M. (1984) Water structure of a hydrophobic protein at atomic resolution: pentagon rings of water molecules in crystals of crambin. *Proc. Natl. Acad. Sci. USA* **81**, 6014–6018.

Thanki, N., Thornton, J.M., & Goodfellow, J.M. (1988) Distributions of water around amino acid residues in proteins. *J. Mol. Biol.*, **202**, 637–657.

Tonelli, A.E. & Brewster, A.I. (1972) The conformational characteristics in solution of the cyclic hexapeptide cyclo-(GlyGlyD-AlaD-AlaGlyGly). *J. Am. Chem. Soc.* **94**, 2851–2854.

van Gunsteren, W.F., Berendsen, H.J.C., Hermans, J., Hol, W.G.J., & Postma, J.P.M. (1983) Computer simulation of the dynamics of hydrated protein crystals and its comparison with X-ray data. *Proc. Natl. Acad. Sci. USA* **80**, 4315–4319.

Vovelle, F. & Goodfellow, J.M. (1989) Modelling of DNA interactions. In: Beveridge, D.L. & Lavery, R. (eds.) *Theoretical chemistry and molecular biophysics: a comprehensive survey*. Adenine Press, New York.

Wako, H. & Gō, N. (1987) Algorithm for rapid calculation of hessian of conformational energy function of proteins by supercomputer. *J. Comp. Chem.* **8**, 625–635.

Warme, P.K., Momany, F.A., Rumball, S.V., Tuttle, R.W. & Scheraga, H.A. (1974) Computation of structures of homologous proteins. α-lactalbumin from lysozyme. *Biochemistry* **13**, 768–782.

Warshel, A. (1979) Calculation of chemical processes in solution. *J. Phys. Chem.* **83**, 1640–1652.

Weiner, S.J., Kollman, P.A., Nguyen, D.T., & Case, D.A. (1986) An all-atom force field for simulation of proteins and nucleic acids. *J. Comp. Chem.*, 7, 230–252.

White, D.N.J., Ruddock, J.N., & Edgington, P.R. (1989). Molecular mechanics. In: Richards, W.G. ed. *Computer-aided molecular design*. IBC Technical Services Ltd.

Whitlow, M. & Teeter, M.M. (1986) An empirical examination of potential energy minimisation using the well-determined structure of the protein crambin. *J. Am. Chem. Soc.* 108, 7163–7172.

Wipff, G., Dearing, A., Weiner, P.K., Blaney, J.M., & Kollman, P.A. (1983) Molecular mechanics studies of enzyme-substrate interactions: the interactions of L- and D-N-acetyltryptophanamide with α-chymotrypsin. *J. Am. Chem. Soc.* 105, 997–1010.

Wong, C.F. & McCammon, J.A. (1986) Dynamics and design of enzymes and inhibitors. *J. Am. Chem. Soc.*, 108, 3830–3832.

Yoshioki, S., Abe, H., Noguti, T., Gō, N., & Nagayama, K. (1983) Conformational change of a globular protein elucidated at atomic resolution. *J. Mol. Biol.* 170, 1031–1036.

7

Computer simulation: techniques and applications

Julia M. Goodfellow and David S. Moss
Department of Crystallography, Birkbeck College, Malet Street,
London WC1E 7HX

1. INTRODUCTION

Computer simulation techniques such as molecular dynamics are now used not only to model the dynamics of macromolecules but also to refine protein or nucleotide structures by using experimental data from X-ray diffraction or NMR spectroscopy and to estimate changes in free energy due to drug binding or conformational changes (Goodfellow 1990a,b). Although the main technique is that of molecular dynamics in which Newton's laws of motion are solved for each atom in the system, the stochastic Monte Carlo technique can also be used in some applications. The main advantages of these simulation methods is that they can provide molecular models where there are limited experimental data such that a complete structural solution is not possible, and that they can be used to correlate structural and energetic changes for a given molecular process.

Computer simulation techniques offer the advantage over energy minimization techniques (see Chapter 6) in that temperature is implicitly included in the calculation either as kinetic energy in the case of molecular dynamics or in the Boltzmann factor in Monte Carlo simulations. Thus, in principle, simulations can be carried out at a realistic temperature for the system under study. The disadvantage is that they require far more computer cpu time than minimization methods. Simulations of macromolecules, especially if surrounded by solvent molecules, may take many tens of hours of cpu time on a supercomputer. Many applications to proteins, nucleotides, and carbohydrates are described below and in Goodfellow (1990c).

2.   METHODS

In this section, we will briefly describe the molecular dynamics and Monte Carlo methods as well as the calculation of free energy differences using perturbation techniques. Further details of these and other simulation methods can be found in the excellent books by Allen & Tildesley (1987) and McCammon & Harvey (1987).

2.1   Molecular dynamics

The basis of the molecular dynamics method is the equation relating the force, F_i, acting on a particle of mass, m_i, and acceleration a_i. When we are simulating molecules, it is usual to consider each atom (or sometimes groups of atoms such as CH_3 groups) as a particle. Thus,

$$F_i = m_i a_i.$$

If we assume that the interaction energy between atoms can be described by using the potential energy functions discussed in Chapter 5, then the force can be calculated as the negative of the gradient of these energy functions. Thus,

$$F_i = -\partial V/\partial r_i$$

where r_i is the vector representing atomic cartesian coordinates (x,y,z) and V is the potential energy. During the simulation, we aim to evaluate the atomic coordinates and velocity for each atom at regular discrete time steps, δt. To do this, we not only need to know the force acting on each particle, as described above, but also to use an approximation to evaluate the acceleration. Using the above equations, we can rewrite the acceleration as

$$a_i = (-\partial V/\partial r_i)/m_i.$$

The acceleration, a_i, is a vector quantity, but each component ax_i, ay_i, and az_i can be written as, for example,

$$ax_i = F_x/m_i$$

where F_x is one component of the force.

Each component of the atomic coordinate at time $t + \delta t$ can be written as a Taylor series expansion involving a previous value of the coordinate at time δt. Thus,

$$x_i(t + \delta t) = x_i(t) + vx_i(t)\delta t + ax_i(t)\delta t^2/2 + \dots$$

and

$$x_i(t - \delta t) = x_i(t) - vx_i(t)\delta t + ax_i(t)\delta t^2/2 + \dots$$

where $vx_i(t)$ and $ax_i(t)$ are the components of velocity and acceleration. The approximation comes in the assumption that this series can be terminated after the third term. These equations (and there is one for each end of the three positional coordinates of each atom) can be solved approximately at each time step (δt) and repeated iteratively for the required number of timesteps. Thus,

$$x_i(t + \delta t) = 2x_i(t) - x_i(t - \delta t) + f_i(t)/m_i$$

and

$$v_i(t) = (x_i(t + \delta t) - x_i(t - \delta t))/2\delta t$$

This solution to the equations is known as the Verlet algorithm (Verlet 1967). Other commonly used algorithms are due to Beeman (1976) and Gear (1971). Frequently for macromolecules a constrained Verlet algorithm, known as SHAKE, is used (van Gunsteren & Berendsen 1977) in which the highest frequency motions (such as those due to bond length vibrations) are constrained. Thus, a larger integration step, δt, can be used and a longer length simulation is achieved for the same number of iterations.

2.2   Monte Carlo method

The Monte Carlo method depends on generating a Boltzmann weighted distribution of states for a given temperature, T. The advantage of this method is that no derivatives are required. One of the most frequently used methods is due to Metropolis (Metropolis *et al.* 1953) in which sampling is considered as part of a Markov chain of configurations. In this method, an initial molecular ensemble is generated and its potential energy, V_0, calculated, using the potential energy functions described in Chapter 5. One particle in the system is chosen at random and is moved a random amount translationally and rotationally and the potential energy recalculated, V_1. The difference in energy between the two states can be calculated as $V_1 - V_0$. If this difference is negative, that is, the new state is energetically more favourable, the move is accepted and the cycle of random moves repeated. If the difference in energy is unfavourable, then the probability of this occurring is calculated as $\exp(-V_0 - V_1)/k_B T$ (where k_B is Boltmann constant and T is the temperature) and compared with a random number between 0 and 1. If the probability is less than the random number the move is again accepted. On the other hand, if the probability is greater than the random number then the move is rejected and the system returns to the initial state. This procedure is repeated many times so that a large number of energetically accessible configurations of the system are generated.

2.3   Free energy perturbation method

A major advance in the use of simulation techniques came from the studies of Tembe & McCammon (1984) in which they developed techniques for estimating free energy differences between related states. The Gibbs free energy, ΔG, is often described as

$$\Delta G = \Delta H - T\Delta S$$

where ΔH is the change in enthalpy and $T\Delta S$ the entropic component.

The free energy difference can be estimated from computer simulations using the following equation which is derived from statistical mechanics:

$$\Delta G = -k_B T \ln \langle \exp -(V_1 - V_0)/k_B t \rangle_0$$

where V_1 and V_0 are the potential energy of two closely related states and the brackets $\langle \rangle$ imply averaging over the initial state. One of the major assumptions in the method is that two states 1 and 0 must be very similar. To tackle problems of interest in which the required changes are likely to be much larger, several changes in free energy are calculated by using a coupling parameter λ. This parameter is used to define the initial state when $\lambda = 0$ and the final state when $\lambda = 1$. The intermediate states are non-physical states used to define windows within which the calculation of ΔG is possible. To estimate the total change in free energy it is necessary to add up the contributions from each window. There is an alternative method, known as slow growth, in which λ changes continuously by very small amounts throughout the simulation. The use of non-physical intermediate states is only possible because the free energy is known to be a path independent quantity. Further details are given in reviews by Beveridge & Dicapua (1989), van Gunsteren (1990), and Williams *et al.* (1990).

3. PRACTICAL CONSIDERATIONS

To use a simulation program in practice, it is necessary to define carefully the system of interest. A fundamental question is whether the simulation should be carried out at constant pressure, p, (which is more relevant to experimental conditions) or at constant volume, V, (which is easier to calculate). It is also necessary to define the temperature, T, of the simulation and the number of atoms, N. Thus, one sees references to NVT or NPT simulations depending on whether the volume or pressure is kept constant.

The molecule itself can be defined by using an all-atom representation, or for large biological molecules it is usual to reduce the number of atom centres by uniting all apolar hydrogen atoms to the nearest carbon atom (the united atom representation). This can save a considerable amount of computer time because of the large number of apolar hydrogen atoms within a protein. As well as the atomic coordinates for all atoms or atomic centres, you may have to define the sequence of amino acids within the protein or bases with the oligonucleotide. The program may then automatically define the molecular topology. For non-standard residues, it will be necessary to define the topology.

A further important consideration is whether the simulation will be performed *in vacuo* or with explicit solvent molecules. For simulations of oligonucleotides, counter-ions can be added to balance the negative charge of the phosphate groups. If the simulation is to include solvent molecules, it is necessary to place the molecule in a 'water bath' and remove overlapping solvent molecules as well as to define the type of water model to be used.

To reduce surface effects, it is usual to apply periodic boundary conditions so that the volume of interest is effectively surrounded by similar cells in all three directions. If an atom is on the edge of the central cell, it will feel the presence of atoms which are close to it but in the next cell. Atoms which move out of the central cell during the simulation can be replaced back in the cell to keep the number of particles constant.

Finally, one needs to assign potential energy parameters to every atom in the molecule. These parameters (described in Chapter 5) will include terms for bond length distortion, bond angle distortion, torsion angle distortion, electrostatic, repulsion, and dispersion terms. Software packages, such as AMBER (Singh *et al.* 1986), provide a number of programs which perform these operations (for example LINK, EDIT, PARM, PREP within AMBER) and generate all the files necessary to begin the minimization and dynamics procedures.

4. PROTEIN DYNAMICS

Many of the initial simulations on macromolecules were carried out on a small protein Bovine Pancreatic Trypsin Inhibitor (BPTI) by McCammon *et al.* (1977) and Levitt (1983). These calculations were performed *in vacuo* (that is, with no explicit solvent molecules surrounding the protein) although solvent effects were approximated to some extent by the use of either a distant dependent dielectric constant or a dielectric constant greater than unity.

The general picture of protein dynamics to emerge from these studies was that atoms close to the surface were moving considerably faster than those in the interior, atoms in secondary structure elements such as alpha helices and beta sheets to move less than those in loop regions, and main-chain backbone atoms to move less than those in the side chains (McCammon & Harvey 1987). Levitt (1983) also found that hydrogen bonds are variable in that they broke and sometimes reformed during his 132 psec simulation of BPTI. He summarized this simulation by describing a model for protein dynamics in which 'the molecule vibrates about a particular conformation but then suddenly changes conformation, jumping over an energy barrier into a new region of conformational space'.

Subsequent studies on BPTI and another peptide Avian Pancreatic Polypeptide, aPP, included solvent either in the crystal or in solution (van Gunsteren & Berendsen, 1984, Kruger *et al.* 1985). Although atomic displacements were very similar when solvent were explicitly included in the calculation, the frequency of the motion of some atoms was lowered. There are still only relatively few dynamics simulations involving a protein with its surrounding solvent (Levitt & Sharon 1988, Ahlstrom *et al.* 1988, Brooks & Karplus 1989, Wodak *et al.* 1989).

We are carrying out a molecule dynamics simulation on an enzyme, ribonuclease A, in solution, using the GROMOS software package (van Gunsteren & Berendsen 1987). Although this is a small enzyme of 13 500 Daltons, the system consists of protein atoms (but hydrogen covalently bonded to carbon atoms are not treated explicitly) and over 3000 surrounding solvent molecules. Even though this system has been energy minimized before the dynamics was started, the system still needs time to equilibrate as can be seen by the plot of energy against length of the simulation in ps (Fig. 1). Another criterion for checking the equilibration of the system is the change in root mean square displacement (rmsd) as the simulation proceeds. This is shown in Fig. 2. Our initial analysis of this simulation used only the configurations generated between 20 and 40 ps.

The plot of rmsd shows that the conformation of the enzyme in solution has slightly changed from that in the crystal, which is not surprising. We can also look

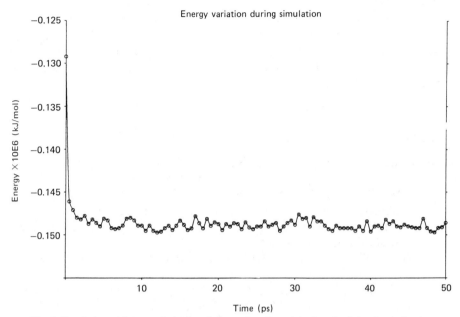

Fig. 1. Total potential energy in kcal mol^{-1} as a function of the length of the simulation in ps for ribonuclease A in solution.

at the motions of atoms by measuring the fluctuations in atomic positions during the simulation. These fluctuations can be directly compared with crystallographic temperature factors which are generated during the refinement of a protein structure. There are some differences in that experimental temperature factors can include both static and dynamic disorder. Both the experimental and simulated fluctuations for ribonuclease A are shown in Fig. 3.

5.   DYNAMICS OF SMALL PEPTIDES

Small biologically active peptides of a dozen or so amino acid residues are conformationally very flexible unless they have cyclic structures. Their active conformations will be of low energy, and it is an objective of rational drug design to be able to synthesize conformationally restricted peptides corresponding to these low-energy structures. Any method that can help to locate the low-energy conformations is invaluable. Here MD simulation techniques can play an important role by identifying possible conformations accessible to the peptide under study. This approach in the past has been under utilized as a tool owing to the cost of these calculations (Brooks 1987). The greater availability of more powerful computers is now making such calculations more feasible.

The first molecular dynamics calculations of peptides were short simulations *in vacuo* of vasopressin (Hagler *et al.* 1985) and gonadotropin-releasing hormone (GnRH) (Struthers *et al.* 1985). From these simulations it was evident that peptides

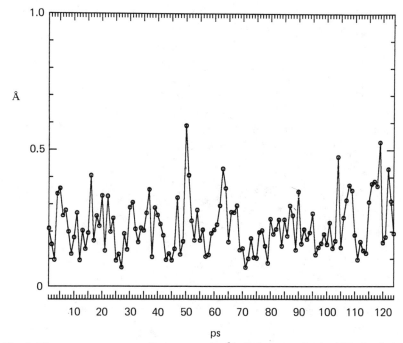

Å

Fig. 2. The root mean square displacement (in Å) of Cα atoms in the MD simulation compared with the crystal structure as a function of the length of the simulation in ps for ribonuclease A in solution.

demonstrate a rich variety of conformations. Since then, molecular mechanics calculations and simulation techniques have been used to investigate other peptides including sulfated CCK8 (Kreissler *et al.* 1989), neuropeptide Y (Mackerell 1988), deamino oxytocin and deamino arginine-vasopressin (Liwo *et al.* 1988), and enkephalin which is used as the most popular test example because of its size (Isogai *et al.* 1977, Purisima and Scheraga 1987, and Zhenqin & Scheraga 1987).

Molecular mechanics calculations suffer from being trapped in local minim, therefore exhaustive starting geometries are required to ensure a reasonable search of conformational space. Molecular dynamics simulations at room temperature are an improvement on molecular mechanics calculations as they can surmount energy barriers of the order of kT.

The inherent ability of molecular dynamics to cross potential energy barriers has been recently used to improve the searching of conformation space. The method is based on work with spin glasses (Sherrington & Kirkpatrick 1978) and has become popularly known as simulated annealing (SA) (Kirkpatrick *et al.* 1983, Bounds 1987, and Press *et al.* 1988). A form of this method has been applied to peptides. To enable the peptide under study to cross high energy barriers that may be blocking its route to the 'global' minima the simulation is carried out at higher temperatures. Minimizing at these temperatures would cause the molecule to be trapped in high-energy minima. To avoid this, the simulation temperature is lowered so that the molecule becomes

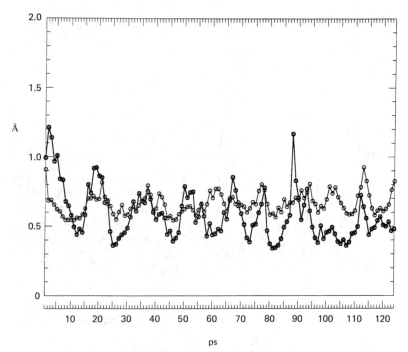

Fig. 3. The root mean square atomic fluctuations in Å for Cα atoms in ribonuclease A
from the MD simulation (heavier line) and calculated from the experimentally derived
crystallographic temperature factors (lighter line).

trapped in a much lower energy well. This method has been incorporated, using both
molecular dynamics (Burt *et al.* 1989, Brooks 1987) and Monte Carlo simulations
(Kawai *et al.* 1989, Wilson *et al.* 1988).

The existence of high-precision crystal structures of some small peptides derived
from X-ray crystallography provides an opportunity to test the accuracy of molecular
dynamics simulations. We have simulated multiple unit cells of deamino-oxytocin
and have compared the mean structure with that derived from X-ray analysis. There
are two symmetry-independent molecules (A and B) in the crystal structure, and the
rms deviations between the MD and X-ray structures are shown in Table 1. It can
be seen that the deviations between the MD and X-ray structures are of the same
order as the deviations between the two molecules. The mean-square displacements
of the atoms about their equilibrium positions may be illustrated in terms of
equiprobability ellipsoids, and these are shown in Fig. 4.

6. CARBOHYDRATE DYNAMICS

There has been a very detailed analysis of the conformation and dynamics of a series
of carbohydrate molecules known as cyclodextrins (Kohler *et al.* 1987a,b, 1988a,b).
These molecules consist of a number of glucose units which are covalently linked via
α-(1-4) glycosidic bonds into a cyclic molecule. The simulations are interesting in that

Table 1. The root mean square differences (Å) between X-ray crystal structures, energy minimized structures (EM) and various time-averaged MD crystal structures of deamino-oxytocin. The upper triangle refers to Cα atoms and the lower triangle refers to side-chain atoms. There are two symmetry independent molecules in the crystal denoted by A and B.

Molecule		X-ray A	X-ray B	E.M. A	E.M. B	6-24ps A	6-24ps B	24-50ps A	24-50ps B	6-50ps A	6-50ps B
X-ray	A	—	0.26	0.08	0.27	0.18	0.34	0.17	0.25	0.17	0.27
	B	0.60	—	0.29	0.06	0.33	0.36	0.29	0.22	0.30	0.27
E.M.	A	0.19	0.63	—	0.29	0.14	0.33	0.14	0.25	0.13	0.27
	B	0.62	0.15	0.66	—	0.33	0.35	0.29	0.22	0.30	0.26
6-20ps	A	0.58	0.78	0.56	0.78	—	0.25	0.10	0.21	0.07	0.21
	B	0.63	0.49	0.62	0.47	0.71	—	0.26	0.17	0.25	0.11
24-50ps	A	0.48	0.72	0.46	0.71	0.28	0.65	—	0.18	0.04	0.20
	B	0.71	0.60	0.72	0.58	0.64	0.49	0.55	—	0.19	0.06
6-50ps	A	0.51	0.73	0.48	0.73	0.18	0.66	0.11	0.57	—	0.20
	B	0.64	0.51	0.65	0.49	0.62	0.32	0.54	0.17	0.56	—

neutron diffraction data are available on some structures so that hydrogen (deuterium) positions can be seen experimentally. Good agreement is found between the results from the molecular dynamics simulations in crystal hydrates and the experimental data.

They have also looked at changes in the conformation and dynamics at low temperature (120 K) compared with the more usual room temperature structure. The cyclodextrin crystals contain a network of hydrogen bonds between the sugar hydroxyl groups and water molecules. The analysis of the simulated systems has included a study of the dynamics of so-called 'flip-flop' hydrogen bonds in which each hydrogen-bond hydrogen atom appears to have two possible locations between the heavy atoms which are alternatively occupied during the simulation. They have also made a detailed comparison of the conformation and dynamics of one molecule in solution compared with that in the crystal. These studies on cyclodextrins have been reviewed by Kohler (1990).

7. MACROMOLECULAR STRUCTURE DETERMINATION

Molecular dynamics algorithms are being used in a very specific way to refine protein and nucleotide structures, given experimental data from X-ray crystallography or NMR spectroscopy (Brunger 1988). In this technique, often called simulated annealing, molecular dynamics is used at elevated temperatures (possibly as high as 3000°C) to explore configuration space given an experimental constraint. In the case of X-ray crystallographic refinement, an X-ray force is calculated as a function of the difference between the experimental and model structure factors and added to the force

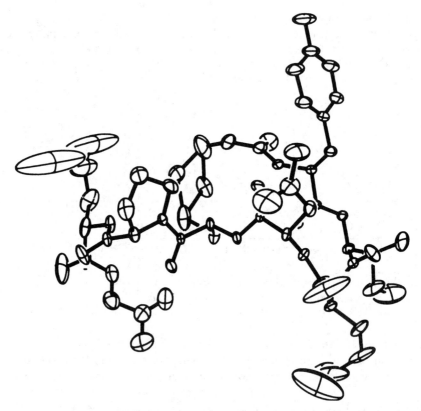

Fig. 4. Mean-square displacements of the atoms of deamino-oxytocin represented as equiprobability ellipsoids. The displacements were derived from a molecular dynamics simulation. Atoms on side groups show larger displacements than those held more firmly in the main chain of the molecule.

calculated by using typical potential energy terms. The simulated annealing protocol allows the molecule to move over energy barriers which would normally be inaccessible at room temperature and, one hopes, reach the conformation which is in best agreement with the experimental constraints.

An example of this use of simulation techniques has been in the refinement of a large protein, rabbit serum transferrin which binds iron. During the refinement of this structure, the XPLOR program of Brunger was used. The method has a larger radius of convergence than that of non-linear least square methods which are traditionally used to refine protein structures.

A related use of molecular dynamics has been in the elucidation of solution structures of small proteins and nucleotides, using two-dimensional NMR nuclear overhauser (NOE) spectroscopy (Clore *et al.* 1986). In this application, the experimental constraints are interproton distances. Simulated annealing protocols are again used, but the total force is now the sum of the traditional molecular dynamics force (that is, the derivative of the potential energy) and an experimental force which is related to the square of the interproton distances. Applications have included the structures of small proteins such as melittin (26 residues), epidermal growth factors (50 residues), insulin-like growth factor IGF-1 (70 residues), and oligonucleotides (Nilsson *et al.* 1986) in solution. Several papers which described the use of restrained molecular dynamics are included in the proceedings of a joint CCP4/CCP5 study weekend (for example Harvey 1989, Nilges *et al.* 1989).

8. NUCLEOTIDE DYNAMICS

As with proteins, the first full molecular dynamics simulations were of nucleotides *in vacuo* but with reduced charges on the phosphate groups (to model the effect of counter-ions) and dielectric constant greater than unity. The analysis of 90 ps calculations on a 12-base pair and 24-base pair DNA double helices (Levitt 1982) showed that the hydrogen bonds between the base pairs were stable and the motions of the torsion angles were small at around 10°. Cooperative bending and twisting motions of large amplitude were seen but with no major effect on the backbone torsion angles. The base-pairs were seen to kink into the minor groove.

A study of a smaller double helical fragment containing only five base-pairs included simulations with and without 'hydrated' counter-ions (Singh *et al.* 1985). Although the average structure from both simulations was very similar, the simulation with counter-ions gave better agreement with a related X-ray structure. Sugar repuckering from C2' endo to C3' endo was seen during the simulation. Seibel *et al.* (1985) continued this study but included both counter-ions and explicit water molecules. In this latter simulation, the overall shape of the double helix was preserved throughout the simulation. The most flexible torsion angles were the glycosidic angle and those related to the sugar pucker.

More recent simulations have attempted to estimate free energy changes associated with 5-methyl cytosine to the B to Z transition (Pearlman & Kollman 1990), with the association of 9-methyladenine and 1-methylthymine bases in water (Dang & Kollman 1990) and with base specificity of drug-DNA interactions (Cieplak *et al.* 1990).

The interactions of drug molecules with DNA are of obvious importance as they are used in the treatment of disease. Unfortunately the experimental structural and dynamics data on some DNA–drug interactions is limited, and so simulating drug/oligonucleotide complexes using molecular dynamics techniques may increase our knowledge of such interactions and provide useful models (Herzyk *et al.* 1991, 1992).

9. FREE ENERGY CHANGES

One of the main applications of free energy perturbation (FEP) techniques has been in the study of drug binding. The method hinges on the fact that it is often important to know not the absolutely free energy of binding of one drug molecule but the relative free energy of binding of two related drug molecules. Tembe & McCammon (1984) pioneered the use of this method which can be illustrated by use of a thermodynamic cycle:

$$
\begin{array}{ccc}
\text{E} + \text{S} \xrightarrow{\quad \Delta G_1 \quad} & & \text{ES} \\
\Big\downarrow \Delta G_3 & & \Big\downarrow \Delta G_4 \\
\text{E} + \text{S'} \quad \Delta G_2 \xrightarrow{\qquad} & & \text{ES'}
\end{array}
$$

where E, S and ES are an enzyme, substrate, and enzyme/substrate complex and S' refers to a modified substrate.

Experimentally, one would measure ΔG_1 (the binding of the first substrate, S, to the enzyme) and ΔG_2 (the binding of the modified substrate to the same enzyme). The difference in binding free energy, $\Delta\Delta B$, is then given by

$$\Delta\Delta B = \Delta G_2 - \Delta G_2.$$

Computationally, however, it is much easier to calculate ΔG_3 and ΔG_4 as these need only two simulations in which in one the substrate is slowly modified from the initial S molecule to S' in solution and secondly the same modification is carried out, but in the complex. Because free energy is a path-independent function, $\Delta\Delta B$ can also be calculated as

$$\Delta\Delta B = \Delta G_4 - \Delta G_3.$$

Wong & McCammon (1986) used this technique to study the binding of benzamidine and benzamidine inhibitors to native and mutant trypsin. The calculated a $\Delta\Delta B$ to be 3.8 kJ mol^{-1} in comparison with an experimental value of 2. kJ mol^{-1}. Subsequent studies have been carried out on a number of systems including inhibitors of thermolysin (Bash *et al.* 1987) and drugs binding to the common cold virus (Pettitt 1989).

This FEP technique has a wide range of applications including the effect of modifying enzymes on the rate of catalysis (Rao *et al.* 1987), the calculation of redox potentials of potential bioreductive agents (Reynolds *et al.* 1988), and the stability of conformational changes in proteins and nucleotides. An example of these latter effects has been the study of the free energy change due to mutating one amino acid to another within a polypeptide chain, that is investigating the effects of protein engineering (Saqi & Goodfellow 1990).

10. PATH INTEGRAL METHODS

Quantum mechanical particles such as electrons cannot be simulated by using classical dynamics techniques. Instead, a technique known as path integral Monte Carlo (PIMC) has been developed. This is based on a formulation of quantum mechanics by Feynman & Hibbs (1965). In this technique, a single quantum particle (for example an electron) is represented by a ring polymer of n particles or beads which are connected to their two neighbours by harmonic springs. It is then necessary to devise a pseudo-potential to represent the interactions between the polymer bead (that is, the quantum particle) and its environment. Monte Carlo methods may then be used to establish the probability of the quantum particle occupying particular locations in the simulated system.

Such effects may not seem immediately relevant to molecular biology, but they are necessary if we are to model electron transfer reactions which occur in photosynthetic and respiratory processes in living organisms. To study these systems of biological interest, there are many technical problems associated with this technique such as the need to model polarizability of atoms because the presence of the electron leads to large inductive effects and to include π-electrons which may be involved in electron transport processes. However, initial calculations have been carried out on ferrocytochrome C (Zheng *et al.* 1988).

11. SUMMARY

There are now several related techniques which can be used to simulate or model the conformation and dynamics of macromolecules and their interactions with small ligands. These techniques are being used by many groups to study both proteins and oligonucleotides. Recent developments include the broadening of simulation techniques to calculate the thermodynamically important free energy difference rather than the traditional potential energy. This is being used to study the relative binding of different drugs and the effect of conformational change. With the increasing power of computers, we expect to see many more applications of these simulation techniques in the area of molecular biology.

ACKNOWLEDGEMENTS

We would like to acknowledge the Science and Engineering Research Council for support from the CSI and MRI initiatives and to thank our collaborator Dr S. Yoskioki.

REFERENCES

Ahlstrom, P., Teleman, O. & Jonsson, B. (1988) Molecular dynamics simulation of interfacial water structure and dynamics in a parvalbumin solution. *J. Am. Chem. Soc.* **110**, 4198–4203.

Allan, M.P. & Tildesley, D.J. (1987) *Computer simulation of liquids*, Clarendon Press, Oxford.

Bash, P.A., Singh, U.C., Brown, F.K., Langridge, R. & Kollman, P.A. (1987) Calculation of relative change in binding free energy of a protein-inhibitor complex. *Science*, **235**, 574–575.

Beeman, D. (1976) Some multistep methods for use in molecular dynamics calculations. *J. Comp. Phys.* **20**, 130

Beveridge, D.L. & Dicapua, F.M. (1989) Free energy via molecular simulation: applications to chemical and biomolecular systems. *Ann. Rev. Biophys. Biophys Chem.*, **18**, 431–492.

Brooks, C.L. & Karplus, M. (1989) Solvent effects on protein motion and protein effects on solvent motion: dynamics of the active site region of lysozyme. *J. Mol. Biol.* **208**, 159–181.

Brunger, A.T. (1988) Crystallographic refinement by simulated annealing. *J. Mol. Biol.* **203**, 803–816.

Cieplak, P., Rao, S.N., Grootenhuis, P.D.J., & Kollman, P.A. (1990) Free energy calculation on base specificity of drug-dna interactions. *Biopolymers* **29**, 717–727.

Clore, G.M., Gronenborn, A.M., Brunger, A.T. & Karplus, M.J. (1986) Structure refinement of an oligonucleotide by molecular dynamics with NOE interproton distance restraints: Application to d(CGTACG)2, *J. Mol. Biol.* **188**, 455–?

Dang, L.X. & Kollman, P.A. (1990) Molecular dynamics simulations study of the free energy of association of 9-methyladenine and 1-methylthymine bases in water. *J. Am. Chem. Soc.* **112**, 503–507.

Feynman, R.P. & Hibbs, A.R. (1965) Quantum mechanics and path integrals, McGraw-Hill, New York.

Gear, C.W. (1971) *Numerical initial value problems in ordinary differential equations.* Prentice-Hall, New York.

Goodfellow, J.M. (1990a) Computer simulations of macromolecules. *Mol. simulation,* **5**, 277–291.

Goodfellow, J.M. (1990b) Computer simulation in molecular biology. *Chemistry in Britain* November 1066–1068.

Goodfellow, J.M. (1990c) *Molecular dynamics: applications in molecular biology,* Macmillan, London.

Goodfellow, J.M., Hendrick, K. & Hubbard, R. (1989) Molecular simulation and protein crystallography. *Proceedings of a joint CCP4/CCP5 study weekend, SERC Daresbury Lab,* DL SC1 R27.

Harvey, T.S. (1989) Molecular simulation and protein cyrstallography. *Proceedings of CCP4/5 study weekend, SERC, Daresbury lab* DL/SCI/R27.

Herzyk, P., Goodfellow, J.M. & Neidle, S. (1991a) Molecular dynamics simulations of dinucleoside and dinucleoside-drug crystal hydrations. *J. Biomol. Structure and Dynamic* **9**, 363–386.

Herzyk, P., Goodfellow, J.M. & Neidle, S. (1992) Conformation and dynamics of drug-DNA intercalation. *Ibid* **10**, 97–140.

Kohler, J.E.H. (1990) *Molecular dynamics simulations of carbohydrates in 'Molecular Dynamics'* (ed. J.M. Goodfellow), Macmillan, London, in press.

Kohler, J.E.H., Saenger, W. & van Gunsteren, W.F. (1987a) A molecular dynamics simulation of crystalline a-cyclodextrin hexahydrate. *Eur. Biophys. J.,* **15**, 197–210.

Kohler, J.E.H., Saenger, W. & van Gunsteren, W.F. (1987b) Molecular dynamics simulation of crystalline b-cyclodextrin dodecahydrate at 293 and 120 K. *Eur. Biophys. J.* **15**, 211–224.

Kohler, J.E.H., Saenger, W. & van Gunsteren, W.F. (1988a) Molecular dynamics simulation of crystalline b-cyclodextrin: the Flip-flop hydrogen bonding phenomenon. *Eur. Biophys. J.* **16**, 153–168.

Kohler, J.E.H., Saenger, W. & van Gunsteren, W.F. (1988b) Conformational differences between a-cyclodextrin in aqueous solution and in crystalline form: a molecular dynamics study. *J. Mol. Biol.* **203**, 241–250.

Kruger, P., Strassburger, W., Wollmer, A. & van Gunsteren, W.F. (1985) A comparison of the structure and dynamics of avian pancreatic polypeptide hormone in solution and in the crystal. *Eur. Biophys. J.* **13**, 77–88.

Levitt, M. (1982) Computer simulation of DNA double-helix dynamics. *Cold Spring Harbour Symposium on quantitative biology* **47**, 261–262.

Levitt, M. (1983) Molecular dynamics of native protein II Analysis and nature of motion. *J. Mol. Biol.*, **168**, 621.

Levitt, M. & Sharon, R. (1988) Accurate simulation of protein dynamics in solution. *Proc. Natl. Acad. Sci. USA* **85**, 7557–7561.

McCammon, J.A. & Harvey, S.C. (1987) *Dynamics of proteins and nucleic acids*, Cambridge University Press, Cambridge.

McCammon, J.A., Gelin, B.R. & Karplus, M. (1977) Dynamics of folded proteins. *Nature* **267**, 585.

Metropolis, N., Rosenbluth, A.W., Rosenbluth, M.N., Teller, A.H. & Teller, E. (1953). Equation of state calculations by fast computing machines. *J. Chem. Phys.* **21**, 1087–1092.

Nilges, M., Gronenborn, A.M. & Clore, G.M. (1989) In Molecular Simulation and Protein Crystallography, *Proceedings of CCP4/5 study weekend*, SERC Daresbury DL/SCI/R27.

Nilsson, L., Clore, G.M., Gronenborn, A.M., Brunger, A.T. & Karplus, M.J. (1986) Structure refinement of an oligonucleotide by molecular dynamics with NOE inter-proton distance restraints: Application to d(CGTACG)$_2$, *J. Mol. Biol.* **188**, 455–?.

Pearlman, D.A. & Kollman, P.A. (1990). The calculated free energy effects of 5-methyl cytosine on the B to Z transition in DNA. *Biopolymers* **29**, 1193–1209.

Pettit, B.M. (1989) Failures, successes and curiosities in free energy calculations in *computer simulation of biomolecular systems* (eds van Gunsteren, W.F. & Weiner, P.) ESCOM, Leiden, 94–100.

Rao, S.N., Singh, U.C., Bash, P.A. & Kollman, P.A. (1987) Free energy perturbation calculations on binding and catalysis on mutating Asn 155 in subtilisin. Nature, **328**, 551–554.

Reynolds, C.A., King, P.M. & Richards, W.G. (1988) Computed redox potentials and the design of bioreductive agents. *Nature* **334**, 80–82.

Saqi, M.A.S. & Goodfellow, J.M. (1990) Free energy changes associated with amino acid substitutions in proteins. *Prot. Engin.*, **3**, 419–423.

Seibel, G.L., Singh, U.C. & Kollman, P.A. (1985). A molecular dynamics simulation of double helical B-DNA including counterions and water. *Proc. Natl. Acad. Sci. USA* **82**, 6537–6540.

Singh, U.C., Weiner, S.J. & Kollman, P.A. (1985) Molecular dynamics simulations of d(CGCCA).d(TCGCG) with and without 'hydrated' counterions. *Proc. Natl. Acad. Sci. USA* **82**, 755–759.

Singh, U.C., Weiner, P.K., Caldwell, J.W. & Kollman, P.A. (1986) AMBER (UCSF 3.0) Department of Pharmaceutical Chemistry, University of California, San Francisco.

Subramanian, P.S., Ravishanker, G. & Beveridge, D.L. (1988) Theoretical considerations on the spine of hydration in the minor groove of d(CGCGAATTCGCG). d(GCGCTTAAGCGC): Monte Carlo computer simulation. *Proc. Natl. Acad. Sci. USA* **85**, 1836–1840.

Tembe, B.L. & McCammon, A.J. (1984) Ligand-receptor Interactions. *Computers in Chemistry*, **8**, 281–283.

van Gunsteren, W.F. (1989) Methods for calculations of free energies and binding constants: successes and problems, in *Computer simulations of biomolecular systems* eds Van Gunsteren, W.F. & Weiner, P., ESCOM, Leiden, 27–59.

van Gunsteren, W.F. & Berendsen, H.J.C. (1977) Algorithms for macromolecular dynamics. *Mol. Phys.* **34**, 1311–1327.

van Gunsteren, W.F. & Berendsen, H.J.C. (1984) Computer simulations as a tool for tracing the conformational differences between proteins in solution and in the crystalline state. *J. Mol. Biol.* **176**, 559–564.

van Gunsteren, W.F. & Berendsen, H.J.C. (1987) *Biomos biomolecular software*, Laboratory of Physical Chemistry, University of Groningen, The Netherlands.

Verlet, L. (1967) Computer experiments on classical fluids. I. Thermodynamical properties of Lennard-Jones molecules. *Phys. Rev.* **159**, 98–103.

Williams, M., Saqi, M.A.S. & Goodfellow, J.M. (1990) in *Molecular dynamics* (ed. J.M. Goodfellow) Macmillan Press, London, In Press.

Wong, C.F. & McCammon, J.A. (1986) Dynamics and design of enzymes and inhibitors. *J. Am. Chem. Soc.* **108**, 3830–3832.

Wodak, S., van Belle, D., Froeyen, M. & Prevost, M. (1989) Molecular dynamics simulations of a solvated protein: analysis of structural and electrostatic properties in *Modelling of molecular structures and properties* (ed J.L. Rivail) Elsevier, Amsterdam

Zheng, C., Wong, C.F., McCammon, J.A. & Wolynes, P.G. (1988) Quantum simulation of ferrocytochrome C. *Nature* **334**, 726–728.

8

Image processing in electron microscopy

Helen Saibil
Department of Crystallography, Birkbeck College, Malet Street,
London WC1E 7HX

1. INTRODUCTION

A major goal of biological electron microscopy (EM) is to visualize protein structures in a native form, that is, with a minimum of disruption caused by specimen preparation and image recording. Image processing is used to extract structural information present in images but obscured by noise or unwanted information.

This chapter introduces the basic theory and application of image processing techniques used to enhance EM images of symmetrical protein structures. More detailed accounts can be found in Misell (1978) and Moody (1991). Biological structures formed of identical subunits in equivalent positions tend to occur in planar lattices or have rotational, helical, or icosahedral symmetry. In some cases it is possible to extract information on secondary structure features and approach atomic resolution from EM images by computer processing, even though this information is not visible on the primary image. More routinely, image processing techniques enhance structural detail to 20–30 Å resolution in two-dimensional (2D) projections, elucidating subunit packing, symmetry, and arrangement of protein complexes. A series of projections taken with different tilt angles can be combined to produce a 3D image, although the resolution obtainable in the third dimension is normally lower.

These methods are important in areas where 3D crystallization and X-ray structure determination are infrequently achieved, such as for membrane and cytoskeletal proteins and viruses. Technical developments in microscopy, specimen conditions, and processing are allowing biological EM to approach the realm of 3D atomic structure determination.

2.   ELECTRON MICROSCOPY OF BIOLOGICAL STRUCTURES

2.1   Image formation
To image a protein structure in the electron microscope, the electron beam must interact with the thin 3D specimen differentially, generating image contrast (areas of light and dark, recorded as optical density on photographic film or intensity on an electronic detector) in a 2D projection. The large depth of field relative to specimen thickness in EM gives a projected image, like a medical X-ray, where all parts of a thin, untilted specimen are at the same level of focus. Electron micrographs are usually recorded on photographic film and digitized in a film scanner. Direct electronic detection in the microscope is still limited by detector resolution.

2.2   Imaging methods for protein
Since biological materials are composed of light elements which have very similar electron scattering amplitudes, they generate little amplitude contrast, and heavy metal stains are employed to increase image contrast and to preserve the specimen in a dehydrated form. Fig. 1(a) shows a side view of a negative stain EM specimen. Negative staining is simple and effective, but problems with the technique are

(a)   (b)

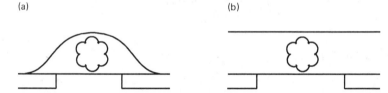

Fig. 1.(a) Diagram of an EM specimen seen from the side, as if in a section. The object is suspended in a film of stain over a hole in the carbon support film. After air drying, it is embedded in a dry layer of negative stain. The electron beam is vertical. (b) Similar view of a specimen embedded in a layer of vitreous ice over a hole in the carbon film, for observation by cryo EM.

dehydration, accuracy of the negative stain replica, and resolution of structures inaccessible to stain, for example in membrane proteins. During drying the sample is exposed to high concentrations of salts and heavy metal stain. Some of these problems can be avoided by drying the sample from a film of glucose or tannin solution. This preserves a more native state, but gives extremely low contrast. Even with negative staining, the main source of image contrast is phase contrast. This arises from interference between transmitted and scattered waves that depend on focus conditions and spherical aberration (see Amos *et al.* 1982), enhancing the contrast generated by slight differences in scattering by protein, lipid, water, or stain.

Another method avoiding dehydration and staining problems is cryo EM, which depends on vitreous, or amorphous, ice (Dubochet *et al.* 1988). If a thin suspension on an EM grid is very rapidly cooled, water crystallization and the associated specimen damage do not occur, and the sample is embedded in a glass-like solid, vitreous ice. When observed at low temperature, the sample remains hydrated in the electron beam. This method allows direct observation of unstained protein density, but gives very low contrast. Fig. 1(b) shows a side view of a cryo EM specimen. With unstained samples, the image is mainly formed by weak phase contrast. For a given specimen, the microscope must be more underfocused than with negative staining to produce phase variations which can generate detectable intensity contrast, necessitating more complicated optical corrections.

2.3 Limitations on image quality

The main problem in biological EM is damage by the electron beam. The radiation dose is the number of electrons incident per unit area of specimen. One twentieth the normal electron dose needed for a photographic exposure is sufficient to destroy high-resolution detail. For crystalline specimens, this can be assessed by loss of intensity in the electron diffraction pattern (see below). A minimal dose is defined as the amount needed to record a normal photograph, with no prior exposure of the specimen area being recorded (this is done by deflecting the beam during alignment and focusing). A subminimal dose is defined as one too low to give a normal optical density on film, and can be only used with crystalline specimens. This leads to the highest obtainable resolution of protein structure by EM, but gives very noise images, so that image analysis and processing provide the only means of extracting the structural information.

Other factors which degrade the image include movement of the specimen, distortion and flattening, and loss of contrast due to scattering by the support film. At present, optimal results are obtained from thin crystalline specimens observed by cryo EM. In addition to the advantage of a hydrated specimen, the rate of radiation damage is slower at low temperature.

3. THE MATHEMATICAL BASIS OF IMAGE ANALYSIS

Once the image has been recorded photographically or electronically, it can be digitized for analysis and processing. An important development in microscopy has been the exploitation of computer power to manipulate images in digital form. Image analysis requires substantial amounts of disk storage, a raster graphics monitor with grey scale display, and a reasonably fast processor to perform 2D and 3D Fourier transforms.

The purpose of image analysis is to determine the symmetry of the structure being imaged, its degree of order, the resolution of structural information in the image and the optical transfer characteristics (defined below) of the image. A branch of applied mathematics ideally suited to this analysis is Fourier analysis, since the imaging process can be formally treated as a Fourier transformation, revealing the spatial frequencies present in an image. In microscopy, the illuminating beam is scattered by the specimen to produce a wave pattern described mathematically by the Fourier transform. This can be observed as a diffraction pattern if the objective lens is removed. In Fourier space the scattered waves are defined by their amplitudes and phases, which are recombined by the objective lens in the inverse Fourier transformation to generate the magnified image.

General references on Fourier transform theory: Bracewell (1986), Brigham (1974), Champeney (1986), Cizek (1986), Steward (1987), Stroud (1984).

3.1 Relation to X-ray diffraction

The atomic scattering factors for electron scattering are similar to, but not identical with, those for X-rays because X-rays are scattered by the electron cloud, while electrons interact with both the electron cloud and the atomic nucleus. Electron scattering rises more slowly with atomic number and falls off more slowly with scattering angle. The lack of high resolution lenses for X-rays means that only the diffraction pattern can be observed. This contains the intensities of the scattered waves but not their relative phases. The central problem in X-ray structure determination is that of determining the missing phases. In principle, a set of EM images could provide all the amplitudes and phases to define a 3D density map, but in practice the image data are also incomplete, particularly for 3D reconstructions, and the resolution is normally much lower.

3.2 Definitions

Image $p(x,y)$, the pattern of optical density related to the number of electrons falling on each area of the photographic film or detector in the electron microscope. This image is related to the 2D projection of the object being observed in the microscope.

3D structure density $\rho(x,y,z)$, electron scattering density of protein or stain. The density projected along the z direction is $\sigma(x,y)$, where x,y are spatial coordinates in the image. X,Y,Z are reciprocal space coordinates in the transform or diffraction pattern.

Fourier transform $FT^-[P(x,y)]$, in general a complex function.

$$FT^-[P(x,y)] = \iint_{\substack{\text{projected} \\ \text{object}}} P(x,y)\exp(-2\pi i(xX + yY))\mathrm{d}x\mathrm{d}y \qquad (1)$$

Inverse Fourier transform $FT^+\{FT^-[P(x,y)]\} = P(x,y)$

$$P(x,y) = \int\int_{-\infty}^{\infty} FT^-[P(x,y)]\exp(2\pi i(xX + yY))\mathrm{d}X\mathrm{d}Y \qquad (2)$$

(note that the sign of the exponential and the location of the 2π factor may vary according to the convention chosen)

Reciprocal relation of coordinates: The image coordinates are considered to be in real space (units of length) and the Fourier transform in reciprocal space (units of spatial frequency). For example, interference between widely separated features in an image will give rise to closely spaced features in the transform (low spatial frequencies), and fine, high-resolution detail in the projected object gives rise to features at large spacings in the transform (high frequencies). Thus a structural feature with a wavelength of 5 Å will give a frequency component in the transform of $2\pi/5$ radians/Å.

Diffraction pattern $|FT^-\ [P(x,y)]|^2$, also called the diffractogram, or power spectrum. It contains the intensities but not the relative phases of the waves. It can be calculated or produced optically from an image. Diffraction patterns may also be generated directly by scattering of electrons (thin specimen in the electron microscope) or X-rays (macroscopic specimen, for example 3D crystals or aligned fibres). Diffraction patterns are used for frequency analysis and processing of image data, and for X-ray structure determination.

Optical transform: A quick way of assessing an image is by optical diffraction of the photographic film with a laser diffractometer. This gives the diffraction pattern of the image, directly equivalent to calculating the Fourier transform and power spectrum of the digitized image.

Electron diffraction pattern: Electron diffraction intensities can be obtained directly in the microscope, by focusing the back focal plane (diffraction plane) of the objective lens onto the film. Much less intensity is needed for recording diffraction intensities than for recording the image, and the diffraction pattern is not affected by specimen drift and optical corrections, but the phase information is not obtained.

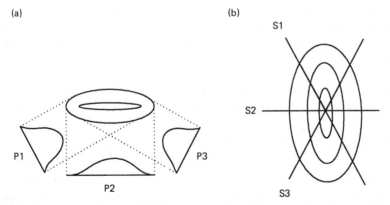

Fig. 2. The projection theorem. (a) Different views of an object are projected onto the plane of the image by tilting the specimen relative to the electron beam. P1–3 represent three different projected views. (b) Each projection is Fourier transformed to give a section inclined at the tilt angle and passing through the origin of the 3D FT (S1–3).

3.3 Projection theorem
The Fourier transform of a projection is a central section (that is, one passing through the origin of reciprocal space) through the 3D transform. This is illustrated in Fig. 2. If

$$F(X,Y,Z) = \iiint\limits_{\text{object}} \rho(x,y,z)\exp(-2\pi i(xX + yY + zZ)\mathrm{d}x\mathrm{d}y\mathrm{d}z \qquad (3)$$

and $\sigma(x,y)$ is the projection of $\rho(x,y,z)$ along z, then

$$FT^{-}[\sigma(x,y)] = \iint\limits_{\substack{\text{projected}\\ \text{object}}} \sigma(x,y)\exp(-2\pi i(xX + yY))\mathrm{d}x\mathrm{d}y = F(X,Y,0) \qquad (4)$$

For clarity, this is shown for the special case of projection along z, but is true for any projection.

3.4   Some properties of Fourier transforms

Addition: $FT[f(x) + g(x)] = FT[f(x)] + FT[g(x)]$
This means that superimposed structures have linear summation of their transforms.

Symmetry: The symmetry of the image is preserved in the transform. For example, a structure with 3-fold rotational symmetry will also have a 3-fold axis in its transform.

Sampling: A continuous function can be reconstructed to a specified resolution from a regularly spaced series of sampled values. When an image is being digitized, the choice of pixel size, or spacing between sampled points, depends on the resolution to which the data will be analysed. The maximum frequency component preserved in the transform of the sampled image is one half the sampling frequency. When an image is being digitized for computer processing, the sampling frequency must be at least twice the highest frequency being analysed. In practice, it is often advantageous to oversample the data, for example to avoid interpolation errors.

Convolution: If the one-dimensional (1D) functions f and g are defined with their Fourier pairs $f(x) \leftrightarrow F(X)$ and $g(x) \leftrightarrow G(X)$, then their convolution is given by

$$f(x) \times g(x) = \int_{-\infty}^{\infty} f(x')g(x - x')\mathrm{d}x'. \qquad (5)$$

The *convolution theorem* states that the Fourier transform of the convolution $f(x) \times g(x)$ is the product of the individual transforms $F(X) \times G(X)$. A convolution of two functions can be considered as the repeating of one function at all the positions of the other. For example, a crystal structure is the convolution of the single unit cell density distribution with the repeating lattice function. A physical equivalent of convolution where both functions are continuous is the instrumental blurring function, where a signal is broadened by the response function of an instrument. The original, undistorted signal can be recovered by deconvolution, if the instrumental response function is known. This can be done by dividing the Fourier transform of the convoluted data by the Fourier transform of the response to a delta function input (the impulse response function), and then inverse transforming to restore the deconvoluted signal. The order of the convolution operation does not matter.

Cross and autocorrelation: For real functions, the cross-correlation is given by

$$f(x) * g(x) = \int_{-\infty}^{\infty} f(x')g(x' + x)dx' \tag{6}$$

and the autocorrelation function is given by

$$f(x) * f(x) = \int_{-\infty}^{\infty} f(x')f(x' + x)\,dx'. \tag{7}$$

This definition looks similar to convolution, but is quite distinct. The cross-correlation detects and locates correlations between different functions, or different parts of the same function (autocorrelation). The sign of the shift between correlated regions depends on the order in which the functions are taken. The Fourier transform of an autocorrelation is the power spectrum, or diffraction pattern of the function. In X-ray crystallography, the autocorrelation function of a structure is called the *Patterson function*, and it is obtained by inverse Fourier transformation of the diffracted intensities.

3.5 Use of Fourier methods in image analysis

Noise (unwanted information in an image) may be additive, or it may operate on the structure information in a known way, for example with optical distortions. In an image, structure information and noise cannot readily be dissociated, but in a diffraction pattern they may be spatially separated, and optical corrections can be applied. This is true when the structure is periodic, for example in a 2D lattice, the best case for EM structure determination. Image analysis, in the form of calculation (or optical production) of the Fourier transform and power spectrum, is used for assessment of resolution and symmetry, which are often not easily visible on noisy images.

3.5.1 Separation of frequency components in diffraction space

Separation of superimposed layers is not possible on the image, but can be obvious on the corresponding diffraction pattern. In Fig. 3(a), the image obtained from superimposed top and bottom layers of a flattened tubular structure (a bacteriophage capsid) is not interpretable in terms of the subunit structure of a single layer. However, in the optical diffraction pattern of the image, the two hexagonal lattices of slightly differing orientation give rise to diffraction peaks separated in reciprocal (frequency) space (Fig. 3(b)). Multiplication of the transform with an appropriate masking function to eliminate one of the lattices, followed by inverse transformation, yields the reconstructed, averaged image of a single layer (Fig. 3(c)). Information from the two sides can thus be processed separately to reveal the subunit lattice of each layer and derive a model for the protein subunit packing (Fig. 3(d)).

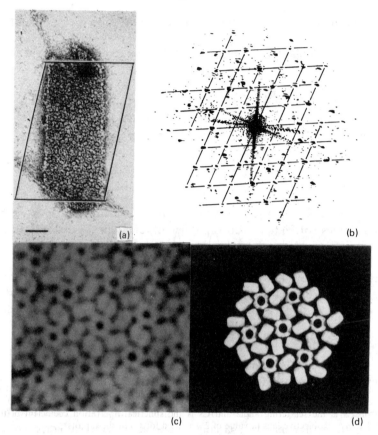

Fig. 3.(a) Negative stain image of a flattened capsid of the bacteriophage ϕCbK (Lake & Leonard, 1974). Top and bottom layers are flattened to form two plane lattices with slightly differing orientations, and they sum to give Moiré patterns. (b) The optical diffraction pattern with peaks from one of the two lattices indexed. (c) The image of a single layer obtained by inverse transformation of only one set of the diffraction peaks. (d) Model of the lattice composed of combinations of large and small protein subunits. Reproduced from Lake & Leonard (1974), by permission of Dr K. Leonard.

3.5.2   *Contrast transfer function (CTF)*
This gives the relation between image density $P(x,y)$ and projected structure density $\sigma(x,y)$. The CTF describes the frequency response of the microscope at the focus used, much as the impulse response function describes the frequency response of a linear system to a delta function input. This can be seen in the diffraction pattern of carbon film, in which a random distribution of point-like carbon grains gives rise to a theoretically constant frequency response which is multiplied by the CTF. Examples of the CTF for two values of defocus are plotted in Fig. 4. Diffraction intensities will be multiplied by the square of this function. To deconvolute this frequency response it is necessary to divide the transform of the image by the CTF at the appropriate level of focus. In images of tilted specimens, the focus level varies across the field of view and the correction is correspondingly more elaborate (Henderson *et al.* 1990).

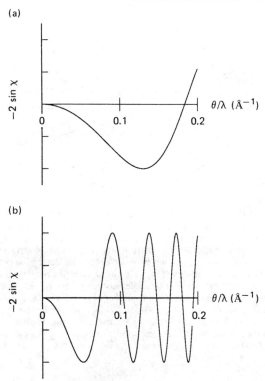

Fig. 4. Phase contrast transfer functions for (a) 800 Å and (b) 5000 Å underfocus at 100 kV, where $\chi = (2\pi/\lambda) (\Delta f\ \theta^2/2 - Cs\ \theta^4/4)$, Δf is the underfocal distance, $\lambda = 0.037$ for 100 kV electrons, θ is the scattering angle and Cs is the spherical aberration coefficient of the objective lens (a value of 2 was used for Cs in these plots).

To record all spatial frequencies at higher resolutions, several images with different levels of defocus are needed, to fill in regions where the CTF passes through a zero.

3.5.3   3D reconstruction from projections (Crowther et al. 1970, Amos et al. 1982, Frank 1992).

This process is equivalent in principle to computed tomography in medical imaging, but in practice different methods are used. In the case of EM, it can be considered in two stages. First, corrected Fourier-transformed data for a set of views (Fig. 2) must be aligned in the same coordinate system, scaled to a common amplitude and origin in transform space. Then the set of sections through the 3D transform must be interpolated to give evenly spaced sample values so that it can be inverse transformed to give the 3D density function. In the EM, images cannot be recorded at tilts greater than 60–70°, resulting in a missing cone of data where the central sections do not sample the 3D transform. As the section planes radiate from the origin of the transform, the transform sampling gets progressively coarser. This puts a limit on the best resolution obtainable from a given number of views (Fig. 5; see discussion in Moody 1991, p. 266). The reverse interpolation is computationally

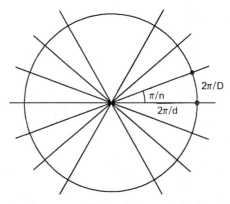

Fig. 5. 3D reconstruction from a set of 2D projections obtained in a tilt series. The circle represents a vertical slice through the 3D Fourier transform of the object to be reconstructed, and the lines are sections obtained by Fourier transformation of tilted images. Because the specimen cannot be viewed at 90° tilt, there is a missing cone of data which cannot be observed in the transform. The spacing between tilt planes determines the resolution to which the transform can be observed. As the radial distance increases, sampling of the transform gets progressively coarser. The angle between successive tilt planes (assuming no missing angles) is given by π/n, where n is the number of views. An indication of the minimum n needed to obtain a spatial resolution d (radius = $2\pi/d$ on the transform) is given by the following construction. The highest frequency fluctuation in the transform will be given by $2\pi/D$, where D is the maximum particle dimension. For small angles, $\sin\theta \approx \theta$, and therefore $2\pi/D/(2\pi/d) = \pi/n$, giving the rule of thumb that $n = \pi D/d$.

demanding, and the choice of coordinate system has important consequences. Crowther (1970) developed a method using a cylindrical polar coordinate system, recently modified by Fuller (1987). An example of this procedure is considered in the section on icosahedral viruses. More recently, developments in computing equipment have allowed more powerful methods to be applied to this problem, for example the use of spherical polar coordinate systems and maximum entropy methods (Provencher & Vogel 1988, Lawrence *et al.* 1989).

4. IMAGE PROCESSING

General reference: Castleman (1979)

The purpose of image processing is to use the information on symmetry and optical transfer characteristics from image analysis to reconstruct an image with an enhanced signal to noise ratio, and also to reconstruct 3D structures from 2D projections. Image processing cannot increase the resolution of an image, only the contrast of selected structural information. It can reveal high-resolution detail present in the original image but buried in noise, that is, present but invisible owing to low contrast. Processing can actually decrease image resolution, by averaging together misaligned or dissimilar structural units, blurring out fine detail.

4.1   Use of symmetry for image enhancement

4.1.1   2D crystals of a membrane protein
The membrane protein bacteriorhodopsin is a light-driven proton pump in the purple membrane of *Halobacterium*. Its structure has been solved to a resolution better than 3 Å in projection and 10 Å in the *z* direction by electron microscopy (Henderson *et al.* 1990). This chromoprotein is found in large 2D crystalline sheets of purple membrane. This protein can be induced to form very large and stable crystals and can be imaged in the electron microscope unstained and embedded in glucose or frozen-hydrated. The electron diffraction pattern of unstained purple membrane is shown in Fig. 6(a) and the optical diffraction pattern of a very low electron dose image is shown in Fig. 6(b).

The higher resolution diffraction peaks are abolished with increasing electron dose. To preserve the high resolution detail, images of large sheets were recorded with an electron dose so low that only statistical fluctuations of the film density could be observed directly on the image. However, the periodic signal was also present, buried in the noise, and Fourier transformation of the scanned film revealed the diffraction peaks shown in Fig. 6(b) above the background level. This is possible because of the very large number of identical unit cells contributing to the diffraction. Inverse transformation of the diffraction maxima, which are present as amplitudes and phases in the complex transform calculated from the image, eliminates most of the noise, by excluding all the regions of the FT outside the peaks. Before calculating a density map, the transform data must be corrected for the CTF and other optical effects, which become more complex as the resolution increases. In addition, small imperfections in the lattice must be detected and corrected for (see correlation averaging section, below). A resulting projection map at 2.8 Å resolution is shown in Fig. 6(c). Averaging the images of some 25 000 unit cells which are individually invisible has increased the contrast of the protein structure to the extent that axially oriented α-helices and bulky side chains are apparent in projection.

By obtaining similar data at a range of tilt angles, the 3D FT is sectioned at various angles. Purple membrane is not crystalline in the *z* direction, but has finite thickness and therefore has a continuously varying FT along the z axis (Fig. 7(a)). Each view gives a section sampling the lattice lines at different heights. A series of images at different tilt angles and different levels of defocus is combined, with appropriate scaling and choice of phase origin, to give the full 3D transform, apart from the missing cone of data, in this case from 45–90° tilt. An example of the 3D data for two diffraction orders is shown in Fig. 7(b). A section of the 3D map obtained by inverse transformation is shown in Fig. 8. By using information from other studies, an atomic model of the bacteriorhodopsin sequence was built into the map.

4.1.2   Helical reconstruction
Many important biological structures are helical, for example the cytoskeletal filaments actin and microtubules, consisting of identical subunits arranged along a helical path. 3D reconstruction is particularly elegant in the case of helical structures as many views about the helix axis are present in a single projection. The resolution

(a)   (b)

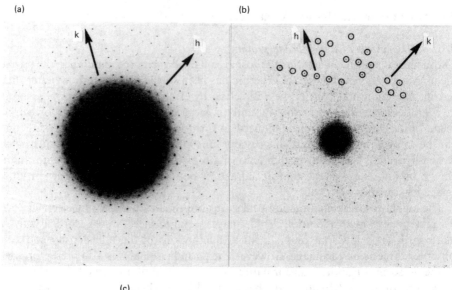

(c)

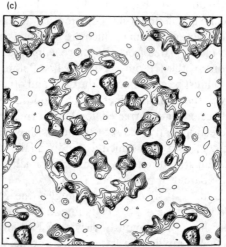

Fig. 6.(a) Electron diffraction pattern of unstained purple membrane, showing the lattice vectors. (b) Optical diffraction pattern of a high resolution cryo EM image of the same material. Some of the higher resolution diffraction spots are circled. (c) The projected density of a bacteriorhodopsin trimer in the purple membrane lattice. Each molecule contains three resolved features known to be α-helices viewed end on, and an arc of density known to contain four other α-helices slightly inclined from the axis of view. Reproduced from Baldwin *et al.* (1988) by permission.

obtainable in a 3D reconstruction from a single view, d, depends on the number of subunits per turn of the helix, N, that is, the number of different subunit views. As for 3D reconstruction from a tilt series, the minimum number of views to give a resolution d is given by $N = \pi D/d$ where D is the subunit diameter (Crowther *et al.* 1970; see Fig. 5).

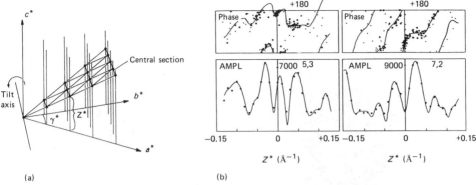

(a)   (b)

Fig. 7.(a) Diagram of part of the 3D FT of a 2D crystal. Lattice lines extend perpendicular to the plane of the crystal. Each projected view of the structure is transformed into a central section (that is, one passing through the origin) of the 3D FT. Reproduced from Amos *et al.* (1982) by permission. (b) Plots of the 5,3 and 7,2 lattice lines from the 3D purple membrane data set. Individual measurements of amplitude and phase are shown fitted by curves obtained by a least squares procedure. Reproduced from Henderson *et al.* (1990) by permission.

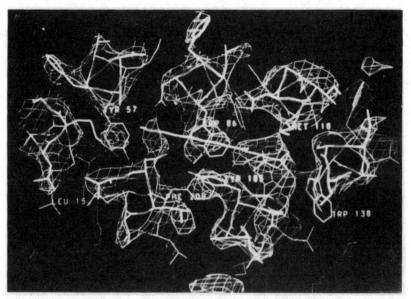

Fig. 8. A 7 Å thick slice through the 3D density map of bacteriorhodopsin with the atomic model superimposed. The seven α-helices surround the retinal chromophore. Reproduced from Henderson *et al.* (1990) by permission.

Diffraction from helices: A continuous helix can be evisaged as a spring. Fig. 9(b) shows a 2D projection perpendicular to the axis of a loosely coiled helix. A helix can be considered as a 1D repeat of a single turn of the coil (Fig. 9(a)). The single coil diffraction pattern (Fig. 9(e)) has the form of an X, and putting this into the 1D repeat causes the transform to be sampled on a series of layer lines whose spacing

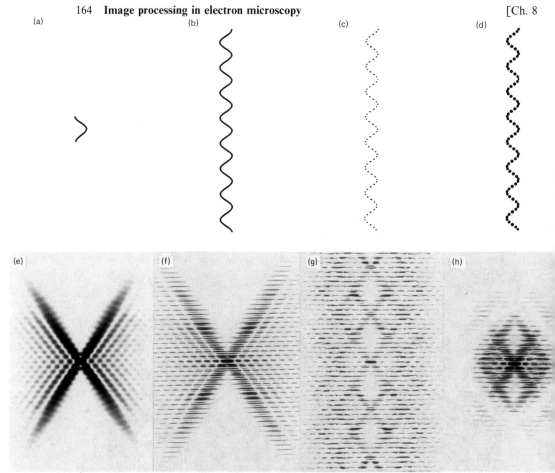

Fig. 9. Diffraction by helices. (a) The projection of a single helical turn. (b) The projection of a continuous helical wire. (c) A discontinuous helix. (d) A discontinuous helix formed of globular subunits. (e) The diffraction pattern of (a). (f) The diffraction pattern of (b). (g) The diffraction pattern of (c). (h) The diffraction pattern of (d).

is inversely related to the pitch of the helix (Fig. 9(f)). A discontinuous helix can be generated by multiplying the continuous function by a grating (Fig. 9(c), and the FT of this product is the convolution of the individual transforms (Fig. 9(g). Finally, the discontinuous point helix is convoluted with a finite subunit to give the model helix made of globular subunits in Fig. 9(d), with the corresponding diffraction pattern in Fig. 9(h). In general, it is possible to identify helical symmetry and subunit arrangement from the transform of a helical structure.

Helical density is most efficiently expressed in cylindrical polar coordinates $\rho(r,\phi,z)$ and its FT as $F(R,\Phi,Z)$. Helices are periodic in z and in ϕ, causing the diffraction pattern to consist of a series of layer lines (Fig. 9(f)). Helical transforms are conveniently expressed in terms of Bessel functions J_n, a series of damped sinusoidal functions. Bessel functions J_0-J_2 are plotted in Fig. 10. The diffraction amplitude along a layer line n is proportional to $J_n(2\pi Rr_0)$, where r_0 is the helix radius (Cochran et al. 1952).

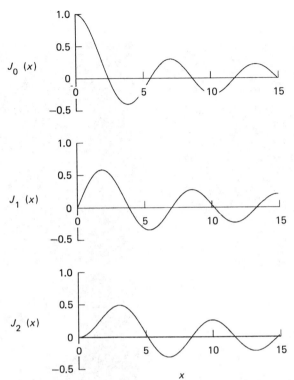

Fig. 10. Plots of the cylindrical Bessel functions $J_n(x)$ for $n = 0,1$ and 2. Note the progressive displacement of the first maximum, which gives rise to the ●ross-shaped intensity of the diffraction pattern (Fig. 9(e)).

Bessel functions have the property that intensities $J^2_n = J^2_{-n}$. Once the symmetry and subunit repeat are known, the 3D density of a helical structure can be calculated from the layer line amplitudes. A clear exposition of helical diffraction theory as it applies to muscle filaments may be found in Squire (1990).

A protein forming helical filaments is the muscle protein, actin. The structure of pure actin filaments has been determined to a resolution of about 40 Å (Trinick *et al.* 1986). A cryo-electron micrograph of frozen hydrated actin filaments is shown in Fig. 11(a). The calculated transform of a straight stretch of filament is shown in Fig. 11(b), showing several layer lines. The strong layer line amplitudes are plotted in Fig. 11(c), along with their Fourier–Bessel transforms, and the 3D reconstruction of filamentous actin is shown in Fig. 11(d). This shows that the long axis of the actin monomer, whose structure has recently been determined, is oriented perpendicular to the filament axis. The orientation of the monomer in the filament is important in determining the interactions between actin filaments and other cellular components.

4.1.3 Icosahedral reconstruction
Spherical viruses usually have icosahedral symmetry with quasi-equivalent packing of identical subunits, one of the classic examples of self assembly in molecular biology

(a)   (b)

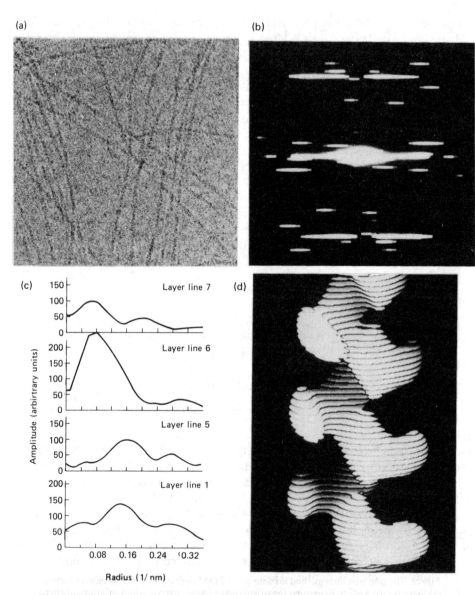

(c)   (d)

Fig. 11(a) Electron micrograph of frozen hydrated actin filaments embedded in a layer of vitreous ice, taken at a defocus of 2.9 μm. Despite the low contrast, structural information is present and can be extracted from this image. Protein density is dark. Magnification 216 000 × . (b) Calculated diffraction pattern of the image of a regular filament, showing layer lines 1, 5, 6 and 7. (c) Layer line amplitudes. (d) 3D reconstruction of an actin filament calculated from the merged transforms of two filaments to a resolution of 40 Å. Reproduced from Trinick *et al.* (1986), by permission.

(Caspar & Klug 1965). Their structures can be solved to about 30 Å resolution by EM, taking advantage of their 60-fold symmetry in 3D reconstructions (Crowther 1971, Fuller 1987). The principle is that the icosahedral symmetry of the structure gives rise to a corresponding icosahedral symmetry in the 3D FT. Each projected view of the virus particle is Fourier transformed to give a central section through the 3D FT. Because of the symmetry elements in the FT, any section will include lines of data related by a symmetry axis, but their positions will depend on the orientation of the particle in 3D (Fig. 12). A search for lines of the same value in the transform can thus be used to determine the orientation of a projection. A search is done through different orientations in 3D, testing the similarity of the predicted common lines for each orientation, until a minimum is found for the sum of squares of the amplitude differences between common lines. The degree of icosahedral symmetry for a particle is given by the phase residual — the average phase difference between nominally identical lines. Different projections will give rise to different central sections of the FT, but these will always intersect in a line which can then be used to assess the degree of similarity between different particles in an image. Once

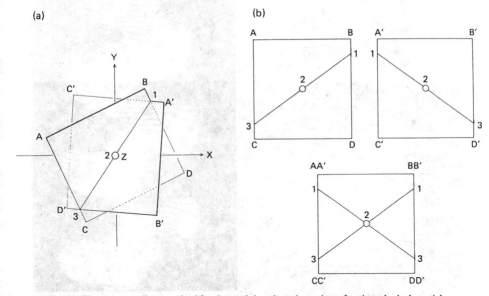

Fig. 12. The common lines method for determining the orientation of an icosahedral particle. (a) Suppose we wish to determine the orientation of a 3-fold axis, at an arbitrary angle to the particle projection. ABCD is a section of the FT calculated from the particle image. The 3-fold axis lies along the z axis, which is perpendicular to the plane of the diagram. This symmetry axis will generate two other symmetry related planes from ABCD, one of which is shown (A'B'C'D'). The two planes intersect along the line 1,2,3, in which they must have common values. (b) Upper panels, the planes ABCD and A'B'C'D' laid flat. The common line at the intersection 1,2,3 occurs in different positions in the two planes. Since these planes are related by the symmetry axis, each plane must contain two copies of the common line, as shown in the lower panel. Therefore, any transform section, derived from an arbitrary projection of a symmetrical particle, will contain identical, or common, lines, whose positions give the orientation of the particle relative to the symmetry axis. Reproduced from Moody (1991), by permission.

the orientations are known, many particle images can be combined to produce a 3D reconstruction. A check on the symmetry is included by imposing only 522 symmetry rather than full 532 icosahedral symmetry, and then assessing the degree of 3-fold symmetry in the reconstruction.

An example of icosahedral reconstruction applied to rotavirus, both in native form and with the Fab fragment of an antibody to the viral protein VP4 bound, is shown

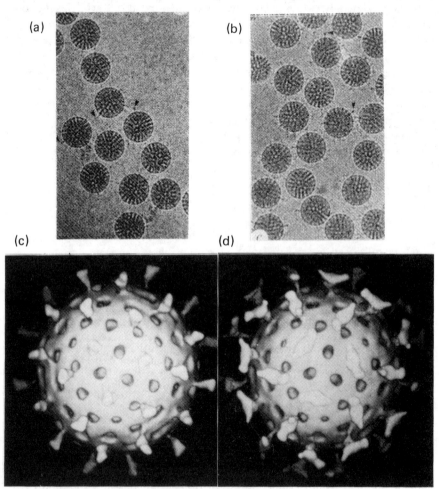

Fig. 13. Cryo electron micrographs of frozen hydrated rotavirus particles (a) and rotavirus complexed with Fab fragments of an antibody to the viral protein VP4 (b). Surface representations of 3D reconstructions of the native virus (c) and the Fab-virus complex (d), showing that VP4 is the viral spike protein. The icosahedral reconstruction was done by the common lines method, using a cylindrical coordinate system. 30 particles were used in each reconstruction, and the resolution was 35 Å. Reproduced from Prasad *et al.* (1990), by permission.

in Fig. 13. The extra density due to the antibody fragment is localized to the tips of the viral spikes, identifying the spike protein as VP4.

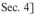

(a)   (b)   (c)

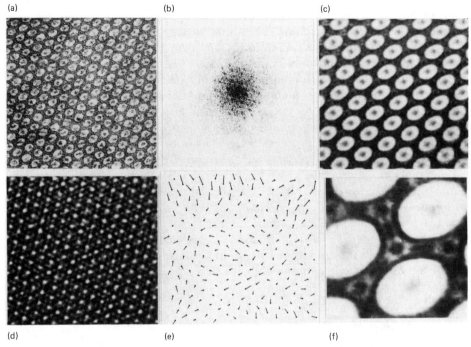

(d)   (e)   (f)

Fig. 14. Lattice correction applied to sections of photoreceptor membranes from the retina of the squid. (a) A section through the lattice of membrane cylinders. Dark features indicate positively stained membrane or protein structures. (b) Diffraction pattern calculated from an image containing about 250 unit cells. Lattice disorder causes the diffraction intensities to become diffuse. (c) The filtered image calculated from the Fourier transform peaks, assuming good lattice order. (d) The correlation map obtained by cross correlation of a single unit cell, or averaged unit cell, with the original image. (e) Positions of the correlation peaks, with 5 x magnified vectors indicating their displacements from ideal lattice positions. (f) Correlation average, taking each unit cell at its position determined from the correlation map. About 200 unit cells were averaged. Note the substantial enhancement of structural detail in the membrane contacts. (Reproduced from Saibil & White (1989), by permission.)

4.1.4 Lattice correction and correlation averaging

A limitation frequently encountered with regular biological specimens is that the repeating lattice structures are imperfectly ordered. Filtering the diffraction patterns of such specimens by the methods described above works poorly for disordered lattices. Methods for correcting deviations from regular lattice order in near-periodic specimens are increasingly being employed to achieve gains in resolution. Crowther & Sleytr (1977) used low-pass filtering of the diffraction pattern to map out the deviations of unit cell positions from their ideal lattice positions. By interpolating the digitized image along lines parallel to the distorted unit cell edges and placing these resampled densities in straightened-out unit cells, they corrected for 'elastic' distortions. Averaging or spatial filtering of the resampled image was then used to obtain the final result. Saxton & Baumeister (1982) used a method which can also be applied to non-crystalline specimens. In their method, a single unit cell of the structure is extracted and its cross-correlation with the whole image is calculated.

This gives a correlation map with a peak at the best fitting position of each similar unit cell. The units at these positions can then be averaged together. The procedure is repeated several times, using a previously determined average as the starting point to avoid bias from the initial selection. In this case the unit cell motif is treated as a displaced, rigid body, with no allowance for distortions. Rotational correlation has been used to bring into register copies of an object viewed from the same direction but rotationally disordered. An example of translational correlation averaging applied to sections of squid photoreceptor microvilli is shown in Fig. 14. The comparison with frequency filtering of the same image illustrates the significant improvement obtained by correlation averaging for this disordered lattice. Lattice correction by interpolation ('unbending') was much less effective than correlation averaging (unpublished results), presumably owing to the nature of the disorder in these sections.

Henderson *et al.* (1986) applied lattice correction to noisy, high-resolution data from large areas of crystalline bacteriorhodopsin. They used a variant of the cross-correlation procedure to locate unit cells and corrected the distortions, which were small compared to the resolution, by resampling. Assumptions about the nature of the distortions become important when the magnitudes of deviations approach the resolution limit.

5. SUMMARY

Computer image processing brings biological EM into the gap between high-resolution crystallography and cell biology, where interesting cellular structures can be characterized at the supramolecular level. Fourier and correlation techniques allow the extraction of desired structural information even in cases where the noise is greater than the signal. For the resolution of macromolecular assemblies, membranes, cytoskeletal filaments, and viruses, electron microscopy is often the most appropriate technique for structural analysis.

REFERENCES

Amos, L.A., Henderson, R. & Unwin, P.N.T. (1982) Three-dimensional structure determination by electron microscopy of two-dimensional crystals. *Prog. Biophys. Molec. Biol.* **39**, 183–231.

Baldwin, J.M., Henderson, R., Beckman, E., & Zemlin, F. (1988) *J. Molec. Biol.* **202**, 585–591.

Bracewell, R. (1986) *The Fourier transform and its applications.* McGraw-Hill.

Brigham, E.O. (1974) *The fast Fourier transform.* Prentice Hall.

Caspar & Klug (1965)

Castleman, K.R. (1979) *Digital image processing.* Prentice Hall, Inc., Englewood Cliffs, N.J., U.S.A.

Champeney, D.C. (1986) *Fourier transforms in physics.* Adam Hilger.

Cizek, V. (1986) *The discrete Fourier transform and its applications.* Adam Hilger

Cochran, W., Crick, F., & Vand, V. (1952) *Acta Crystallogr.* **4**, 581–586.

Crowther, R.A. (1971) Procedures for three-dimensional reconstruction of spherical viruses by Fourier synthesis from electron micrographs. *Phil. Trans. Roy. Soc. B* **261**, 221–230.

Crowther, R.A., DeRosier, D.J., & Klug, A. (1970) The reconstruction of a three-dimensional structure from projections and its application to electron microscopy. *Proc. Roy. Soc. Lond. A* **317**, 319–340.

Crowther, R.A. & Klug, A. (1975) *Ann. Rev. Biochem.* **44**, 161–182.

Crowther, R.A. & Sleytr, U.B. (1977) An analysis of the fine structure of the surface layers from two strains of *Clostridia*, including correction for distorted images. *J. Ultrastruct. Res.* **58**, 41–49.

Dubochet, J., Adrian, M., Chang, J.-J., Homo, J.C., Lepault, J., McDowall, A.W., & Schultz, P. (1988) Cryo-electron microscopy of vitrified specimens. *Quart. Rev. Biophys.* **21**, 129–288.

Frank, J. (Ed.) (1992) *Electron tomography: Three-dimensional imaging with the transmission electron microscope*. Plenum Press, New York.

Fuller, S. (1987) The $T = 4$ envelope of Sindbis virus is organized by interactions with a complementary $T = 3$ capsid. *Cell* **48**, 923–934.

Henderson, R., Baldwin, J.M., Ceska, T.A., Zemlin, F., Beckmann, E., & Downing, K.H. (1990) Model for the structure of bacteriorhodopsin based on high-resolution electron cryo-microscopy. *J. Molec. Biol.* **213**, 899–929.

Lake, J.A. & Leonard, K. (1974) Structure and protein distribution for the capsid of *Caulobacter crescentus* bacteriophage ϕCbK. *J. Molec. Biol.* **86**, 499–518.

Lawrence, M.C., Jaffer, M.A., & Sewell, B.T. (1989) The application of the maximum entropy method to electron microscopic tomography. *Ultramicrosc.* **31**, 285–302.

Milligan, R.A. & Flicker, P.F. (1987) Structural relationships of actin, myosin and tropomyosin revealed by cryo-electron microscopy. *J. Cell Biol.* **105**, 29–39.

Misell, D.L. (1978) Image analysis, enhancement and interpretation. *Practical methods in electron microscopy* Vol 7, A.M. Glauert, Ed. North Holland Publishing Co.

Moody, M.F. (1991) Image analysis of electron micrographs, in *Electron microscope imaging and analysis for biologists*, eds. Hawkes P.W. & Valdrè U., Academic Press.

Prasad, B.V.V., Burns, J.W., Marietta, E., Estes, M.K., & Chiu, W. (1990) Localization of VP4 neutralization sites in rotavirus by three-dimensional cryo-electron microscopy. *Nature* **343**, 476–479.

Provencher, S.W. & Vogel, R.H. (1988) Three-dimensional reconstruction from electron micrographs of disordered specimens. *Ultramicrosc.* **25**, 209–222.

Saibil, H.R. & Hewat, E.A. (1987) Ordered transmembrane and extracellular structure in squid photoreceptor microvilli. *J. Cell Biol.* **105**, 19–28.

Saxton, W.O. & Baumeister, W. (1982) The correlation averaging of a regularly arranged bacterial cell envelope protein. *J. Microsc.* **127**, 127–138.

Steward, E.G. (1987) *Fourier optics. An introduction*, 2nd ed., Ellis Horwood Ltd., Chichester, UK.

Stroud, K.A. (1984) *Fourier series and harmonic analysis*. Stanley Thornes Ltd, Cheltenham, UK.

Squire, J. (1981) *The structural basis of muscular contraction*. Plenum Press, New York.

Trinick, J., Cooper, J., Seymour, J., & Egelman, E. (1986) Cryo-electron microscopy and three-dimensional reconstruction of actin filaments. *J. Microsc.* **141**, 349–360.

9

Enzyme kinetics

Christopher M. Topham
Laboratory of Molecular Biology, Department of Crystallography

1. INTRODUCTION

An understanding of the remarkable catalytic effectiveness of enzymes is one of the most challenging problems in modern biology. The advent of site-directed mutagenesis (see for example Knowles, 1987, Leatherbarrow & Fersht 1987, Anthony-Cahill *et al.* 1989) and the production of catalytic antibodies (Blackburn *et al.* 1989, Powell & Hansen 1989, Schultz 1989) have provided much of the recent impetus toward the discovery of the molecular origins of enzyme catalysis.

Enzymes work by lowering the activation barriers of the corresponding reactions in water, and rate enhancements of 10^{10} or more (over the acid- or base-catalysed reactions, for example) are not uncommon (Jencks 1975, Kraut 1988, Burbaum *et al.* 1989, Warshel *et al.* 1989). Much effort has been devoted by structural enzymologists to the characterization of the binding interactions between an enzyme and its substrate (ground state) and between the enzyme and transition state: the free energy difference between the ground state and the transition state relative to the same system in water lies at the heart of catalysis.

Effective catalysis depends upon a complex interplay of factors acting in concert. These include electrostatic effects and the coupling of binding interactions with catalytic-site chemistry. Through site-directed mutagenesis the hope is to determine the contribution of individual amino acid residues to the catalytic activity of the enzyme. The relationship between enzyme structure and function has been further aided by major advances in physical techniques such as X-ray crystallography (Eisenberg & Hill 1989, Hajdu *et al.* 1988), two-dimensional nmr (Wüthrich 1989, Wright 1989, Williamson 1991), resonance Raman and Fourier transform infrared spectroscopy (Wharton 1986), and time-resolved fluorescence spectroscopy (Szabo 1990). Theoretical approaches such as molecular dynamics and semi-empirical quantum mechanics are playing an increasingly important role as well (for recent examples see Arad *et al.* 1990, Daggett & Kollman 1990, Hirono & Kollman 1991, Warshel 1991, 1992).

The focus of this chapter is on the kinetic aspects of strategies for studying structure–activity relationships. A core of knowledge about the theory and practice of kinetics is essential to an understanding of the subtleties of mechanisms by which the free energy of binding may be utilized to bring about the rate accelerations characteristic of enzyme–catalysed reactions. Enzyme kinetics is a dauntingly large subject in its own right, and to provide a balanced distillate in a short review is a difficult task. For more extensive treatments with differing emphases the texts by Fersht (1985), Wharton & Eisenthal (1981), Roberts (1977), and Cornish-Bowden (1979) can be recommended. The shorter monographs by Engel (1981) and Cornish-Bowden & Wharton (1988) are valuable introductions to the subject.

2.   THE MICHAELIS–MENTEN EQUATION: AN OVERVIEW

2.1   Basics
A characteristic feature of enzyme–catalysed reactions is that they exhibit saturation. Nearly all enzyme-catalysed reactions show a first-order dependence of rate (v) on substrate concentration ([S]) at very low concentrations, but instead of increasing indefinitely as the concentration of substrate increases, v approaches a limit (V) at which v is independent of [S], and the reaction becomes zero-order with respect to substrate. The hyperbolic dependence of v on [S] (Fig. 1) may be described more formally by the Michaelis–Menten equation:

$$v = \frac{V[S]}{K_m + [S]} = \frac{k_{cat}[E]_0[S]}{K_m + [S]} \tag{1}$$

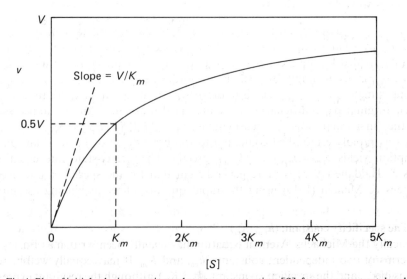

Fig. 1. Plot of initial velocity v against substrate concentration, [S], for an enzyme-catalysed reaction obeying the Michaelis–Menten equation.

where $[E]_0$ is the total enzyme concentration and k_{cat} and K_m are constants characteristic of a particular enzyme-catalysed reaction. The first-order rate constant k_{cat} $(= V/[E]_0)$ is often referred to as the catalytic constant or turnover number, defining the number of catalytic processes (or 'turnovers') that the enzyme catalyses per unit time. The dimensions of k_{cat} are reciprocal time. The other parameter of the Michaelis–Menten equation is called the Michaelis constant (K_m). K_m is best defined in an operational way as the substrate concentration at which the initial rate (v) is one-half of the maximum velocity $(0.5V)$. By definition, therefore, K_m has the dimensions of concentration. The kinetic parameters k_{cat} and K_m may be more precisely defined in terms of mechanism-dependent assemblies of individual rate constants (and concentrations of species such as H^+ and other effectors of enzyme activity). There are an infinite number of enzyme mechanisms which give rise to rate equations of the form of the Michaelis–Menten equation and for which precise definitions of k_{cat} and K_m can be derived. The simplest of these is the following two-step, single-intermediate mechanism in which the substrate (S) combines reversibly with the free enzyme (E) to form an enzyme–substrate (Michaelis) complex (ES) which in turn breaks down irreversibly to release the product (P) and the free enzyme:

$$E + S \underset{k_{-1}}{\overset{k_{+1}}{\rightleftharpoons}} ES \overset{k_{+2}}{\rightarrow} E + P \qquad (2)$$

Application of the steady-state treatment of Briggs & Haldane (1925) to this mechanism leads to the Michaelis–Menten equation with

$$K_m = \frac{(k_{-1} + k_{+2})}{k_{+1}} \text{ and } k_{cat} = k_{+2} \qquad (3)$$

The steady-state assumption is that the rate of production of ES is balanced by its rate of decay (that is, $d[ES]/dt = 0$). Thus K_m is the sum of two first-order rate constants divided by the second-order rate constant for the combination of E with S, while k_{cat} is given simply by a single first-order rate constant. If $k_{+2} \ll k_{-1}$, then K_m approximates to k_{-1}/k_{+1}, that is to the dissociation constant (K_s) for the substrate. In their original paper Michaelis & Menten (1913) assumed (in fact unnecessarily) that the first step was a quasi-equilibrium $([E][S]/[ES] = K_s = k_{-1}/k_{+1})$ which was rapidly established compared to the breakdown of ES to E and P. This assumption yields $K_m = K_s(= k_{-1}/k_{+1})$ directly. The steady-state rate equation of Briggs & Haldane (1925) is more general than that for the special case derived by Michaelis & Menten (1913) using the rapid quasi-equilibrium binding assumption.

2.2 The specificity constant: (k_{cat}/K_m)

Historically the Michaelis–Menten equation has usually been written as Eq. (1), that is in terms of two independent constants, k_{cat} and K_m. It may equally well be recast in terms of k_{cat} and the specificity constant, (k_{cat}/K_m), although the resultant expression does not have quite such a tidy appearance.

$$v = \frac{k_{\text{cat}}(k_{\text{cat}}/K_m)[S][E]_0}{k_{\text{cat}} + (k_{\text{cat}}/K_m)[S]} \tag{4}$$

The specificity constant is an apparent second-order rate constant for an enzyme-catalysed reaction at very low substrate concentrations, that is it defines the rate at those concentrations (see Fig. 1). This can readily be shown by application of the condition $[S] \ll K_m$ to the Michaelis–Menten equation. Eq. (1) collapses to give:

$$v = (k_{\text{cat}}/K_m)[S][E]_0 \tag{5}$$

The specificity constant is not a true microscopic rate constant except for the case in which the rate-determining step in the reaction is the encounter of enzyme and substrate (see section 4B). At low substrate concentrations almost all of the enzyme exists as the free enzyme (E), and Eq. (5) may be rewritten as:

$$v = (k_{\text{cat}}/K_m)[S][E] \tag{6}$$

In fact Eq. (6) holds not just at low values of $[S]$ but for all values (Fersht 1985, pp 104–112); $[E]_0$ may be equated with $[E](1 + [S]/K_m)$ and so substitution for $[E]_0$ in the numerator of the Michaelis–Menten equation yields Eq. (6). The importance of (k_{cat}/K_m) is that it relates the overall enzyme-catalysed reaction rate to the concentration of free, rather than total, enzyme. As for all second-order rate constants, the units of (k_{cat}/K_m) are (concentration^{-1}.time^{-1}).

The term specificity constant is particularly appropriate as it is the ratio of the individual (k_{cat}/K_m) values for two (or more) different (alternative) substrates that determines an enzyme's ability to distinguish between them. Thus the relative rate of competing reactions (v_A/v_B) when two substrates (A and B) are mixed with enzyme is given by (see for example Cornish-Bowden 1979, pp 82–85):

$$\frac{v_A}{v_B} = \frac{(k_{\text{cat}}/K_m)_A[A]}{(k_{\text{cat}}/K_m)_B[B]} \tag{7}$$

where $(k_{\text{cat}}/K_m)_A$ and $(k_{\text{cat}}/K_m)_B$ are the specificity constants for A and B, respectively. It should be emphasized that Eq. (7) holds true for any values of $[A]$ and $[B]$, not necessarily low concentrations. The crucial point here is that specificity is governed by the ratio of (k_{cat}/K_m) values for the two substrates and not by ratios of either the individual turnover numbers $(k_{\text{cat(A)}}/k_{\text{cat(B)}})$ or Michaelis constants (K_{mA}/K_{mB}) alone; (k_{cat}/K_m) is the fundamental parameter to be considered in discussions of enzyme specificity. Unlike K_m the specificity constant is not affected by non-productive binding (Bender & Kézdy 1965), a phenomenon that can sometimes complicate mechanistic studies of reactions of enzymes with analogue substrates.

2.3   Graphical representation of the Michaelis–Menten equation

Data sets comprising a series of initial velocity measurements determined at different constant substrate concentrations are not normally displayed as hyperbolic plots of v against $[S]$ according to the Michaelis–Menten equation, but are transformed and plotted by using one of three possible linear transforms of the Michaelis–Menten equation. The most popular transform is to take reciprocals of both sides of Eq. (1):

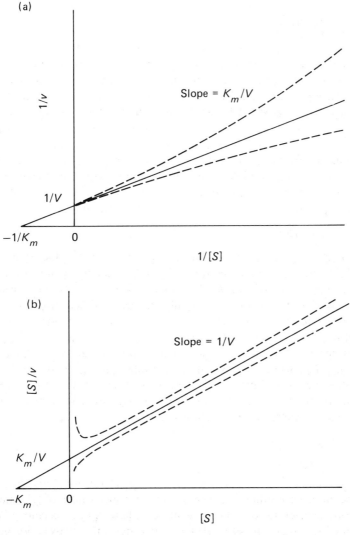

Fig. 2. (a) Plot of $1/v$ against $1/[S]$ (Lineweaver–Burk or double-reciprocal plot). The error envelope was constructed with error values of $\pm 0.05V$ in v.
(b) Plot of $[S]/v$ against $[S]$ (sometimes called a Hanes plot). The error envelope was constructed with error values of $0.05V$ in v.

$$\frac{1}{v} = \frac{1}{V} + \frac{K_m}{V} \cdot \frac{1}{[S]} \tag{8}$$

A double-reciprocal plot of $(1/v)$ versus $(1/[S])$ is a straight line with a slope of K_m/V, an intercept on the ordinate axis of $1/V$, and an intercept on the abscissa of $-1/Km$ (Fig. 2a). Unfortunately this plot grossly distorts the appearance of any experimental error in primary observations of v: for small values of v, small errors in v lead to enormous errors in $1/v$; but for large values of v the same errors in v

lead to barely perceptible errors in $1/v$. Unweighted linear regression (that is, with each data point equally weighted) of $1/v$ on $1/[S]$ should not therefore be used for kinetic parameter determination. The same argument applies to attempts to fit the data by eye, since it is virtually impossible to judge the amount of weight to be given to individual points. It will be noted that this line of reasoning holds true irrespective of the actual error structure involved [In principle, these difficulties can be overcome by use of suitable weights for the dependent variable, $(1/v)$, in the linear regression analysis; for example weights $\alpha \ v^4$ for rate measurements subject to a constant standard deviation or $\alpha \ v^2$ for measurements of v with a constant coefficient of variation (Wilkinson 1961)].

The second transform can be generated by multiplying both sides of Eq. (8) by $[S]$:

$$\frac{[S]}{v} = \frac{K_m}{V} + \frac{1}{V} \cdot [S] \tag{9}$$

Thus a plot of $[S]/v$ against $[S]$ is also a straight line with slope equal to $1/V$ and intercepts of K_m/V and $-K_m$ on the ordinate and abscissa, respectively (Fig. 2b). In this case constant errors in v are better reflected in $[S]/v$ (cf. Fig. 2a), although some distortion is still apparent. For this reason the plot of $[S]/v$ against $[S]$ should be preferred to the double-reciprocal plot.

In addition to its undeniable popularity, the double-reciprocal plot has a certain advantage, however, in providing the framework for the systematic treatment of multi-substrate enzyme kinetics introduced initially for two-substrate reaction mechanisms by Dalziel (1957):

$$\frac{[E]_0}{v} = \phi_0 + \frac{\phi_A}{[A]} + \frac{\phi_B}{[B]} + \frac{\phi_{AB}}{[A][B]} \tag{10}$$

$$= \left[\phi_0 + \frac{\phi_B}{[B]} \right] + \left[\phi_A + \frac{\phi_{AB}}{[B]} \right] \cdot \frac{1}{[A]}$$

where $[A]$ and $[B]$ are the substrate concentrations and the ϕ coefficients are mechanism-dependent assemblies of rate constants. Primary plots of $[E]_0/v$ versus $1/[A]$ (or $1/[B]$) for several fixed values of $[B]$ (or $[A]$) are linear and non-parallel (except if $\phi_{AB} = 0$). Secondary plots of the slopes and intercepts against the reciprocal of the fixed substration are also linear. The four Dalziel ϕ coefficients are identified with the slopes and intercepts of these secondary plots. Dalziel later extended the treatment to three-substrate reactions (Dalziel 1969, 1975). The symbolism lends itself well to descriptions of product and other types of multi-substrate enzyme inhibition when used in conjunction with Cleland's (1963) rules (see for example Engel 1981, pp 68–72).

The third linear plot of the Michaelis–Menten equation is obtained by multiplying both sides of Eq. (9) by $vV/[S]$ and rearrangement.

$$v = V - K_m \frac{v}{[S]} \tag{11}$$

However, plots of v against $v/[S]$ according to Eq. (11) are not widely used; errors in v are present in both axes, making this linear transformation inappropriate both for the visual representation of data and regression analysis.

3. DERIVATION STEADY-STATE RATE EQUATIONS

3.1 The traditional approach

3.1.1 Briggs–Haldane kinetics

In principle the steady-state rate equation for any enzyme-catalysed reaction may be obtained by solution of the set of simultaneous equations resulting from the combination of the enzyme conservation and the steady-state rate expressions for all the enzyme-containing intermediates. The well-known three-step acyl enzyme mechanism may be used as an illustrative example of how to derive a steady-state rate expression.

$$
\begin{array}{ccccc}
k_{+1} & k_{+2} & k_{+3} \\
E + S \rightleftharpoons & ES & \rightarrow & ES' & \rightarrow & E + P_2 \\
k_{-1} & & + & \\
& & P_1
\end{array}
\tag{12}
$$

This mechanism represents a minimal kinetic model for serine proteinase (Fersht 1985 pp. 195–208, Fink 1987, Polgár 1987) and cysteine proteinase (Baker & Drenth 1987, Brocklehurst *et al.* 1987, Polgár 1989) catalysed hydrolyses of amides and esters. Following the formation of a reversible enzyme–substrate (ES) complex, an acyl-enzyme intermediate (ES') is formed with rate constant k_{+2}. The free enzyme (E) is then regenerated in a deacylation step with rate constant k_{+3}. Acylation is accompanied by the concomitant release of the first product, P_1. Structure–function relationships in these proteinases have been studied experimentally using synthetic peptide-derived substrates containing a chromophoric leaving group. This enables the reaction to be followed spectrophotometrically by monitoring the release of the chromophore P_1, typically the p-nitrophenolate ion or the p-nitroanilinium cation. The rate of appearance of P_1 is given by the steady-state concentration of ES multiplied by the rate constant for acylation:

$$
v = \frac{d[P_1]}{dt} = k_{+2}[ES]
\tag{13}
$$

The steady-state concentrations of the other enzyme species (E and ES') are worked out below in terms of $[ES]$. However, this choice is abitrary, as Eq. (13) could equally well have been written as $v = d[P_2]/dt = k_{+3}[ES']$, and the steady-state expressions developed in terms of $[ES']$. It will be noted also that the reverse reactions ($E + P_2 \rightarrow ES'$ and $ES' + P_1 \rightarrow ES$) have been omitted in the reaction mechanism shown in Eq. (12). This is justified during the early stages of the reaction when the concentrations of the products are small unless one or both have been deliberately included in the reaction mixture.

To derive the steady-state rate equation it is assumed that the total concentration of substrate is much greater than the total enzyme concentration ($[S]_0 \gg [E]_0$). It follows that the total concentration of all forms of enzyme-bound substrate must be negligible compared to $[S]_0$. Provided too that only a small fraction of the substrate is converted to products during the initial stages of reaction, the total and free concentrations of substrate may be equated ($[S] \approx [S]_0$). By using the Briggs–Haldane assumption, a steady-state is established soon after the mixing of enzyme with substrate and the concentrations of all the enzyme species remain constant throughout the period of observation. Accordingly, steady-state expressions for $[ES]$ and $[ES']$ may be written as:

$$\frac{d[ES]}{dt} = k_{+1}[E][S] - (k_{-1} + k_{+2})[ES] = 0$$

$$\frac{d[ES']}{dt} = k_{+2}[ES] - k_{+3}[ES'] = 0$$

from which

$$[E] = \frac{(k_{-1} + k_{+2})}{k_{+1}} \frac{[ES]}{[S]} \tag{14}$$

and

$$[ES'] = \frac{k_{+2}}{k_{+3}}[ES] \tag{15}$$

Substitution for $[E]$ and $[ES']$ into Eq. (16), the enzyme conservation equation:

$$[E]_0 = [E] + [ES] + [ES'] \tag{16}$$

yields

$$[E]_0 = [ES]\left[\frac{k_{-1} + k_{+2}}{k_{+1}[S]} + 1 + \frac{k_{+2}}{k_{+3}}\right] \tag{17}$$

Equation 17 may be algebraically rearranged to make $[ES]$ the subject. Substitution for $[ES]$ in Eq. (13) results in the Michaelis–Menten equation:

$$v = \frac{\dfrac{k_{+2}k_{+3}}{(k_{+2} + k_{+3})}[E]_0[S]}{\dfrac{k_{+3}(k_{-1} + k_{+2})}{k_{+1}(k_{+2} + k_{+3})} + [S]} \tag{18}$$

The kinetic parameters k_{cat} and K_m are now more complex assemblies of rate constants than for the two-step single-intermediate mechanism (cf. Eq. (3)):

$$k_{cat} = \frac{k_{+2}k_{+3}}{(k_{+2} + k_{+3})} \tag{19}$$

$$K_m = \left(\frac{k_{-1} + k_{+2}}{k_{+1}}\right) \cdot \left(\frac{k_{+3}}{k_{+2} + k_{+3}}\right) = K_{m(Acyl)} \left(\frac{k_{+3}}{k_{+2} + k_{+3}}\right) \tag{20}$$

and

$$\frac{k_{cat}}{K_m} = \frac{k_{+1} k_{+2}}{k_{-1} + k_{+2}} = \frac{k_{+2}}{K_{m(Acyl)}} \tag{21}$$

where $K_{m(Acyl)}$ is the K_m for the overall acylation process.

3.1.2 Michaelis–Menten kinetics

If instead of applying the Briggs–Haldane steady-state assumption, the quasi-equilibrium assumption for the binding of S to the free enzyme had been made, then $K_{m(Acyl)}$ in Eqs (20) and (21) is replaced by K_s $(= [E][S]/[ES] = k_{-1}/k_{+1})$. The specificity constant in this case becomes (k_{+2}/K_s). K_m/k_{cat} is related to K_s/k_{+2} by Eq. (22).

$$\frac{K_m}{k_{cat}} = \frac{1}{k_{+1}} \cdot \left(1 + \frac{k_{-1}}{k_{+2}}\right) = \frac{K_s}{k_{+2}} + \frac{1}{k_{+1}} \tag{22}$$

Accordingly, if an independent estimate of K_s/k_{+2} could be obtained for a catalysis where the steady-state specificity constant $(k_{cat}/K_m) \neq (k_{+2}/K_s)$, this would permit calculation of k_{+1}, the second-order rate constant for the encounter of enzyme and substrate. Christensen *et al.* (1990) have suggested that a comparison of steady-state and single-turnover transient kinetic data might therefore provide a value for k_{+1}. This argument is flawed, however, for the simple reason that for a given catalysis both methods of kinetic analysis yield the same quantity $k_{+2}/K_{m(Acyl)}$, whether or not this happens to approximate closely to (k_{+2}/K_s) (Brocklehurst & Topham 1990).

The conventional criterion for quasi-equilibrium is $k_{+2} \ll k_{-1}$, whence $K_{m(Acyl)} = K_s = k_{-1}/k_{+1}$. The difficulty of attempting to use this inequality in practice is that it is not always possible to assess the relative values of k_{+2} and k_{-1}. Fortunately the condition $(k_{cat}/K_m) \ll k_{+1}$ (that is, $k_{+2}/K_{m(Acyl)} \ll k_{+1}$) also provides that $K_{m(Acyl)} \approx K_s$ (Brocklehurst 1979, Brocklehurst & Topham 1990). This is clear from a transformation of Eq. (21),

$$\frac{k_{+2}}{k_{-1}} = \frac{(k_{cat}/K_m)/k_{+1}}{1 - [(k_{cat}/K_m)/k_{+1}]} \tag{23}$$

since $k_{+2} \ll k_{-1}$ is a necessary consequence of the condition $(k_{cat}/K_m) \ll k_{+1}$. The latter inequality is of more use than the conventional criterion, since probable values for k_{+1} are $\geq 10^6$ M^{-1} s^{-1}, and so the quasi-equilibrium binding assumption is reasonable for enzyme catalyses characterized by values of the specificity constant (k_{cat}/K_m), $\leq 5 \times 10^5$ M^{-1} s^{-1}.

3.2 The determinant method

The procedure outlined in section 3A(i) for obtaining the concentrations of the various enzyme forms in the irreversible three-step acyl enzyme mechanism (Eq. (12)) in terms of the measurable concentrations of substrate and total enzyme is equivalent to solving the following matrix equation.

$$
\begin{vmatrix}
0 & k_{+2} & -k_{+3} \\
k_{+1}[S] & -(k_{-1}+k_{+2}) & 0 \\
1 & 1 & 1
\end{vmatrix}
\begin{vmatrix}
[ES'] \\
[ES] \\
[E]
\end{vmatrix}
=
\begin{vmatrix}
0 \\
0 \\
[E]_0
\end{vmatrix}
\tag{24}
$$

This may be done by applying Cramer's rule either manually, or using computer programs such as those described by Herries (1984) and Ishikawa *et al.* (1988) for the automatic derivation of steady-state rate equations.

3.3 King–Altman schematic method

Any manual method of deriving steady-state rate equations is, however, likely to be tedious and prone to human error for all but the simplest kinetic mechanisms. The derivation of steady-state rate equations was therefore greatly facilitated by the introduction of a schematic method by King & Altman (1956) and the publication a decade later of rule-based modifications by Volkenstein & Goldstein (1966), using the theory of flow graphs. The King–Altman method is based on the determinant method and is, in effect, a set of geometric rules designed to simplify an algebraic procedure. Several automated versions of the method are now available (see, for example, Lam & Priest 1972, Lam 1981, Cornish-Bowden 1977, Olavarria 1986). However, much of the value of the King–Altman method to the enzymologist lies in the insights it provides into the kinetic properties of mechanisms rather than as a tool for actually deriving rate equations.

Taking again the three-step acyl enzyme mechanism as an example, the first stage is to represent the mechanism by a scheme that shows all of the enzyme species and the reactions between them.

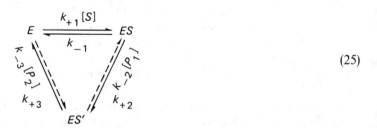

$$\tag{25}$$

All of the reactions are treated as first-order reactions. This means that second-order reactions such as $E + S \rightarrow ES$ must be given a pseudo-first-order rate constant ($k_{+1}[S]$). Next a master pattern is drawn, representing the skeleton of the scheme, in this case a triangle. It is then necessary to find every pattern that (a) consists only of lines from the master pattern, (b) connects every enzyme species, and (c) contains no closed loops. Each pattern will contain one line fewer than the number of enzyme species. Here there are three such patterns:

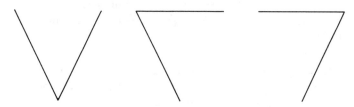

For each enzyme species arrowheads are drawn on the lines of the patterns such that each pattern leads to the species considered, regardless of the starting point. Thus for E the three vector diagrams are:

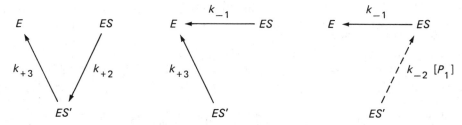

The rightmost vector diagram can be discarded if the steady-state treatment is restricted to the irreversible mechanism of Eq. (12) in the absence of products, since it comprises a step utilizing P_1 ($P_1 + ES' \rightarrow ES$). This leaves two vector diagrams, and the fraction of the total enzyme concentration ($[E]_0$) existing as E in the steady state is given by:

$$\frac{[E]}{[E]_0} = (k_{+2}k_{+3} + k_{-1}k_{+3})/\sum \tag{26}$$

The fractional concentrations of ES and ES' are similarly obtained in the absence of products after discarding two vector diagrams for each species:

$$\frac{[ES]}{[E]_0} = (k_{+1}k_{+3}[S])/\sum \tag{27}$$

$$\frac{[ES']}{[E]_0} = (k_{+1}k_{+2}[S]/\sum \tag{28}$$

The denominator $\sum$ is the sum of all three numerators, that is, the sum of the four terms remaining after the removal of a total of five vector diagrams involving $[P_1]$ or $[P_2]$.

$$\sum = [(k_{+2}k_{+3} + k_{-1}k_{+3}) + (k_{+1}k_{+3} + k_{+1}k_{+2})[S]] \tag{29}$$

The Michaelis–Menten equation (18) can now be simply derived by substitution of $[ES]$ from Eqs. (27) and (28) in the rate equation [Eq. (13)]. From an analytical perspective one of the main strengths of the method is the immediacy with which ratios of the relative concentrations of different enzyme species can be obtained. For example, the partitioning of ES and ES' in the steady state is governed by the ratio $k_{+3}/k_{+2}(= [ES]/[ES'])$. This can be seen by combining Eqs. (27) and (28). In an analogous way $K_{m(Acyl)} = [E][S]/[ES] = (k_{-1} + k_{+2})/k_{+1}$ can be directly obtained from Eqs. (26) and (27).

3.4   Cha's combined quasi-equilibrium and steady-state treatment

The rigorous application of steady-state assumptions, however, often leads to the generation of initial-rate equations of such complexity as to be of limited value in cases of practical interest. This prompted Cha (1968) to propose a simplification of the full King–Altman method for analysing mechanisms in which some steps are considered as quasi-equilibria whilst steady-state assumptions are retained for others. In outline, the Cha method treats each assembly of enzyme forms at quasi-equilibrium as a single form, and each rate constant (k_i) leading away from the composite form is weighted $(f_i k_i)$ according to the fraction (f_i) of reactive molecules in the quasi-equilibrium mixture. If there is more than one reactive species within the composite form, then the rate constant is the sum of the reduced rate constants for the parallel reactions. This follows from rule (a) of Volkenstein & Goldstein (1966) which relates to the addition of two or more parallel branches interconverting a particular pair of enzyme forms.

Cha's method may be applied to any mechanism where there are steps which are considered to be at quasi-equilibrium. It ensures that thermodynamic boxes are treated correctly with all interconversions explicitly recognized (see Topham & Brocklehurst 1992). The method is particularly useful in the analysis of pH-dependence (see, for example, Brocklehurst & Dixon 1976, 1977) since such rapid equilibrium assumptions may be justified for ionization reactions by the exceptionally high rate of hydron (proton) transfer steps in buffered aqueous solutions (Jencks 1969, pp. 207–211). For in-depth treatments of pH-dependence in enzyme kinetics, review articles by Knowles (1976) and Tipton & Dixon (1979) are highly recommended.

4.   ENZYME CATALYSIS

4.1   Transition-state theory

Most theories of enzyme catalysis are based on the transition-state theory (see for example, Page 1987, Kraut 1988). Transition-states (or activated complexes) are unstable species occurring along the reaction coordinate (or minimum energy path) through which a reactant must pass in order to be successfully converted to product. Transition-state theory (or absolute reaction rate theory) stems from the application of statistical mechanics to reactants and activated complexes. It was published almost simultaneously by Eyring and by Evans & Polanyi in 1935. Several accounts of the theory are available in the secondary literature (see, for example, Moore & Pearson 1981, pp. 137–191, Atkins 1986, pp. 745–758, Laidler 1987, pp. 89–136).

The theory rests on two main assumptions. The first is that the reaction rate is controlled by the decomposition of an activated transition-state complex. The second asserts that the system can be treated as though the transition-state complex is in (quasi-) equilibrium with the reactants. Imagining therefore a reaction between A and B as proceeding through the formation of an activated complex $C^{\neq}$ which breaks down to yield products (P) with a rate constant $k^{\neq}$,

$$\frac{d[P]}{dt} = k[A][B] = k^{\neq}[C^{\neq}] \tag{30}$$

where k is an experimentally observable rate constant for the reaction. The motion through the saddlepoint (or col) on the potential energy surface corresponding to the activated complex $(C^{\neq})$ can be treated as a very loose vibration with frequency v; that is, there is no restoring force and so a vibration of $C^{\neq}$ tips it through the transition state. It is possible that not every oscillation along the reaction coordinate takes the complex through the transition state, and so it is supposed that the rate of passage is proportional to the vibration frequency along the reaction coordinate:

$$k^{\neq} = \kappa v \tag{31}$$

where κ is called the transmission coefficient, the fraction of forward crossings leading to product. The transmission coefficient may be viewed as a combined correction factor for barrier re-crossing, quantum mechanical tunnelling, and solvent frictional effects.

The equilibrium between the two reactants A and B and the activated complex may be expressed by:

$$K_c^{\neq} = \frac{[C^{\neq}]}{[A][B]} \tag{32}$$

where $K_c^{\neq}$ is a concentration equilibrium constant. Eqs. (30)–(32) may be combined to give:

$$k = \kappa v K_c^{\neq} \tag{33}$$

$K_c^{\neq}$ may now be expressed in terms of the partition functions q_A, q_B and $q^{\neq}$:

$$K_c^{\neq} = \frac{q^{\neq}}{q_A q_B} \cdot e^{-E_0/k_B T} \tag{34}$$

where k_B is the Boltzmann constant, T is the absolute temperature, and E_0 is the difference between the molar zero-point energy of the activated complex and that of the reactants (that is, the hypothetical activation energy of the reaction at absolute zero). The partition function for the activated complex $(q^{\neq})$ is replaced by $q_{\neq} \dfrac{k_B T}{hv}$:

$$K_c^{\neq} = \frac{k_B T}{hv} \frac{q_{\neq}}{q_A q_B} \cdot e^{-E_0/k_B T} \tag{35}$$

where h is Planck's constant. The new partition function $(q_{\neq})$ is a special type of partition function for the activated complex, in which the factor relating to the actual motion over the col is omitted. The partition function for this vibration is $(1 - e^{-hv/k_BT})$, but for a loose vibration the value of the function can be calculated in the limit at which v approaches zero by expanding the exponential and taking only the first term (k_BT/hv). The rate constant k is given below after substitution for $K_c^{\neq}$ from Eq. (35) into Eq. (33) and cancellation of the unknown frequency v:

$$k = \kappa \frac{k_BT}{h} \frac{q_{\neq}}{q_Aq_B} \cdot e^{-E_0/k_BT} \tag{36}$$

In the original derivation of Eq. (36) [Evans & Polanyi (1935), Eyring (1935)], the motion over the col was not expressed as a vibrational motion but as a translational motion. The relationship between the partition functions $q^{\neq}$ and $q_{\neq}$ is different in this case. However, a common factor again cancels, and the final result, the Eyring equation, is the same.

For most purposes it is convenient to express rate constants in terms of thermodynamic quantities instead of partition functions, since the former are easier to estimate is aqueous media. Thus Eq. (36) may be rewritten as:

$$k = \kappa \frac{k_BT}{h} K_c^{\neq\prime} \tag{37}$$

Note that the equilibrium constant $K_c^{\neq\prime}$ is a modified quasi-equilibrium constant; it includes all possible modes in which the transition-state complex may contain energy except for the one factored out. If $K_c^{\neq}$ is now expressed in terms of $\Delta^{\neq}G^0$ $(= -RT\ln K_c^{\neq\prime})$, the change in standard Gibbs energy when the activated complex is formed from reactants, the result is:

$$k = \kappa \frac{k_BT}{h} e^{-\Delta^{\neq}G^0/RT} \tag{38}$$

where R is the gas constant. The importance of Eq. (38) is that it relates the rate of reaction to the difference in Gibbs energy between the transition state and the ground state.

4.2   The theory applied to the origin of enzyme catalysis and the evolution of catalytic power

Elementary transition state theory can be applied to enzyme catalysis by using the conceptual device of a thermodynamic cycle linking the binding of substrate (S) and the transition state ($S^{\neq}$) to the enzyme (E), through the intermediacy of interconvertible enzyme–substrate (ES) and enzyme–transition-state ($ES^{\neq}$) complexes (Kraut 1988):

$$
\begin{array}{c}
\overset{K_n^{\neq}}{E + S \rightleftharpoons E + S^{\neq}} \searrow \\
K_s \quad\quad K_T \quad\quad E + P \\
ES \rightleftharpoons ES^{\neq} \nearrow \\
K_e^{\neq}
\end{array}
\tag{39}
$$

The upper pathway of Eq. (39) represents the non-enzymatically catalysed conversion of S to product, P, and the lower pathway represents the enzyme–catalysed reaction. Equation (31) can be used to compare the first-order rate constants for the simple two-step enzyme-catalysed reaction met earlier (Eq. (2)) and for the same uncatalysed reaction (k_e/k_n):

$$\frac{k_e}{k_n} = \frac{\kappa_e v_e K_e^{\neq}}{\kappa_n v_n K_n^{\neq}} \tag{40}$$

The subscripts e and n denote the enzymic and non-enzymic reactions, respectively. The rate constant for the enzyme-catalysed reaction (k_e) corresponds to k_{cat} ($=k_{+2}$ in Eq. (2)). Using the thermodynamic identity ($1/K_n^{\neq}$). $K_T = (1/K_e^{\neq}).K_s$, the ratio of transition-state formation constants ($K_e^{\neq}/K_n^{\neq}$) may be equated with the ratio of dissociation constants for substrate and transition-state (K_s/K_T):

$$\frac{k_e}{k_n} = \frac{\kappa_e v_e K_s}{\kappa_n v_n K_T} \approx \frac{K_s}{K_T} \tag{41}$$

Setting aside the complication that the ratio $\kappa_e v_e/\kappa_n v_n$ might differ from unity (Kraut 1988), it can be seen that the magnitude of the acceleration in rate of an enzyme-catalysed reaction (k_e/k_n) is governed by the relative strength of binding to the enzyme of the transition state and the substrate in its ground state. Thus if the enzyme recognizes and binds the transition state more tightly than it binds the substrate ground state, the rate of reaction is increased.

Pauling (1948) advanced the view that the structure of an enzyme should be complementary to the transition-state structure rather than to that of the substrate (or product) so that the substrate is strained toward the unstable transition state (strain theory). This followed earlier suggestions by Haldane (1930) that enzymes can use the binding energy of their substrates to increase the rate of catalysis by distorting the substrate to the structure of the products. A more modern view of the concept of transition-state stabilization is not that the substrate is distorted but rather than the transition state makes better contacts with the enzyme than the substrate does (Fersht 1985, p 331).

The principle of transition-state stabilization may be illustrated schematically by reference to a Gibbs energy profile for the two-step enzyme-catalysed reaction (Fig. 3) with $K_m = K_s$. Free energy profiles can be constructed, using standard-state concentrations for substrate of 1M, but often the ambient substrate concentration that an enzyme experiences *in vivo* is chosen. The profile shown in Fig. 3a is for an enzyme exposed to a substrate concentration much greater than its K_m. Under these conditions the reaction rate is $v = k_{cat}[E]_0$ where $k_{cat} = k_{+2}$ (Eq. (3)). From transition-state theory the magnitude of k_{cat} is determined by the difference in Gibbs energy levels between the transition state, $ES^{\neq}$, and the enzyme–substrate (ES) complex ($\Delta G^{\neq}$). The substrate dissociation constant K_s is proportional to ΔG_s, the difference in free energy levels of the ES complex and $E + S$ ($\Delta G_s = +RT\ln K_s$; the positive sign on the right-hand side of the equation takes into account the fact that the equilibrium constant for the *binding* process is K_s^{-1}).

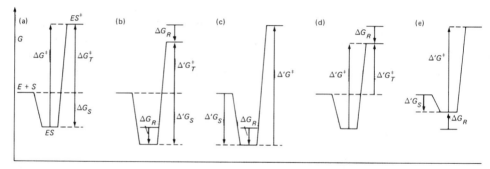

Fig. 3. Effect of a hypothetical mutational event on the free energy profile of a simple enzyme-catalysed reaction when $[S] > K_m$. (a) Schematic Gibbs free energy profile for

$$E + S \overset{K_m}{\rightleftharpoons} ES \overset{k_{cat}}{\rightarrow} E + P$$

(E, enzyme; S, substrate; ES, enzyme-substrate complex; $ES^{\pm}$, enzyme-transition-state complex; P, product). K_m ($= K_s$, the substrate dissociation constant) is proportional to ΔG_s (algebraically negative); k_{cat} is proportional to $\Delta G_T^{\pm}$ (algebraically positive). The rate of reaction, $v = k_{cat}[E]_0$ where $[E]_0$ is the total enzyme concentration. (b)–(e) Equal stabilization of ES and $ES^{\pm}$ (b) by ΔG_R (algebraically negative); Stabilization of ES (c) and $ES^{\pm}$ (d) individually by ΔG_R (algebraically negative); (e) Destabilization of ES by ΔG_R (algebraically positive). Values of ΔG_s, $\Delta G^{\pm}$, $\Delta G_T^{\pm}$ that change as a result of the mutation are indicated by a prime ('). Differences in free energy levels that remain the same as in (a) have been omitted for clarity. See text and Table 1 for further details.

It will be recalled from Eq. (6) that the specificity constant, (k_{cat}/K_m), relates the reaction rate to the concentration of free enzyme and free substrate at any substrate concentration. The activation energy of (k_{cat}/K_m) is therefore proportional to the free energy difference between $E + S$ and the transition state $ES^{\pm}$ ($\Delta G_T^{\neq}$). The $\Delta G_T^{\neq}$ term can be expressed as the sum of the energetically unfavourable (algebraically positive) term $\Delta G^{\neq}$ due to the activation energy of the chemical steps of bond making and breaking and the compensating (algebraically negative) substrate binding energy term ΔG_S.

$$\Delta G_T^{\neq} = \Delta G^{\neq} + \Delta G_s \tag{42}$$

Substitution of Eq. (42) into Eq. (38) derived from transition-state theory shows the relation between these two energy terms and the specificity constant (with κ set equal to unity):

$$RT\ln\left(\frac{k_{cat}}{K_m}\right) = RT\ln\frac{k_B T}{h} - \Delta G^{\neq} - \Delta G_s \tag{43}$$

Binding energy is provided by interactions between the enzyme and the substrate and transition state of the reaction. A hypothetical mutational event could contribute some additional binding energy (ΔG_R) through, for example, the formation of an extra hydrogen bond. In the case that the extra binding energy is realized equally well in the enzyme–substrate (ES) and enzyme–transition-state ($ES^{\pm}$) complexes (Fig. 3b), the free energies of the 'bound-states' are lowered by the same amount (ΔG_R) with respect to the 'free states' ($E + S$). This type of interaction has been termed

Table 1. Summary of changes in free energy differences ($\Delta\Delta G$) in Fig. 3: effect on the rate of the enzyme-catalysed reaction when $[S] > K_m$

$\Delta\Delta G$	Stabilization[1] of			Destabilization[2] of
	ES and $ES^{\neq}$	ES	$ES^{\neq}$	ES
	Case b	Case c	Case d	Case e
$\Delta\Delta G^{\neq}(= \Delta'G^{\neq} - \Delta G)$	0	$-\Delta G_R$	ΔG_R	$-\Delta G_R$
$\Delta\Delta G_s(= \Delta'G_s - \Delta G_s)$	ΔG_R	ΔG_R	0	ΔG_R
$\Delta\Delta G_T^{\neq}(= \Delta'G_T^{\neq} - \Delta G_T^{\neq})$	ΔG_R	0	ΔG_R	0

[1] ΔG_R is algebraically negative.
[2] ΔG_R is algebraically positive.
The effect of the mutation on the rate of reaction ($v = k_{cat}[E]_0$) is governed by the change in activation energy ($\Delta G^{\neq}$) that is, $\Delta\Delta G^{\neq} = (\Delta'G^{\neq} - \Delta G^{\neq}) = \Delta\Delta G_T^{\neq} - \Delta\Delta G_s$. An algebraically negative value for $\Delta\Delta G^{\neq}$ (Cases d and e) corresponds to an increase in rate by a factor $\exp(-\Delta\Delta G^{\neq}/RT)$. An algebraically positive value of $\Delta\Delta G^{\neq}$ (Case c) corresponds to a reduction in rate and a value of zero (Case b) indicates that the reaction rate is unaffected by the mutation.

'uniform-binding' by Knowles and Albery (Albery & Knowles 1976, 1977, Knowles & Albery 1977). The net effect when $[S] \gg K_m$ is to lower K_m but to leave k_m unchanged, and so the rate of reaction is not increased (Table 1). The specificity constant is increased owing to a favourable change in the ΔG_s term of Eq. (43). This, however, is accompanied by a compensating reduction in the free enzyme concentration ($[E]$), and an examination of Eq. (6) confirms that the reaction rate remains the same. If the enzyme achieves tighter interaction with the substrate alone, the free energy of ES is decreased by ΔG_R but the free energy of $ES^{\neq}$ is unchanged (see Fig. 3c, Table 1). The result of this is that K_m is decreased, k_{cat} is decreased and since ES is more stable $[E]$ decreases. The overall effect is a reduction in rate since the effects upon K_m and k_{cat} compensate; $\Delta G_T^{\neq}$ remains the same (Table 1).

Tighter binding of the transition state alone, leaving the interactions of the enzyme with the substrate unchanged, increases k_{cat} by reducing the activation energy $\Delta G^{\neq}$ (Fig. 3d). K_m and $[E]$ are unchanged, but (k_{cat}/K_m) is increased as a consequence of the reduction of the $\Delta G^{\neq}$ component of Eq. (43) by ΔG_R (Table 1). This phenomenon is frequently referred to as transition-state stabilization and leads directly to an increase in catalytic power. It is informative to consider the converse of transition-state stabilization, namely ground-state destabilization. If having achieved optimal transition-state binding, the rate of reaction may be enhanced (through compensatory increases in k_{cat} and K_m) by mutational events leading to a weakening of the interaction of the enzyme with the substrate ground state in the Michaelis (ES) complex. As a consequence of the destabilization of ES by ΔG_R (Fig 3e, Table 1), the concentration of free enzyme is increased, and a simple calculation using Eq. (16) reveals the considerable acceleration in rate that can be gained from an increase in K_m at constant (k_{cat}/K_m) when $[S] \gg K_m$ (see, for example, Fersht 1985, pp 325–327). The evolutionary pressure on K_m to increase rapidly falls away, however, as K_m becomes greater than $[S]$. Knowles and co-workers (Burbaum et al. 1989) have pointed out that 'transition-state stabilization' and 'ground-state destabilization' are not in fact conceptually different since they both refer to a decrease in the activation energy for an elementary step which is shared between the ground state and the transition state. Binding interactions that preferentially discriminate between the substrate (or product) and the transition state characterize the theme referred to by Knowles and Albery as 'catalysis of an elementary step' (Albery & Knowles 1976, 1977, Knowles & Albery 1977).

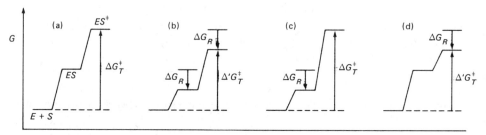

Fig. 4. Effect of a hypothetical mutational event on the free energy profile of a simple enzyme-catalysed reaction when $[S] < K_m$.
(a) Schematic Gibbs free energy profile for $E + S \underset{\rightleftharpoons}{\overset{K_m}{\longrightarrow}} ES \overset{k_{cat}}{\longrightarrow} E + P$ The rate of reaction, $v = (k_{cat}/K_m)[E]_0[S]$. The activation energy (ΔG_T^*) is for $E + S \rightarrow ES^*$. (See Fig. 3 legend for full details of symbols.) (b)–(d) Extra binding energy ΔG_R (algebraically negative) used to stabilize ES and ES^* (b); ES alone (c); or ES^* alone (d). $\Delta\Delta G_T^* = (\Delta'G_T^* - \Delta G_T^*) = \Delta G_R$ for cases (b) and (d) indicating an increase in rate. ΔG_T^* is unchanged in case (c) and so v is unaffected.

Figure 4(a) shows a Gibbs energy profile when the K_m for the enzyme is greater than the ambient substrate concentration. The free energy of ES is greater than that of $E + S$, and the reaction rate is $v = (k_{cat}/K_m)[E]_0[S]$ (Eq. (5)). The activation energy $(\Delta G_T^{\neq})$ is lowered by ΔG_R on the stabilization of $ES^{\neq}$ alone (catalysis of an elementary step) or ES and $ES^{\neq}$ together (universal binding) [see Figs 4c and 4d]. Stabilization of ES does not affect $\Delta G_T^{\neq}$, and there is no increase in rate (Fig. 4(b)).

The maximum value that (k_{cat}/K_m) can attain is the rate constant for a diffusion-controlled encounter between enzyme and substrate ($\sim 10^8 - 10^9 \mathrm{M}^{-1}\mathrm{s}^{-1}$). The Briggs–Haldane definition of (k_{cat}/K_m) for the simple two-step enzyme-catalysed reaction is given by $k_{+1}k_{+2}/(k_{-1} + k_{+2})$. The specificity constant is at its diffusion-controlled limit ($= k_{+1}$) when $k_{+2} \gg k_{-1}$. An unfavourable equilibrium constant for the reaction, over which an enzyme cannot exert any influence, may however impose a thermodynamic constraint on the upper limit for (k_{cat}/K_m) of less than the rate constant for a diffusion-controlled encounter (Fersht 1985, pp. 336–337). Fully evolved enzymes catalysing multi-step reactions whose fluxes cannot be increased any further are said to be diffusion-limited or diffusion-controlled. For these enzymes the chemical interconversion steps are extremely rapid and the highest barrier between $E + S$ and $E + P$ is either that for substrate binding or product release. The reaction catalysed by the glycolytic pathway enzyme triosephosphate isomerase has been confirmed to be diffusion-controlled (Blacklow *et al.* 1988).

In order that diffusional limitation should occur, the maximum barrier heights among the internal (enzyme-bound) states in a multi-step reaction must be similar to that for the diffusional process. Optimization of the free energies of the internal ground states (intermediates) and transition states ensures that no enzyme intermediate species accumulates to such an extent as to trap the enzyme in a thermodynamic pit.

Burbaum *et al.* (1989) have made a detailed analysis of the energetics of a reversible one-substrate/one-product reaction ($E + S \rightleftharpoons ES \rightleftharpoons EP \rightleftharpoons E + P$) comprising three transition states. The evolutionary optimization of the internal states was described in terms of uniform binding, catalysis of an elementary step, and a third type of binding interaction, 'differential binding'. Differential binding refers here to mutational events affecting the differential binding of substrate and product in the internal states (ES and EP) flanking the transition state for a single chemical step (Albery & Knowles 1976, 1977, Knowles & Albery 1977). Note that the relative free energies of ES and EP influence the energy level of the transition state between them. Changes in the internal equilibrium constant (K_{int}) between ES and EP can be related to changes in the kinetic barrier that joins them through the use of Brønsted-type rate-equilibrium relationships (see section 4.3). Alterations in the enzyme structure which lead to an optimization of the differential binding are viewed to be less probable (more discriminating) than those leading to the optimization of uniform binding, but are less discriminating than mutations which permit recognition of the fine structural and electronic differences between a transition state and flanking ground states (catalysis of an elementary step). For enzymes operating at equilibrium *in vivo* the optimum value for K_{int} is unity, that is when the free energy levels of ES and EP are equal. For an enzyme that operates far from equilibrium *in vivo*, K_{int} assumes a value that ensures that the rate of chemical transformation matches the rate of product release. The internal equilibrium constant for the amino acid activation step of the amino acylation of tRNA^{Tyr} catalysed by tyrosyl t-RNA synthetase (see Eq. (47)) is close to unity ($K_{int} = 2.3$). This compares to an equilibrium constant for the free substrates ([Tyr-AMP][PPi]/[Tyr][ATP]) of 4×10^{-7} (Wells and Fersht 1986). Tighter binding by the enzyme of the highly reactive Tyr-AMP compared to Tyr and ATP prevents its diffusion into solution where it would otherwise rapidly hydrolyse or acylate protein side chains (Fersht *et al.* 1986a).

4.3 Site-directed mutagenesis and linear free energy relationships (LFER)

The rational alteration of amino acid side chains by site-directed mutagenesis can be used to provide estimates of the energetic contributions of a particular residue to the overall catalytic power of the enzyme. Measurements of rate constants and dissociation constants along an enzyme reaction pathway are used to construct free energy profiles or kinetic barrier diagrams for the wild type and mutant enzymes. The general strategy is to make side chain replacements such that the molecular interactions of interest are effectively removed in the mutant protein. The substitutions should not cause disruptive structural changes in the enzyme molecule. Knowles (1987) has warned too of the dangers that substitutions may cause an alteration in the reaction mechanism through a change in the transition state of the rate-limiting step. The effect of the mutation should be localized and independent of other changes. For limited data sets the independence of two different substitutions can be established by making the double mutant (Carter *et al.* 1984).

With these caveats in mind, a comparison of the free energy profiles for the wild type and mutant enzymes enables the apparent energetic contributions (ΔG_{App}) of the interaction to binding and catalysis to be calculated for each ground-state intermediate and transition state along the reaction pathway. Loss of steric contacts (van der Waals' interactions) with the substrate may be achieved by side-chain shortening. Hydrogen-bonding interactions may be removed by replacement with shorter or isoteric residues lacking the functional groups capable of forming hydrogen bonds (for example Tyr → Phe or Ser → Ala). In general, however, the incremental energy of a hydrogen bond (ΔG_{Bind}) is not measured by ΔG_{App} (Fersht 1988, Fersht *et al.* 1985). This is because removal by mutagenesis of a side chain engaged in hydrogen bond formation with a substrate may leave an unpaired charged or uncharged hydrogen bond donor or acceptor on the substrate if water is unable to gain access to the cavity in the mutant enzyme. Furthermore, even if the substrate can be solvated, the properties of water in the active-site region may differ somewhat from those of bulk water, and so ΔG_{App} may still not be an accurate measure of ΔG_{Bind}. Fersht (1988) has suggested, however, that values of the changes in ΔG_{App} ($\Delta\Delta G_{App}$) as the reaction proceeds can often be used to measure the true changes in binding energies ($\Delta\Delta G_{Bind}$) in the corresponding states.

The classical approach to probing transition-state structure in the reactions of simple organic molecules has been to use linear free energy relationships (LFER) such as the Brønsted and Hammet plots. The Brønsted equation (Brønsted & Petersen 1924) relates the rates of similar reactions to equilibrium constants in a systematic way through the exponent, β:

$$k = A K_{eq}^{\beta} \tag{44}$$

where A is a constant, and K_{eq} and k are the equilibrium and rate constants respectively, for a series of related reactions in which a substituent has affected the rate and equilibrium but not the mechanism. A plot of log k against log K_{eq} is a straight line with slope β when Eq. (44) holds:

$$\log k = constant + \beta K_{eq} \tag{45}$$

From transition-state theory log k is proportional to the free energy of activation of the reaction $\Delta G^{\neq}$ (see Eq. (38)), and from equilibrium thermodynamics log K_{eq} is proportional to the free energy change for the equilibrium, ΔG_{eq}. Eq. (45) is equivalent to

$$\Delta G^{\neq} = constant + \beta \Delta G_{eq} \tag{46}$$

The exponent β may be experimentally evaluated and used in relating the transition state and reactant or product ground states. For example, measurements could be made of the second-order rate constants (k) for the attack of a series of nucleophiles on a particular ester or for general base-catalysed ester hydrolysis by different buffer systems. Values of β can then be obtained from the slopes of linear Brønsted plots of log k against the pK_as of the nucleophiles or bases. Similar Brønsted relationships are found when the rate constants for the attack of a particular nucleophile on a series of esters with differing leaving groups are plotted against the pKa's of the leaving groups.

For general base-catalysed reactions values of β are always between 0 and 1, and for ester hydrolysis usually in the range 0.3–0.5. The value of β may be interpreted in terms of the degree of hydron (proton) transfer that has occurred (or charge developed) in the transition state of the reaction. For complete transfer $\beta = 1$, and this represents specific catalysis. A value of zero, corresponding to no hydron transfer, indicates that the reaction is insensitive to general catalysis. The same considerations apply in the interpretation of Brønsted plots of nucleophilic reactions in which the catalytic species becomes directly attached to the substrate molecule. For those reactions, however, the value of β can be outside of the range 0–1.

Fersht et al. (1986b, 1987) have applied LFERs in the form of Eq. (44) to changes in binding energies that occur in hydrogen-bond deletion mutants of tyrosyl t-RNA synthetase. The enzyme catalyses the formation of enzyme-bound tyrosyl-adenylate (E.Tyr-AMP) and free pyrophosphate (PPi) from tyrosine and ATP through the intermediacy of an E.Tyr-AMP.PPi ternary complex:

$$
\begin{array}{ccccccc}
Tyr & & ATP & & k_3 & & K_{pp} \\
E & \rightleftharpoons E.Tyr & \rightleftharpoons & E.Tyr.ATP & \rightleftharpoons & E.Tyr-AMP.PPi & \rightleftharpoons E.Tyr-AMP \quad (47) \\
K_t & & K_a & & k_{-3} & &
\end{array}
$$

The catalysis utilizes substrate binding energy alone without the apparent involvement of classical general acid–base or covalent catalysis (Fersht 1987a). Kinetic data for the formation of E.Tyr-AMP.PPi from E.Tyr.ATP reported by Fersht et al. (1986b, 1987) for non-disruptive mutations of residues Tyr 34, Cys 35, His 48, Thr 41, and Tyr 169 in the binding sites for tyrosine and for the ATP ribose ring are reproduced in Fig. 5a as a plot of log k_3 against log (k_3/k_{-3}). The data conform to the relationship:

$$
k_3 = A(k_3/k_{-3})^\beta \tag{48}
$$

where A and β are constants. Fersht et al. (1986b, 1987) calculated a value of 0.79 for β, corresponding to the slope of the plot shown in Fig. 5a. This was interpreted quantitatively as indicating that 79% of the binding energy change on going from E.Tyr.ATP to E.Tyr-AMP.PPi is realized in the transition state $(E.[Tyr.ATP]^{\neq})$ for the reaction. In qualitative terms this means that the transition state resembles the product ground state (E.Tyr-AMP.PPi) far more closely (but not entirely) than it does the E.Tyr.ATP complex with respect to the pattern of hydrogen bonding interactions involved. As previously mentioned in section 4.2, tyrosyl t-RNA synthetase binds tyrosyl-adenylate and pyrophosphate more tightly than tyrosine and ATP (Wells & Fersht 1986).

This type of binding interaction provides an example of 'differential' binding (Albery & Knowles 1976, 1977, Burbaum et al. 1989) and can be achieved through the agency of groups on the enzyme surface that bind non-reacting parts of the substrate more tightly in the enzyme-product complex than in the enzyme–substrate and enzyme–transition-state complexes. Fersht et al. (1987), using several different Brønsted plots to systematize kinetic and thermodynamic equilibria data for mutants predominantly affecting the binding of the ribose ring, were able to quantify the progressive utilization of the binding energy of adenosine as the reaction proceeds from E.Tyr to E.Tyr-AMP (see Eq. (47)); β values were used to measure the fractional changes in binding energy for particular processes.

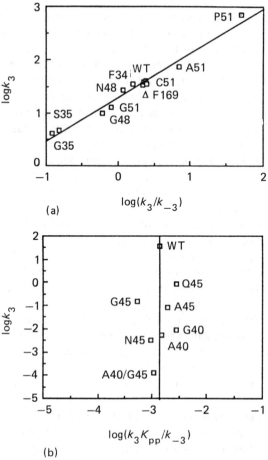

Fig. 5. (a) Linear free energy plot for mutations in the binding site for tyrosine (Y34F, Y169F) and the ribose of ATP (C35G, C35S, H48G, H48N, T51G, T51A and T51C) in tyrosyl t-RNA synthetase. (b) Linear free energy plot for mutations in the transition-state binding site for the λ-phosphate of ATP (T40A; H45G, H45A, H45N, H45Q) in tyrosyl t-RNA synthetase (reproduced with permission from Fersht *et al.* 1987).

The applicability of LFERs to the analysis of such site-directed mutagenesis experiments has, however, been questioned by Straub & Karplus (1990). They concluded that when mutants differ solely through the formation or deletion of a hydrogen bond away from the seat of reaction, a LFER is to be expected only in limiting cases for which the Brønsted exponent is 0, 1 or ∞, and that fractional values of β are not permissible. Their argument is based on the reasoning that because the energy of a hydrogen bond varies non-linearly with distance or orientation (see, for example, Baker & Hubbard 1984), there is no guarantee of a simple relation between the reaction coordinate and the Brønsted exponent for mutations removed from the active-centre. Straub & Karplus (1990) interpreted the value of $\beta \sim 0.8$ obtained by Fersht *et al.* (1986b,1987) as being sufficiently close to unity for linearity to be observed over the experimental range (see Fig. 5a). According to this interpretation both E.[Tyr.ATP]$^{\neq}$ and the product (E.Tyr-AMP.PPi) ground state are equally stabilized by these hydrogen bonds.

In reply, Fersht & Wells (1991) claim that the fractional value obtained for β of ~ 0.8 is genuine, and the probability of it being 1.0 is <0.01 (see section 6A, Fersht 1987b, Wells & Fersht 1989). Indeed, the difference free energy diagrams for individual mutants (see Fersht *et al.* 1986a, Leatherbarrow & Fersht 1987) support the view that the binding energy of many of the side chains is only partly realized in the E.[Tyr.ATP]$^{\neq}$ transition state. Moreover, Fersht & Wells (1991) point out that LFERs do not in general require a linear relationship between bond energies and bond distances.

To illustrate this they have used a simple model to describe differential binding. In the model each of a set of (i) non-covalent interactions in an enzyme-substrate (*ES*) intermediate changes in strength by ΔG_i (relative to *ES*) on formation of the enzyme–product(s) complex. If, as the reaction proceeds through the enzyme–transition-state complex, the gain in strength of each bond is $\beta_i \Delta G_i$ (again relative to *ES*), then a LFER in binding interactions in non-reacting parts of the substrate can arise when each member of the set contributes the same fraction of the final energy change in the transition-state complex; that is, when the value of β_i is the same (β) for each bond. The value of β from such LFERs measures the fraction of the energy of the non-covalent interactions manifested in the transition state, and need not be limited to 0, 1, or ∞. However, Fersht & Wells (1991) emphasize that interactions in enzyme–substrate complexes are often unique (that is, belong to a set with only one member $i = 1$) and so the results of mutagenesis are specific to that mutation.

Figure 5b shows an LFER for a second set of deletion of mutants of Thr 40 and His 45 in tyrosyl t-RNA synthetase (Fersht *et al.* 1986b, 1987). Mutation of these residues markedly affects the rate constant k_3, whilst the equilibrium constant between E.Tyr.ATP and E.Tyr-AMP is hardly changed. Here the interpretation of the experimentally observed Brønsted plot slope value ($\beta = \infty$) is more straightforward as it constitutes a limiting case (Straub & Karplus 1990). Thus residues Thr 40 and His 45 bind the transition state strongly but do not contribute any stabilization energy to the ground states ('catalysis of an elementary step'). Earlier model building studies (Leatherbarrow *et al.* 1985) had predicted that these residues would hydrogen bond with the γ phosphate of ATP in the penta-coordinate transition state but not in the ground-state (E.Tyr.ATP).

5. TRANSIENT KINETICS OF SYSTEMS FAR FROM EQUILIBRIUM

5.1 Enzyme-catalysed reactions

The transient or pre-steady state phase of an enzyme-catalysed reaction is, as its name suggests, the period after the mixing of enzyme and substrate but before the concentrations of all the enzyme species reach their steady-state levels. Steady-state kinetic measurements are limited in their ability to provide information about individual steps along an enzyme reaction pathway necessary for the construction of free energy profiles. However, the detection of intermediates and measurements of rate constants can often be achieved on the ms time scale by using rapid mixing techniques (Fersht 1985, pp. 121–124) such as stopped-flow (Gibson & Milnes 1964) and pulsed-quenched flow (Fersht & Jakes 1975) to monitor reactions far from equilibrium. In steady-state experiments observations of the reactants or products are made, but in transient kinetic experiments the observed events occur on the enzyme itself, so much larger enzyme concentrations are required, typically in the range 10^{-6}–10^{-5} M.

Integrated-rate equations describing the time course of enzyme intermediate and product formation during the transient phase are obtained by solution of the set of differential rate equations for the reaction mechanism. Analytical solutions can be derived by assuming that the substrate is present in excess over the total enzyme concentration ($[S]_0 \gg [E]_0$), thus enabling the (free) substrate concentration to be treated as a constant. Alternatively, in the case of single-turnover kinetics it is the enzyme which is in excess ($[E]_0 \gg [S]_0$). One of the most convenient methods for the manual solution of a set of differential rate equations is the Laplace–Carson operator method (Roberts 1977, pp. 279–284), an extension of the ordinary Laplace transform. In this method an integral operator transform is obtained for each species, the solution of which can be found from mathematical tables. Zhang et al. (1989) have described a computer program for the solution of transient kinetic equations using the Laplace transform. Integrated-rate equations for many common enzyme mechanisms are available in the literature, and Varón et al. (1990) have outlined procedures for the derivation of transient phase equations as special cases of equations already known for more complex kinetic mechanisms.

The time-dependence for the formation of the first product (P_1) in the irreversible three-step acyl enzyme mechanism (Eq. (12)), under conditions of substrate excess ($[S] \gg [E]_0$) is well known (see, for example, Roberts 1977, pp. 146–167):

$$[P]_1 = \frac{k_{cat}[S][E]_0}{K_m + [S]} \cdot t + \sum_{i=1}^{2} \alpha_i (1 - e^{-\lambda_i t}) \tag{49}$$

where the first-order rate constants are (λ_i) are:

$$\lambda_i = [A + \sqrt{(A^2 - 4B)}]/2$$

$$\lambda_2 = [A - \sqrt{A^2 - 4B}]/2$$

$$A = (k_{+1}[S] + k_{-1} + k_{+2} + k_{+3}) = (\lambda_1 + \lambda_2)$$

$$B = k_{+1}(k_{+2} + k_{+3})(K_m + [S]) = \lambda_1 \lambda_2$$

and the corresponding amplitudes (α_i):

$$\alpha_i = \frac{(k_{+1} k_{+2}[S][E]_0(\lambda_i - k_{+3})}{\lambda_i^2(\lambda_j - \lambda_i)} j = 1,2; \ i \neq j$$

The two amplitudes (α_1 and α_2) have opposite sign. Their sum (π) is often referred to as the 'burst-size' and is given by:

$$\pi = \sum_{i=1}^{2} \alpha_i = \frac{k_{+2}[S][E]_0(k_{+1}k_{+2}[S] - k_{+3}^2)}{k_{+1}(k_{+2} + k_{+3})^2(K_m + [S])^2} \tag{50}$$

Equation (49) describes a biphasic exponential approach to a linear steady-state rate $v = k_{cat}[S][E]_0/(K_m + [S])$. The definitions of k_{cat} and K_m are as given previously in Eqs. (19) and (20). In general, if there are n enzyme species then there will be $(n-1)$ transients (Pettersen 1978). Analogous integrated-rate expressions may be derived for the second product, P_2 and the three enzyme species (E, ES and ES'). These can be found in Roberts (1977, pp. 152–154). The equations for the various enzyme species do not contain a term in t, however, since their concentrations are independent of time during the steady-state period after the decay of the two exponential terms.

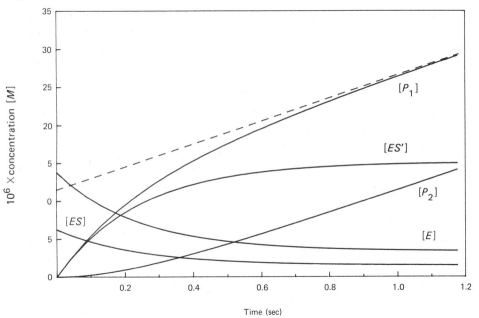

Fig. 6. Transient kinetics of the 3-step acyl enzyme mechanism [eqn. (12)] with $S] \gg [E]_0$. The time courses of formation of the products P_1 and P_2 and the various enzyme species for the approach to the steady-state phase of the reaction are shown. The set of differential rate equations describing the mechanism were solved numerically by means of a variable-order, variable-step formulation of the method of Gear (see Hall & Watt 1976) for stiff systems of differential equations using the NAG FORTRAN subroutine DO2EBF (PC50 Library, Release 1). Values for the initial concentrations and kinetic parameters were as follows: $[E]_0 = 2.0 \times 10^{-5}$M; $[S] = 2.273 \times 10^{-3}$M $(5K_m)$; $k_{+1} = 1.0 \times 10^{-7}$M^{-1}s^{-1}; $k_{-1} = 5.0 \times 10^4$s^{-1}; $k_{+2} = 10.0$ s^{-1}; $k_{+3} = 1.0$ s^{-1}. The dashed line was constructed as $[P_1] = \pi + vt$ and represents the linear steady-state rate extrapolated back to zero-time. The burst-size (π) is 1.148×10^{-5}M or 57.4% of the total enzyme concentration ($[E]_0$).

Figure 6 shows the time courses of formation of the products and enzyme species under conditions of substrate excess with a rate-limiting deacylation step ($k_{+3} \ll k_{+2}$, k_{-1} and $k_{+1}[S]$). The enzyme exists predominantly as the acyl-enzyme intermediate (ES') in the steady state. It is not necessary for ES' to be formed before P_1 is released, and so in the transient phase P_1 can be formed at a rate much greater than the steady-state rate giving rise to a 'burst' when the linear portion of the progress curve is extrapolated back to zero time. The formation of the second product, P_2, on the other hand displays a 'lag'. For a positive burst size ($\pi > 0$) as in Fig. 6, it can be seen from Eq. (50) that $k_{+1}k_{+2}[S] \gg k_{+3}^2$, If, however, $k_{+1}k_{+2}[S] \gg k_{+3}^2$, then this equation reduces to:

$$\pi = \frac{k_{+2}^2[E]_0[S]^2}{(k_{+2} + k_{+3})^2(K_m + [S])^2} \tag{51}$$

If in addition $[S] \gg K_m$ and $k_{+2} \gg k_{+3}$, π collapses to $[E]_0$ or the total concentration of enzyme active sites. This provides an effective method for titrating enzymes. Schonbaum *et al.* (1961) found that *trans*-cinnamoylimidazole reacts rapidly at pH 5.5 with chymotrypsin to give imidazole (P_1) and *trans*-cinnamoyl-chymotrypsin (ES'), but no further reaction occurs readily, that is, $k_3 \approx 0$. Measurement of the amount of release imidazole provides a measure of the amount of active enzyme. Suitable titrants for a number of other enzymes have also been found (see, for example, Bender *et al.* 1966).

Although the time courses shown in Fig. 6 were constructed by using numerical integration they could equally well have been drawn by using Eq. (49) and the corresponding exact analytical solutions for the other species. In practice, however, the first fast transient of Eq. (49) is not normally observable. In mathematical terms this means that the (real) roots of the secular equation (λ_1, λ_2) differ considerably in magnitude (Pettersson 1976,1978): $\lambda_1 \gg \lambda_2$, $\pi = \alpha_2 \gg |\alpha_1|$, and Eq. (49) can be approximated by:

$$[P_1] = vt + \pi(1 - e^{-k_{App}t}) \tag{52}$$

where k_{App} is a substrate concentration-dependent rate constant describing a single exponential approach to the steady state. This rate constant can be defined as:

$$k_{App} = \frac{k_{+1}(k_{+2} + k_{+3})(K_m + [S])}{k_{+1}[S] + k_{-1} + k_{+2} + k_{+3}} = \frac{X_1(K_m + [S])}{X_2 + [S]} \tag{53}$$

where X_1 and X_2 are constants:

$$X_1 = (k_{+2} + k_{+3})$$
$$X_2 = (k_{-1} + k_{+2} + k_{+3})/k_{+1}.$$

The dependence of k_{App} on $[S]$ may be exploited experimentally, and estimates of X_1 and X_2 obtained by non-linear regression analysis (section 6) assuming a knowledge of K_m from steady-state measurements. It will be noted that in the limit $[S] \to 0$,

$$\underset{[S]\to 0}{k_{App}} = \frac{k_{+3}(k_{-1} + k_{+2})}{(k_{-1} + k_{+2} + k_{+3})} = \frac{X_1 K_m}{X_2} \tag{54}$$

and so $X_1 K_m/X_2$ approximates to k_{+3} when $k_{+3} \ll (k_{-1} + k_{+2})$ [cf. Bender *et al.*

1966, Aducci et al. 1988, Ascenzi et al. 1989]. It is likely that this inequality will hold in many cases of practical interest. More generally, individual estimates of k_{+2} and k_{+3} may be determined from estimates of X_1 and k_{cat} provided that the latter is known:

$$k_{+2}, k_{+3} = [X_1 \pm \sqrt{(X_1^2 - 4k_{cat}X_1)}]/2 \tag{55}$$

In theory there is also sufficient available information to be able to determine k_{-1} (and hence k_{+1}) from Eq. (56).

$$k_{-1} = \frac{K_m X_1^2 - k_{+2}k_{+3}X_2}{k_{+3}X_2 - X_1 K_m} \tag{56}$$

However, in practice small errors in the measured parameters will lead to enormous errors in k_{-1}. A more reliable way to determine k_{+1} is from the dependence of K_m/k_{cat} on viscosity (see Hardy & Kirsh, 1984, Blacklow et al. 1988, Christensen et al. 1990).

5.2 Partial reactions
Transient kinetic measurements of rate constants in enzyme mechanisms are not restricted to complete catalyses. Partial reactions may be studied as well. An example of this is the ligand displacement method (Gibson & Roughton, 1955, Kvassman & Pettersson 1979) to determine 'off' rate constants for ligands (L_1) from their complexes with the free enzyme (EL_1). In the case of enzymes which catalyse multi-substrate reactions the ligand could be a substrate or a coenzyme since catalytic turnover cannot occur in the absence of the other substrate(s). Enzyme and ligand L_1 are pre-incubated and the equilibrium mixture placed in one syringe of the stopped-flow apparatus. The other syringe is filled with a high concentration of a second displacing ligand (L_2) and the contents of the two syringes rapidly mixed. Provided that some suitable spectroscopic signal is available, an apparent rate constant, r_{App}, may be determined from the observed time course of the displacement reaction at each of several fixed concentrations of L_2.

$$EL_1 \underset{k_1}{\overset{k_1}{\rightleftharpoons}} E \overset{\substack{L_2 \\ \downarrow k_2}}{\underset{k_{-2}}{\rightleftharpoons}} EL_2 \tag{57}$$

$$\Big\downarrow{\scriptstyle k_1}$$
$$L_1$$

Strictly speaking the time course will be biphase $[(n-1) = 2]$, but often the fast transient will not be seen and its amplitude will be negligible. If both ligands are present in large excess over the enzyme, such that their free and total concentrations can be equated, then according to Kvassman & Pettersson (1979):

$$\frac{1}{r_{App}} = \frac{1}{k_{-1}} \cdot \left[1 + \frac{k_1[L_1]}{k_2[L_2])} \right] \tag{58}$$

When Eq. (58) applies, a plot of $1/r_{App}$ versus $1/[L_2]$ will be a straight line. The ordinate intercept is equal to $1/k_{-1}$ (or the reciprocal 'off' rate constant) and the slope provides direct information about the ratio of the two 'on' rate constants (k_1/k_2).

The displacement method has been used to determine the 'off' rate constants for the dissociation of the coenzyme NADPH from the respective complexes formed with the NADP$^+$-linked oxidative decarboxylases, isocitrate dehydrogenase (Fatania et al. 1982), and 6-phosphogluconate dehydrogenase (Topham et al. 1986). The fluorescence of NADPH is enhanced in binary complexes formed with these enzymes. The displacement of NADPH (L_1) by NADP$^+$ $(L_2$ which has no intrinsic nucleotide fluorescence) can therefore be followed in a stopped-flow fluorimeter. However, it is not practical to use a large excess of free NADPH over enzyme-bound NADPH, and so Eq. (58) does not apply. Computer simulation studies were used to investigate the deviations from this equation that occur when equimolar concentrations of enzyme and reduced coenzyme are used (Fatania et al. 1982). These showed that over a range of relatively low concentrations of the displacing agent (NADP$^+$), r_{App} was either an overestimate or an underestimate of k_{-1} (k_{off}) depending on the values of the rate constants in the reaction mechanism shown in Eq. (57). In all cases, however, r_{App} approached k_{off} as the level of [NADP$^+$] was increased in the numerical integration analysis.

6.   KINETIC PARAMETER DETERMINATION AND MODEL DISCRIMINATION

6.1   Least-squares procedures

Parameter estimation in enzyme kinetics is commonly achieved by fitting a set of experimental data to a model (for example, the Michaelis–Menten equation), using weighted non-linear regression analysis (Mannervik 1981, Leatherbarrow 1990a). Most procedures use the principle of least squares according to which the regression function Y is iteratively minimized:

$$Y = \sum_{i=1}^{n} w_i(x_i - \hat{x}_i)^2 \tag{59}$$

where x_i and $\hat{x}_i$ are the observed and calculated values of the dependent variable of the ith measurement, and w_i is a weighting factor to compensate for unequal variance in the experimental data. The initial rate, v, is the dependent variable in the Michaelis–Menten equation. The difference $(x_i - \hat{x}_i)$ is called the residual. The calculated (or predicted) value is a function of the independent variable(s) (substrate concentration in the case of the Michaelis–Menten equation) and the current estimates of the model parameters (that is, K_m and V). Minimization of Y by searching for optimal combinations of parameter values is continued until some (arbitrary) convergence criterion between successive iterations is met. Several computer programs are available for non-linear regression analysis with facilities for specifying the regression function directly, thus avoiding the difficulties of defining partial derivatives with respect to each parameter. These include the AR program from the BMDP statistical software package (Dixon *et al.* 1988) and Leatherbarrow's ENZfitter (1987) and GraFit (1990b) programs.

After convergence the value of Y is referred to as the residual sum of squares (SS) and is a measure of the goodness of fit of the model to the data set. A model with p parameters has $(n - p)$ degrees of freedom and a mean sum of squares (Q^2) for n data points:

$$Q^2 = SS/(n - p) \tag{60}$$

The four principal assumptions that must be satisfied for least-squares calculations to provide minimum variance parameter estimates are (Cornish-Bowden 1981): (i) only the dependent variable is subject to error; (ii) errors are random rather than systematic; (iii) the correct weights, w_i are known; (iv) errors in the dependent variable are normally distributed.

The first assumption is probably reasonable for many purposes in enzyme kinetics since typical independent variables such as substrate concentration, time, pH, etc. can all be reasonably accurately measured. In such cases the ratio of the error variances on the Y axis, and the X axis tends to infinity. One obvious exception to this situation is for data used to construct linear free energy relationships such as those shown in Fig. 5. Here the error variance ratio can often be close to unity (Wells & Fersht 1989), and there is said to be a functional relationship between the two variables. Wells & Fersht (1989) have outlined a regression analysis procedure to find the maximum likelihood estimator, b, for the slope β. An expression is also given for calculating confidence limits for b. The second assumption depends ultimately on good experimental design for which no amount of statistical manipulation can compensate.

The calculation of weighting factors (assumption (iii)) is dependent upon a knowledge of the experimental variance since it is seldom reasonable to assume kinetic data to be homoscedastic (that is, to have equal variance or constant absolute error) when wide ranges of the dependent variable are measured. The error structure may be investigated by making replicate measurements of the dependent variable. However, this requires many replicates and in any event the estimated variance so obtained in such artificial experiments may be too small and not representative of the error in normal kinetic experiments lacking replicates (Mannervik *et al.* 1979, Cornish-Bowden 1981). An alternative approach is the analysis of residuals (Mannervik *et al.* 1979, Mannervik 1981,1982). Residuals obtained from a preliminary unbiased least-squares fit to a model, preferably an over-determined equation, are taken to represent the experimental error. Neighbouring residuals (q_i) are ordered into groups of 5 or 6 (m), and the local variance ($\sigma_{(x)}^2$) taken as the sum of their mean-squared values:

$$\frac{1}{m} \sum_{i=1}^{m} q_i^2 \tag{61}$$

The error structure of initial-rate measurements (v) in enzyme kinetics has attracted particular interest, and several empirical models have been described in the literature (see, for example, Askelöf et al. 1976, Cornish-Bowden & Endrenyi 1981, Mannervik 1981, Mannervik et al. 1988). These models can be tested by regression analysis of the local experimental error, $\sigma_{(v)}$ (that is, $\sigma_{(x)}$), as a function (of the median values) of the corresponding predicted (calculated) initial-rates for each of the (m) groups. One such empirical error function is shown in Eq. (62) where K_1 and K_2 are parameters:

$$\sigma_{(v)} = K_1 v^{K_2} \qquad (62)$$

This error function provides for each of the two most common assumptions about error structure as particular cases, that is, a constant absolute error structure when $K_2 = 0$ and thus $\sigma_{(v)} = K_1$, and a constant relative error structure when $K_2 = 1$ and thus $\sigma_{(v)} = K_1 v$. The value of K_2 is not constrained to be either 0 or 1, although a simple physical significance of other situations is not obvious. The error function Eq. (63) treats experimental error as the sum of constant absolute error and constant relative error components, and is more easily understood therefore in physical terms.

$$\sigma_{(v)} = K_1 + K_2 v \qquad (63)$$

Recent studies of error structure in steady-state enzyme kinetic experiments by Mannervik et al. (1986) and Danielson & Mannervik (1988) suggest that, contrary to the general view, error (in v) is not governed by the measured dependent variable (that is, v), but by independent variables (such as concentration of substrate or added inhibitor, etc.). Investigations using residual analysis of the error structure describing the pH-dependence of (k_{cat}/K_m) for the papain-catalysed hydrolysis of N^α-benzoyl-L-arginine p-nitroanilide (L-Bz-Arg-NH-Np) in alkaline media support this view (C.M. Topham, E. Salih, and K. Brocklehurst, unpublished). Better regression fits (as judged by small values of Q^2 in Eq. (60)) of the estimated experimental error in (k_{cat}/K_m) were obtained for two pH error functions (see Fig. 7)) than for four empirical error functions of (k_{cat}/K_m) including the two given above in Eqs. (62) and (63) (with v replaced by (k_{cat}/K_m)).

Having established an appropriate error function describing the experimental variance, weighting factors in the regression equation (Eq. (59)) can be calculated. The weights are inversely proportional to the experimental variance of the dependent variable, x:

$$w_i \propto 1/\sigma_{(x_i)}^2 \qquad (64)$$

Figure 8 shows the results of a weighted non-linear regression analysis of kinetic data for the pH-dependence of (k_{cat}/K_m) for the hydrolysis of L-Bz-Arg-NH-Np by papain in alkaline media. The analysis clearly demonstrates the existence of two kinetically influential ionizations (Scheme 1) with pKa values of 8.0 and 9.6, rather than a single ionization as is generally supposed. The difficulty in distinguishing some overlapping double ionizations from a single ionization has been discussed by Brocklehurst et al. (1983).

Statistical procedures can be helpful in discriminating between alternative kinetic models. These include the F-test and the examination of residuals for systematic

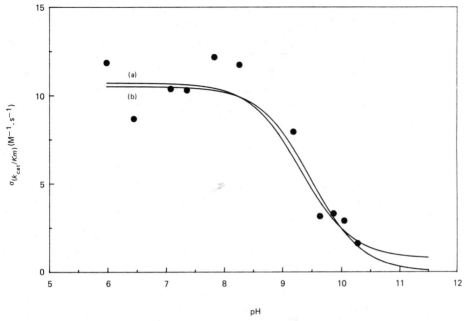

Fig. 7. Estimated experimental error in (k_{cat}/K_m) for the pH-dependent kinetics of the papain-catalysed hydrolysis of L-Bz-Arg-NH-Np in alkaline media plotted as a function of pH. The local error $(\sigma_{(kcat/Km)})$ was determined by residual analysis (Mannervik *et al.* 1979) of the experimental data (C.M. Topham, E. Salih, and K. Brocklehurst, unpublished) shown in Fig. 8. Data were fitted to two error functions using weighted non-linear regression analysis:

(a) $$\sigma_{(k_{cat}/K_m)} = \frac{K_1}{1 + K_2/[H^+]} + K_3$$

and

(b) $$\sigma_{(k_{cat}/K_m)} = \frac{K_1}{1 + K_2/[H^+]}$$

The solid curves were drawn by using best-fit estimates of the parameters: $k_1 = 9.95 \pm 0.93$ $M^{-1}s^{-1}$, $K_2 = 4.91 \pm 1.85 \times 10^{-10}M$, and $K_3 = 0.76 \pm 0.56$ $M^{-1}s^{-1}$ (curve a) and $K_1 = 10.50 \pm 0.82$ $M^{-1}s^{-1}$ and $K_2 = 3.32 \pm 0.58 \times 10^{-10}M$ (curve b). Curve (a) is a slightly better fit to the data.

trends (Mannervik 1981,1982, Ellis & Duggleby 1978). However, Mannervik (1982) has drawn attention to certain limitations in the application of the F-test. One caveat is that the significance levels calculated by use of the F-statistic are fully reliable only for models which (unlike most rate equations) are linear in the parameters. Secondly, the test is apppropriate only for distinguishing between kinetic models that are interconvertible by addition or elimination of terms.

6.2   Biweight regression: a robust version of least squares
The fourth assumption about least-squares analysis to be considered (assumption (iv) in section 6.1 above) relates to departures from the assumed normal distribution of errors in the dependent variable. One such example is the presence of outliers which

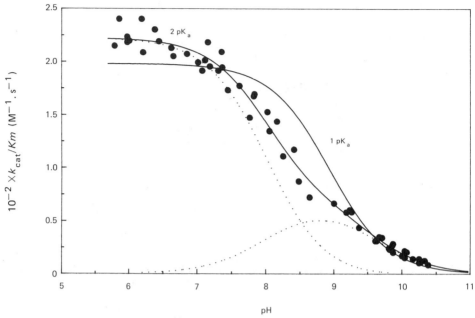

Fig. 8. pH-dependence of (k_{cat}/K_m) for the hydrolysis of L-Bz-Arg-NH-Np catalysed by papain in alkaline media. Experimental data (C.M. Topham, E. Salih, and K. Brocklehurst, unpublished) were fitted to two kinetic models (A and B of Scheme 1) using weighted non-linear regression analysis. The weighting scheme used was based on pH error function (a) of Fig. 7 with weights $\alpha \ \sigma_{(k_{cat}/K_m)}^{-2}$). The continuous solid line denoted 1 pK_a is theoretical for:

$$(k_{cat}/K_m) = \frac{\tilde{k}_{EHS}/\tilde{K}_{EHS}}{1 + K_{EH}/[H^+]}$$

corresponding to the single kinetically influential pK_a model (A) of Scheme 1. The line was constructed by using best-fit estimates of $\tilde{k}_{EHS} = 198.1 \pm 5.2 \ M^{-1}s^{-1}$ and p$K_{EH} = 8.93 \pm 0.04$. The solid line donated 2pK_a is theoretical for:

$$(k_{cat}/K_m) = \frac{\tilde{k}_{EH_2S}/\tilde{K}_{EH_2S}}{1 + \dfrac{K_{EH_2}}{[H^+]} + \dfrac{K_{EH}K_{EH_2}}{[H^+]^2}} + \frac{\tilde{k}_{EHS}/\tilde{K}_{EHS}}{1 + \dfrac{K_{EH}}{[H^+]} + \dfrac{[H^+]}{K_{EH_2}}}$$

and corresponds to the two pK_a model (B) shown in Scheme 1. The line was drawn by using best-fit of $\tilde{k}_{EH_2} = 222.6 \pm 3.3 \ M^{-1}s^{-1}$, $\tilde{k}_{EHS} = 66.70 \pm 8.9 \ M^{-1}s^{-1}$, p$K_{EH} = 9.60 \pm 0.08$ and p$K_{EH2} = 8.00 \pm 0.08$. The dotted-line curves show the two constituent components.

are poor observations occurring at a higher frequency than allowed for by the normal distribution (Cornish-Bowden *et al.* 1978, Atkins & Nimmo 1980, 1981). This can have a serious effect on the residual sum of squares in the regression analysis. A more robust approach is to employ a biweight regression procedure (Cornish-Bowden 1981, Cornish-Bowden & Endrenyi 1981, Mosteller & Tukey 1977). Weights (w_i) used in the first iteration are replaced in subsequent iterations by a modified set of weights (W_i) successively adjusted in accordance with the magnitudes of deviations found in the previous iteration. Thus, W_i is approximately the same as w_i for

Scheme 1.   Single (A) and double (B) active ionization state kinetic model for the acylation of papain (E) by L-Bz-Arg-NH-NP (S) in alkaline media.

A

$$
\begin{array}{ccc}
& \tilde{K}_{EHS} & \tilde{k}_{EHS} \\
EH + S & \rightleftharpoons\ EHS & \rightarrow\ EHS' + P_1 \\
K_{EH}\ \updownarrow & \updownarrow & \\
E + S & \rightleftharpoons\ ES &
\end{array}
$$

B

$$
\begin{array}{ccc}
& \tilde{K}_{EH_2} & \tilde{k}_{EH_2S} \\
EH_2 + S & \rightleftharpoons\ EH_2S & \rightarrow\ EH_2S' + P_1 \\
K_{EH_2}\ \updownarrow & \updownarrow & \\
& \tilde{K}_{EHS} & \tilde{k}_{EHS} \\
EH + S & \rightleftharpoons\ EHS & \rightarrow\ EHS' + P_1 \\
K_{EH}\ \updownarrow & \updownarrow & \\
E + S & \rightleftharpoons\ ES &
\end{array}
$$

EH_2S and EHS are adsorptive complexes that lead to the production of acyl enzyme intermediates EH_2S' and EHS' respectively with concomitant formation of p-nitroaniline (P_1). The relative stoichiometries in hydrons (protons) of the enzyme states are indicated, although the relative ionic charges have been omitted. When acylation is rate-determining, as in the case of the catalysed hydrolysis of L-Bz-Arg-NH-Np, the regeneration of enzyme forms from the acyl-enzyme intermediates (not shown) is rapid.

observations with small or moderate residuals, but small or zero weights are given to observations with large residuals.

6.3   The median method: a robust alternative to least squares
The median method is a statistical method for curve fitting that makes fewer assumptions than least squares about the nature of the underlying error (Cornish-Bowden 1981, Atkins & Nimmo 1981). A specific application of the median method for fitting a straight line is the direct-linear plot of the Michaelis–Menten equation in parameter space (Eisenthal & Cornish-Bowden 1974, Cornish-Bowden & Eisenthal 1974, 1978, Porter & Trager 1977, Cornish-Bowden et al. 1978, Cornish-Bowden 1981). In its original form the axes of the direct-linear plot refer to the parameters

to be estimated (that is, K_m and V), and each observation of $[S]_i$ and v_i is represented by a straight line rather than a point. Each pair of lines intersects to provide an estimate $K_{m(ij)}$ of K_m and an estimate $V_{(ij)}$ of V. The medians of the two series are taken as best estimates. In the revised version of the direct-linear plot the axes are K_m/V and $1/V$, but median estimates of $1/V$ and K_m/V can readily be converted into the corresponding estimates of V and K_m. In practice the method is essentially computational rather than graphical, and Henderson (1985) has published a FOR-TRAN program of the algorithm.

There is a requirement that errors in v be uncorrelated with one another and as likely to be positive as negative. In addition the values of $[S]$ should be in their correct rank order. There is no need for weighting, and the presence of outliers should make little difference to the median parameter estimates. The direct-linear plot compares well in Monte Carlo trials with least squares methods, particularly when outliers are present or the least squares calculations are performed by using the wrong weights (Cornish-Bowden 1981). Median methods can be applied to other two-parameter models, but cannot be easily extended to models with more parameters.

REFERENCES

Aducci, P., Ascenzi, P., Amiconi, G. & Galbio, A. (1988) *J. Mol. Catalysis* **47**, 343–350.

Albery, W.J. & Knowles, J.R. (1976) *Biochemistry* **15**, 5631–5640.

Albery, W.J. & Knowles, J.R. (1977) *Agnew Chem. Int. Ed. Engl.* **16**, 285–293.

Anthony-Cahill, S.J., Griffith, M.C., Noren, C.J., Suich, D.J. & Schultz, P.G. (1989) *TIBS* **14**, 400–403.

Arad, D., Langridge, R. & Kollman, P.A. (1990) *J. Am. Chem. Soc.* **112**, 491–502.

Ascenzi, P., Menegatti, E., Guarneri, M. & Amicone, G. (1989) *Biochim. Biophys. Acta* **998**, 210–214.

Askelöf, P., Korsfeldt, M. & Mannervik, B. (1976) *Eur. J. Biochem.* **69**, 61–67.

Atkins, G.L. & Nimmo, I.A. (1980) *Anal. Biochem.* **104**, 1–9.

Atkins, G.L. & Nimmo, I.A. (1981) in *Kinetic data analysis: design and analysis of enzyme and pharmacokinetic experiments* (Endrenyi, L. ed.), pp. 121–135, Plenum Press, New York.

Atkins, P.W. (1986) *Physical chemistry* (3rd ed.) Oxford University Press, Oxford.

Baker, E.N. & Drenth, J. (1987) in *Biological macromolecules and assemblies* (Jurnak, F. & McPherson, A. eds.) 313–368, John Wiley and Sons, New York.

Baker, E.N. & Hubbard, R.E. (1984) *Prog. Biophys. Mol. Biol.* **44**, 97–179.

Bender, M.L., Begué-Cantón, M.L., Blakeley, R.L., Brubacher, L.J., Feder, J., Gunter, C.R., Kézdy, F.J., Killheffer, J.V. Jr., Marshall, T.H., Miller, C.G., Roeske, R.W. & Stoops, J.K. (1966) *J. Am. Chem. Soc.* **88**, 5890–5913.

Blacklow, S.C., Raines, R.T., Lim, W.A., Zamore, P.D. & Knowles, J.R. (1988) *Biochemistry* **27**, 1158–1167.

Blackburn, G.M., Kang, A.S., Kingsbury, G.A. & Burton, D.R. (1989) *Biochem. J.* **262**, 381–390.

Briggs, G.E. & Haldane, J.B.S. (1925) *Biochem. J.* **19**, 338–339.

Brocklehurst, K. (1979) *Biochem. J.* **181**, 775–778.

Brocklehurst, K. & Dixon, H.B.F. (1976) *Biochem. J.* **155**, 61–70.

Brocklehurst, K. & Dixon, H.B.F. (1977) *Biochem. J.* **167**, 859–862.

Brocklehurst, K. & Topham, C.M. (1990) *Biochem. J.* **270**, 561–563.

Brocklehurst, K., Willenbrock, S.J.F. & Salih, E. (1983) *Biochem. J.* **211**, 701–708.

Brocklehurst, K., Willenbrock, F. & Salih, E. (1987) *New Compr. Biochem.* **16**, 39–158.

Brønsted, J.N. & Petersen, J. (1924) *Z. Phys. Chem.* **108**, 185–235.

Burbaum, J.J., Raines, R.T., Albery, W.J. & Knowles, J.R. (1989) *Biochemistry* **28**, 9293–9305.

Carter, P.J., Winter, G., Wilkinson, A.J. & Fersht, A.R. (1984) *Cell* **38**, 835–840.

Cha, S. (1968) *J. Biol. Chem.* **243**, 820–825.

Christensen, J., Martin, M.T. & Waley, S.G. (1990) *Biochem. J.* **266**, 853–861.

Cleland, W.W. (1963) *Biochim. Biophys. Acta* **67**, 188–196.

Cornish-Bowden, A. (1977) *Biochem. J.* **165**, 55–59.

Cornish-Bowden, A. (1979) *Fundamentals of enzyme kinetics* Butterworths, London-Boston.

Cornish-Bowden, A. (1981) in *Kinetic data analysis: design and analysis of enzyme and pharmacokinetic experiments* (Endrenyi, L. ed.) 105–119.

Cornish-Bowden, A. & Eisenthal, R. (1974) *Biochem. J.* **139**, 721–730.

Cornish-Bowden, A. & Eisenthal, R. (1978) *Biochim. Biophys. Acta* **523**, 268–272.

Cornish-Bowden, A. & Endrenyi, L. (1981) *Biochem. J.* **193**, 1005–1008.

Cornish-Bowden, A. & Wharton, C.W. (1988) *Enzyme kinetics* IRL Press, Oxford.

Cornish-Bowden, A., Porter, W.R. & Trager, W.F. (1978) *J. Theor. Biol.* **74**, 163–175.

Daggett, V. & Kollman, P.A. (1990) *Protein Engineering* **3**, 677–690.

Dalziel, K. (1957) *Acta Chem. Scand.* **11**, 1706–1723.

Dalziel, K. (1969) *Biochem. J.* **114**, 547–556.

Dalziel, K. (1975) in *The enzymes* (3rd ed.) **11**, 1–60.

Danielson, U.H. & Mannervik, B. (1988) *Biochem. J.* **250**, 705–711.

Dixon, W.J., Brown, M.B., Engelman, L., Hill, M.A. & Jennrich, R.I. (1988) *BMDP Statistical Software Manual* Vol. 1, 389–417, University of California Press, Berkeley.

Eisenberg, D. & Hill, C.P. (1989) *TIBS* **14**, 260–264.

Eisenthal, R. & Cornish-Bowden, A. (1974) *Biochem. J.* **138**, 715–720.

Ellis, K.J. & Duggleby, R.G. (1978) *Biochem. J.* **171**, 513–517.

Engel, P.C. (1981) *Enzyme kinetics: the steady-state approach* Chapman and Hall, London and New York.

Evans, M.G. & Polanyi, M. (1935) *Trans. Faraday Soc.* **31**, 875–894.

Eyring, H. (1935) *J. Chem. Phys.* **3**, 107–115.

Fatania, H.R., Matthews, B., & Dalziel, K. (1982) *Proc. R. Soc. Lond. B.* **214**, 369–387.

Fersht, A.R. (1985) *Enzyme structure and mechanism* (2nd ed.) Freeman and Co., New York.

Fersht, A.R. (1987a) *Biochemistry* **26**, 8031–8037.

Fersht, A.R. (1987b) *Protein Engineering* **1**, 442–445.

Fersht, A.R. (1988) *Biochemstry* **27**, 1577–1580.

Fersht, A.R. & Jakes, R. (1975) **14**, 3350–3356.

Fersht, A.R. & Wells, T.N.C. (1991) *Protein Engineering* **4**, 229–231.

Fersht, A.R., Shi, J.P., Knill-Jones, J.W., Lowe, D.M., Wilkinson, A.T., Blow, D.M.,Brick, P., Carter, P., Waye, M.M.Y. & Winter, G. (1985) *Nature* **314**, 235–238.

Fersht, A.R., Leatherbarrow, R.J. & Wells, T.N.C. (1986a) *TIBS* **11**, 321–325.

Fersht, A.R., Leatherbarrow, R.J. & Wells, T.N.C. (1986b) *Nature* **322**, 284–286.

Fersht, A.R., Leatherbarrow, R.J. & Wells, T.N.C. (1987) *Biochemistry* **26**, 6030–6038.

Fink, A.L. (1987) in *Enzyme mechanisms* (Page, M.I. & Williams, R.A., eds.) 159–177, Royal Society of Chemistry, London.

Gibson, Q.H. & Milnes, L. (1964) *Biochem. J.* **91**, 161–171.

Gibson, Q.H. & Roughton, F.J.W. (1955) *Proc. R. Soc. Lond. B.* **143**, 310–334.

Hajdu, J., Acharya, K.R., Stuart, D.I., Barford, D. & Johnson, L.N. (1988) *TIBS* **13**, 104–109.

Haldane, J.B.S. (1930) *Enzymes* Longmans Green, London.

Hall, G. & Watt, J.M. (eds.) (1976) *Modern numerical methods for ordinary differential equations* Clarendon Press, Oxford.

Hardy, L.W. & Kirsch, J.F. (1984) *Biochemistry* **23**, 1275–1282.

Henderson, P.J.F. (1985) in 'Techniques in the Life Sciences' (Tipton, K.F. ed.) BI/II Supplement, *Protein and Enzyme Biochemistry* **BS114**, 1–48, Elsevier, Ireland.

Herries, D.G. (1984) *Biochem. J.* **223**, 551–553.

Hirono, S. & Kollman, P.A. (1991) *Protein Engineering* **4**, 233–243.

Ishikawa, H., Maeda, T., Hikita, H. & Miyatake, K. (1988) *Biochem. J.* **251**, 175–181.

Jencks, W.P. (1969) *Catalysis in chemistry and enzymology* McGraw-Hill, New York.

Jencks, W.P. (1975) *Adv. Enzymol.* **43**, 219–410.

King, E.L. & Altman, C. (1956) *J. Phys. Chem.* **60**, 1375–1378.

Knowles, J.R. (1976) *CRC Crit. Rev. Biochem.* **4**, 165–173.

Knowles, J.R. (1987) *Science* **236**, 1252–1258.

Knowles, J.R. & Albery, W.J. (1977) *Acc. Chem. Res.* **10**, 105–111.

Kraut, I (1988) *Science* **242**, 533–540.

Kvassman, J. & Pettersson, G. (1979) *Eur. J. Biochem.* **100**, 115–123.

Laidler, K.J. (1987) *Chemical kinetics* (3rd ed.) Harper and Row, New York.

Lam, C.F. (1981) *Techniques for the analysis and modelling of enzyme kinetic mechanisms.* 1–62, Research Studies Press, Chichester.

Lam, C.F. & Priest, D.G. (1972) *Biophys. J.* **12**, 248–256.

Leatherbarrow, R.J. (1987) *Enzfitter* Elsevier Biosoft.

Leatherbarrow, R.J. (1990a) *TIBS* **15**, 455–458.

Leatherbarrow, R.J. (1990b) *GraFit* (Version 2.0) Erithacus Software.

Leatherbarrow, R.J. & Fersht, A.R. (1987) in *Enzyme mechanisms* (Page, M.I. & Williams, R.A., eds.), 78–96 Royal Society of Chemistry, London.

Leatherbarrow, R.J., Fersht, A.R. & Winter, G. (1985) *Proc. Natl. Acad. Sci. USA* **82**, 7840–7844.

Mannervik, B. (1981) in *Kinetic data analysis: design and analysis of enzyme and pharmacokinetic experiments* (Endrenyi, L. ed.), 235–270, Plenum Press, New York.

Mannervik, B. (1982) *Methods Enzymol.* **87**, 370–390.

Mannervik, B., Jakobson, I. & Warholm, M. (1979) *Biochim. Biophys. Acta* **567**, 43–48.

Mannervik, B., Jakobson, I. & Warholm, M. (1988) *Biochem. J.* **235**, 797–804.

Michaelis, L. & Menten, M.L. (1913) *Biochem. Z.* **49**, 333–369.

Moore, J.W. & Pearson, R.G. (1981) *Kinetics and mechanism: a study of homogeneous chemical reactions* (3rd ed.) John Wiley and Sons, New York.

Mosteller, F. & Tukey, J.W. (1977) *Data analysis and regression* 333–379, Addison-Wesley, Reading, M.A.

Olavarria, J.M. (1986) *J. Theor. Biol.* **122**, 269–275.

Page, M.I. (1987) in *Enzyme mechanisms* (Page, M.I. & Williams, R.A. eds.), 1–13, Royal Society of Chemistry, London.

Pauling, L. (1948) *Am. Sci.* **36**, 51–58.

Pettersson, G. (1976) *Eur. J. Biochem.* **69**, 273–289.

Pettersson, G. (1978) *Acta Chem. Scand.* **B32**, 437–446.

Polgár, L. (1987) *New Compr. Biochem.* **16**, 159–200.

Polgár, L. (1989) in *Mechanism of protease action* (Polgár, L. ed.), 122–155, CRC Press, Florida.

Powell, M.J. & Hansen, D.E. (1989) *Protein Engineering* **3**, 69–75.

Porter, W.R. & Trager, W.F. (1977) *Biochem. J.* **161**, 293–302.

Roberts, D.V. (1977) *Enzyme kinetics* Cambridge University Press, Cambridge.

Schonbaum, G.R., Zerner, B. & Bender, M.L. (1961) *J. Biol. Chem.* **236**, 2930–2935.

Schultz, P.G. (1989) *Agnew Chem. Int. Ed. Engl.* **28**, 1283–1444.

Straub, J.E. & Karplus, M. (1990) *Protein Engineering* **3**, 673–675.

Szabo, A.G. (1990) in *Protein engineering: approaches to the manipulation of protein folding* (Narang, S.A. ed.) Butterworths, Boston.

Tipton, K.F. & Dixon, H.B.F. (1979) *Methods Enzymol.* **63**, 183–234.

Topham, C.M. and Brocklehurst, K. (1992) *Biochem. J.* **282**, 261–265.

Topham, C.M., Matthews, B. & Dalziel, K. (1986) *Eur. J. Biochem.* **156**, 555–567.

Varón, R., Havsteen, B.H., Garcia, M., Valero, E. & Garcia Cánovas, F. (1990) *J. Theor. Biol.* **143**, 251–268.

Volkenstein, M.V. & Goldstein, B.N. (1966) *Biochim. Biophys. Acta* **115**, 471–477.

Warshel, A. (1991) *Computer modeling of chemical reactions in enzymes and solutions.* John Wiley and Sons, New York.

Warshel, A. (1992) *Curr. Opin. Struct. Biol.* **2**, 230–236.

Warshel, A., Szabo-Naray, G., Sussman, F. & Hwang, J-K. (1989) *Biochemistry* **28**, 3629–3637.

Wells, T.N.C. & Fersht, A.R. (1986) *Biochemistry* **25**, 1881–1886.

Wells, T.N.C. & Fersht, A.R. (1989) *Biochemistry* **28**, 9201–9209.

Wharton, C.W. (1986) *Biochem. J.* **233**, 25–36.

Wharton, C.W. & Eisenthal, R. (1981) *Molecular enzymology* Blackie and Son, Glasgow.

Wilkinson, G.N. (1961) *Biochem. J.* **80**, 324–332.

Williamson, M.P. (1991) *Chem. Brit.* **27**, 335–337.

Wright, P.E. (1989) *TIBS* **14**, 255–260.
Wüthrich, K. (1989) *Science* **243**, 45–50.
Zhang, X.-Z., Stroud, A. & White, H.D. (1989) *Anal. Biochem.* **176**, 427–431.

10

Protein structure databases: design and applications

Janet M. Thornton, Stephen P. Gardner, and E. Gail Hutchinson
Biomolecular Structure and Modelling Unit, Department of Biochemistry and
Molecular Biology, University College, Gower Street, London WC1E 6BT

1. INTRODUCTION

The three-dimensional structure of a protein is essential for its biological function, and it allows an understanding of how interactions and reactions occur at the molecular level. The first protein structure was solved in the early 1960s, and since then the number of structures has gradually increased, with a rapid acceleration over the last few years as the techniques of data collection and processing have improved (Eisenberg & Hill 1989). However, comparison with the number of protein sequences (Fig. 1) shows that there are still many proteins for which the sequence is known, but no three-dimensional information is available. Therefore the problem of predicting structure from sequence has become one of the major goals of modern molecular biology.

Since the work of Anfinsen and colleagues on refolding proteins, it has been known that the sequence of a protein is sufficient to determine its structures (Richards 1991). This is true for small monomeric proteins, although it now appears that larger multimeric proteins may need assistance from molecular chaperonins (Ellis 1990). With the increased number of structures, coupled with the failure of *ab initio* methods, attempts to predict structure from sequence have recently concentrated on recognizing previously observed structures or substructures. This knowledge-based approach to prediction is extremely powerful if there is evidence of sequence homology. It is known that if two proteins have more than 25% sequence identity spread over the whole sequence, they will almost certainly have the same overall topology. Further-more, it is increasingly observed that sequences with no significant homology adopt the same structures. For example the pharmacologically important cytokine

Number of sequences/structures

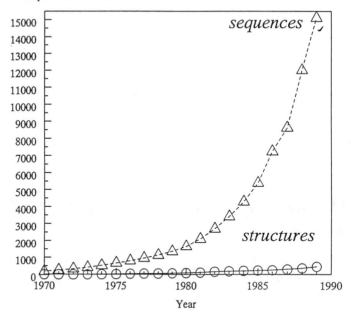

Fig. 1. Increase in the number of known protein sequences and structures. These data were derived from the PIR sequence database and the Brookhaven Protein Data Bank.

interleukin 1β has only 6 residues out of 170 identical with soybean trypsin inhibitor and yet its structure is remarkably similar (Priestle *et al.* 1988).

Progress toward prediction by recognition requires good organization of protein structural data. Traditionally, protein structures have been examined by eye, using sophisticated computer graphics software. Although these systems are excellent for studying individual proteins in detail, they can be very time consuming if many structures are to be scanned. Four factors therefore have led to the requirement for protein structure databases:

(1) The increasing number of known protein structures, currently over 400.
(2) Data derived from the atomic coordinates, such as secondary structure and hydrogen bonding, are invaluable for prediction. Such data should be calculated once, and stored for instant retrieval.
(3) The data need to be rationalized, so that properties are defined consistently over all structures. Algorithms which can be applied without bias to all structures must be designed in order to obtain a consistent set of data.
(4) A requirement for easy access to all structures and their derived properties, using a simple query system.

2. RELATIONAL DATABASE MANAGEMENT SYSTEMS

To fulfil these requirements several laboratories around the World have been setting up protein structure databases. A database consists of a shell structure (database management system) into which data in the form of flat files (TABLES) can be loaded. The data can then be rapidly accessed by using a simple query language.

Most groups have chosen a relational database management system (RDBMS) such as the commercially available Oracle RDBMS (Oracle Corporation UK Ltd, Bristol, UK). The relational approach was suggested by E.F. Codd (1970). It has proved simple to use and understand, and has provided the required facilities for design, implementation, and update of the database. It can handle large volumes of data fairly quickly via indexing systems, although a great deal of care needs to be exercised in the choice of indices.

A RDBMS views a logical database as a collection of two-dimensional TABLES or RELATIONS made up of ROWS and COLUMNS. Each column contains a different type of information, e.g. X, Y, Z coordinates. A row contains all the data for one particular atom, residue, protein, etc., depending on the table.

Data can be extracted from the database with little or no programming knowledge by using a high-level language such as SQL (Structured Query Language). This is a non-procedural language with which the user can simply state what data he needs without having to specify the procedural steps required to access the data. SQL consists of English-like constructs, taking a simple standard form as illustrated in Fig. 2.

```
SELECT      column(s)
FROM        table(s)
WHERE       conditions met      [optional]
GROUP BY    field(s)            [optional]
ORDER BY    field(s)            [optional]
```

Fig. 2. SQL query form.

Data from more than one table can be cross-correlated or JOINED via a common key. Since the order of rows within a table is undefined in a relational database, joining is also required to extract sequential information from a single table, for example information about two consecutive residues within a protein. This is called a SELF-JOIN.

At Birkbeck and University College we have established two protein structure databases. The original database BIPED (Akrigg *et al.* 1988), Islam & Sternberg 1989), later redesigned as STEP (Smith *et al.* 1991), is based on the Oracle RDBMS outlined above. Subsequently an in-house DBMS (IDITIS) has been designed to cope with the specific requirements of protein structure analysis. These databases are described below.

3. THE PROTEIN STRUCTURE DATA-VALIDATION AND CONSISTENCY

The source of the raw data for the database is the Brookhaven Laboratory (Bernstein *et al.* 1977) which collects and distributes the protein structure data derived by crystallographers. The files consists primarily of protein sequence and coordinate data, but also contain some bibliographic and crystallographic information. These data are deposited by the authors with only minor checks for internal consistency and errors. In establishing a database, however, it is essential that the files are as consistent and error free as possible. Hence the raw Brookhaven files are first run through a 'clean-up' program (BRKCLN) which checks for potential errors and inconsistencies and generates new 'clean' Brookhaven format files.

The most commonly occurring 'error' in the Brookhaven files is non-standard labelling of side-chain atoms. Standard labelling is clearly defined by the IUPAC-IUB Commission (1970, 1975), but is not always adhered to in Brookhaven files. In particular, labelling of arginine, aspartic and glutamic acids, phenylalanine, and tyrosine is often incorrect. For example, in arginine (Fig. 3), the guanidine group is

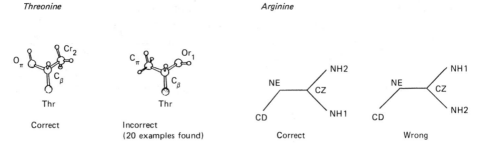

Fig. 3. Correct and incorrect labelling of threonine and arginine residues.

planar, and it is always possible to distinguish the NH1 and NH2 groups. 13% of the arginines in the original Brookhaven files were found to be wrongly labelled. These were correctly labelled in the 'clean' files, and the original atom labels included in an additional column to indicate which residues had been changed.

For the other side chains, correct labelling depends on identifying which atom defines the smallest value of the appropriate side-chain dihedral angle; for example, in tyrosine CD1 is defined as the atom which gives the lowest value of $\chi 2$. Since, for these residues, the labelling actually changes as the conformation of the side chain changes, this labelling can be considered rather arbitrary, and around 50% of Phe, Tyr, Asp, and Glu residues were found to be incorrectly labelled in the Brookhaven files. For the sake of consistency, however, all these residues have been relabelled in the 'cleaned up' files.

Threonine and isoleucine are also occasionally mislabelled. In these cases the chirality of the side chain must be correct. Out of a total of 6374 threonines, 20 were relabelled because of incorrect chirality. All the isoleucines had the correct chirality, but 2 were incorrectly labelled.

Other errors found by the BRKCLN program include chain breaks, missing atoms, and clashes caused by two atoms being closer together than the sum of their van der Waals' radii. These cannot actually be corrected, as this would entail changing the actual coordinates of the atoms or adding in new ones. This is impossible without access to the original electron density maps, and so such errors are simply flagged in the 'cleaned-up' files.

4. DERIVATION OF THE DATA FOR THE DATABASE TABLES

The 'clean' files generated by the BRKCLN program contain the raw coordinate data for the database. Although these coordinates hold all the information, protein structures are more easily understood by considering secondary and supersecondary structures or motifs. These derived data are calculated by a suite of programs which are run on the new coordinate files. Like the BRKCLN program, these programs calculate parameters, such as secondary structure according to established algorithms, so that the data are self-consistent. For example Kabsch and Sander's DSSP program (Kabsch & Sander 1983) has become the standard means of defining secondary structure, and a slightly modified implementation of this algorithm was used to generate the secondary structures for the database. The files of derived data then form the database tables. Table 1 gives a brief description of the major programs used to derive the data.

Table 1. Summary of the major programs used to generate the database tables, their function, and the tables for which each is used.

PROGRAM	FUNCTION	TABLES
BRKCLN	cleans up Brookhaven files	all tables
ACCESS	calculates solvent accessibilities	ATOM, AMINO ACID, CHAIN
SSTRUC	assigns secondary structures	AMINO ACID, CALPHA, DISULF, CHAIN
EFIMOV	classifies residue main chain dihedral angles (modified Efimov (1986))	AMINO ACID
ATOM	combines coordinate and accessibility data	ATOM
AMINO	combines secondary structure, accessibility and Efimov regions	AMINO ACID
CALPHA		CALPHA
TURN, HELIX, SHEET	extract and classify secondary structural features	TURN, HELIX, HELIXINT, SHEET, STRAND
DISULF		DISULPHIDE
HYDROGEN, NEIGHBOUR, SALT		HYDROGEN BOND, NEIGHBOUR, SALT
LIGAND		LIGAND, WATER
CHAIN	extracts chain data from Brookhaven and accessibility files	CHAIN
PROTIN	extracts relevant data from bibliographic records and manually extracted data	PROTEIN
SITE	classifies active sites	SITE

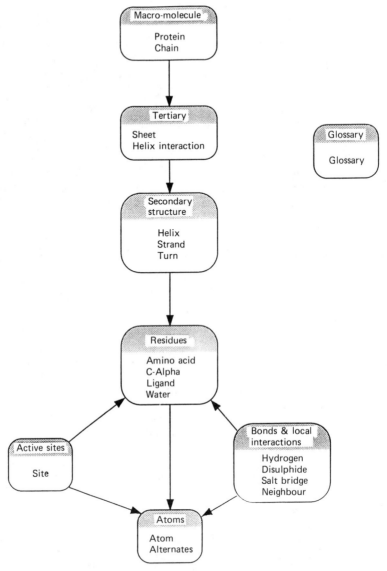

Fig. 4. Logical arrangement of the tables in the database.

The logical arrangement of tables in the database is shown in Fig. 4. Information about the protein is held at different levels, corresponding to the hierarchical manner in which protein structure is organized. For example, at the lowest (**ATOM**) level, the ATOM table holds the coordinate data for each atom, and other parameters such as B-values and solvent accessibilities. The tables at the **RESIDUE** level give details of the various groups of atoms, for example for each amino acid the AMINO ACID table stores information such as secondary structure, dihedral angles, and accessibility. Hydrogen bonding partners calculated by using a distance criterion only can be extracted from the HYDROGEN table at the **BONDS AND LOCAL INTERACTIONS** level. Active sites which have been described in the Brookhaven files by the authors are listed and classified in the SITE table.

Higher order protein structures are represented by the five tables at the **SECONDARY STRUCTURE** and **TERTIARY STRUCTURE** levels. As an example, the HELIX table includes information such as sequence, length, and various geometrical parameters for each helix. Finally, the PROTEIN and CHAIN tables at the **MACROMOLECULE** level contain more general information such as resolution, crystallographic R factor, number of residues, etc. for each protein.

5. EXTRACTING DATA FROM THE DATABASE

Having read the data into the Oracle RDBMS and established a consistent database, the query language SQL outlined above may be used to extract the required information. This may be from one particular table, or may combine data from several tables. The following examples illustrate the types of enquiry which can be made.

At the **MACROMOLECULE** level we can, for example, search for all proteins which bind zinc. We can add the constraint that we require only well-resolved proteins at resolutions of 2.0 Å or better. The query in Fig. 5 will extract this information from the database in 6 seconds. All this information is held in the PROTEIN table, and no JOINS are required.

```
SQL>    SELECT brcode,pname,resol,ligs
   2    FROM protein
   3    WHERE resol < = 2.0 and ligs like '%ZN%'
```

BRCO	PNAME	RESOL	LIGS
1PPT	AVIAN PANCREATIC POLYPEPTIDE	1.3	/ ZN ZN1 + +/
5CPA	CARBOXYPEPTIDASE 1 = ALPHA =	1.5	/ ZN ZN1 + +/
1INS	INSULIN	1.5	/ ZN1 ZN1 + +/ ZN2 ZN
3TLN	THERMOLYSIN (E.C.3.4.24.4)	1.6	/CA 4 (CA1 + +)/ ZN Z
2CAB	CARBONIC ANHYDRASE FORM B	2	/ZN ZN1 + +/
1CAC	CARBONIC ANHYDRASE FORM C	2	/ZN ZN1 + +/
3CPA	CARBOXYPEPTIDASE A = ALPHA =	2	/ZN ZN1 + +/
2SOD	CU, ZN SUPEROXIDE DISMUTASE	2	/ CU 4 (CU1 + +)/ ZN 4

8 records selected

Fig. 5. Query to extract all zinc-binding proteins with resolution ≤ 2.0 Å from the PROTEIN table. BRCO is the four-letter Brookhaven code for the protein. PNAME is the protein name and RESOL is the resolution. The LIGS column contains the ligands attached to each protein.

At the **RESIDUE** level we can extract for example all prolines in α helices plus information on the residues preceding them (Fig. 6).

At the **BONDS AND LOCAL INTERACTIONS** level we can extract all examples of a disulphide bridge connection between two α helices (Fig. 7). These are relatively rare, and only 13 non-homologous examples were found in 300 structures.

```
SQL>   select brookid, aminoid, seqm3, seqm2, seqm1, name1, mksm3, mksm2,
       mksm1, mks2ds
  2    from amino
  3    where name1 = 'P'
  4    and (mks2ds = 'H' or mks2ds = 'h');
```

BROO	AMINOID	S	S	S	N	M	M	M	M
1CRN	1CRN/−0022−	P	G	T	P	T	T	t	h
1CTS	1CTS/−0121−	A	A	L	P	h			h
1FDH	1FDH/A0095−	R	V	D	P	t		t	h
1FDH	1FDH/G0100−	H	V	D	P	t		t	h
1HBS	1HBS/B0100−	H	V	D	P	t		t	h
1HBS	1HBS/D0100−	H	V	D	P	t		t	h
1HBS	1HBS/F0100−	H	V	D	P			t	h
1HBS	1HBS/H0100−	H	V	D	P	t		t	h
1HCO	1HCO/A0095−	R	V	D	P			t	h
1HDS	1HDS/B0057−	M	N	N	P	H	H	h	h
.	.	.	.	.	.	.	.	.	.
.	.	.	.	.	.	.	.	.	.
.	.	.	.	.	.	.	.	.	.
8CAT	8CAT/A0486−	D	V	H	P	H	H	h	H
8CAT	8CAT/B0161−	L	L	F	P	G	h	H	H
8CAT	8CAT/B0178−	L	K	D	P	S		h	H
8CAT	8CAT/B0358−	F	A	Y	P	H	H	H	H
8CAT	8CAT/B0486−	D	V	H	P	H	H	h	H
9PAP	9PAP/−0068−	G	G	Y	P	t		h	H

573 records selected.

> Fig. 6. Query to extract all prolines in α-helices from the AMINO table. BROO is the four letter Brookhaven code for the protein. AMINOID is the unique identifier for the residue, S, S, S are the one letter codes for the 3 preceding residues, N is the one letter code for the current residue (*i*). M, M, M, M are the secondary structures of residues *i*-3 to *i*.

At the **ATOM** level we can extract, for example, the B values for all buried α carbon atoms in a given protein (see Fig. 8).

Structural motifs can also be extracted either from the AMINO ACID table by defining the relevant geometrical constraints, or from a secondary structure if one is available. For example, β-turns can be extracted from the AMINO ACID table by selecting 4 residues where the separation between the end α-carbons is less than 7 Å and the central two residues are not helical (Fig. 9). To do this, the table must be joined to itself twice so that sequential residues are selected and the internal ϕ and ψ angles can be extracted. This is time consuming. Alternatively, the TURNS table stores this information directly, making the query both simpler and faster to run (Fig. 10).

Higher order structural motifs may also be extracted from the **SECONDARY** and **TERTIARY STRUCTURE** tables. In particular, the SHEETS and STRANDS tables allow simple β sheet motifs to be extracted. For example, one commonly occurring simple motif is a beta-hairpin (Fig. 11), which consists of two adjacent antiparallel

```
Select all disulphide bridges occurring between two
residues in alpha helical conformation

1   SELECT BRCODE,SEQNO,SEQNOP,STRK,STRKP,GAP,CADIST
2   FROM DISULPHIDE
3*  WHERE STRK='H' AND STRKP='H'

    BRCO  SEQNO    SEQNOP  S S  GAP   CADIST
    ----  ------   ------  - -  ----  ------
    1CRN    16       26   H H   10    5.80
    1HMG   144      148   H H    4    5.19
    1PP2    28       44   H H   16    5.34
    1PP2    43       95   H H   52    5.80
    1PP2    49      122   H H   73    5.35
    1PP2    50       88   H H   38    5.60
    1PP2    57       81   H H   24    6.09
    2ACT    56       98   H H   42    4.66
    2GRS    58       63   H H    5    4.65
    2HFL    30      115   H H   85    6.23
    2LYM    30      115   H H   85    6.12
    2PAD    56       95   H H   39    4.57
    2TGP     5       55   H H   50    5.67

    13 records selected.
```

Fig. 7. Query and response from the DISULPHIDE table. SEQNO is the logical number of the first Cys residue. SEQNOP is the logical number of partner Cys residue. S S are the columns holding secondary structure assignments for the two Cys residues. GAP is the number of residues separating the two Cys residues in the protein, CADIST is the distance (in Å) between the C-alpha atoms of the two residues. The figure is taken from Thornton & Gardner (1989).

SQL>   SELECT uniqid,name,atmnam,b,relm
  2   FROM atom
  3   WHERE atmnam=' CA' and relm <=30

UNIQID	NAM	ATMN	B	RELM
351C.0.0003.0.0.0.0.0	PRO	CA	14.59	0
351C.0.0004.0.0.0.0.0	GLU	CA	10.06	13.7
351C.0.0006.0.0.0.0.0	LEU	CA	11.56	0
351C.0.0007.0.0.0.0.0	PHE	CA	3.99	0
351C.0.0008.0.0.0.0.0	LYS	CA	5.17	0
. .	.	.	.	.
. .	.	.	.	.
. .	.	.	.	.
351C.0.00 72.0.0.0.0.0	GLN	CA	4.23	0
351C.0.00 74.0.0.0.0.0	LEU	CA	5.38	0
351C.0.00 75.0.0.0.0.0	ALA	CA	6.76	0
351C.0.00 78.0.0.0.0.0	VAL	CA	6.36	0
351C.0.00 79.0.0.0.0.0	LEU	CA	10.35	0

Fig. 8. Query and response from the ATOM table. UNIQID represents the unique identifier assigned to each atom. NAM is the three letter name for the corresponding residue. ATMN corresponds to the atom name. B represents *B*-values and RELM the solvent accessibility for each atom.

beta-strands. According to the notation of Richardson (1981) the connection between these two strands has a 'topological linkage number' of 1. The notation assigns a

```
SQL>   run
   1     SELECT    a.aminoid, a.name1, a.seqp1, a.seqp2,
   2               a.seqp3, a.cadp3, a.mks2ds, a.mksp1,
   3               a.mksp2, a.mksp3, b.phi phip1,
   4               b.psi psip1, c.phi phip2, c.psi psip2
   5     FROM      amino a, amino b, amino c
   6     WHERE     (a.mksp1 !='H' and a.mksp1 !='G' and
   7               a.mksp2 !='H' and a.mksp2 !='G' and
   8               a.cadp3 < 7.0 and a.brookid = '1GCR' and
   9               a.brookid = b.brookid and
  10               a.brookid = c.brookid and
  11               b.ordernum = a.ordernum + 1 and
  12*              c.ordernum = a.ordernum +2
```

AMINOID	N	S	S	S	CADP3	M	M	M	M	PHIP1	PSIP1	PHIP2	PSIP2
1GCR/−0008−	D	R	G	F	6.5	E	T	T	T	−77.3	168.2	66.2	24.3
1GCR/−0009−	R	G	F	Q	6.0	T	T	T	E	66.2	24.3	69.2	33.2
1GCR/−0022−	C	P	N	L	6.5	B	S	t		−66.7	−24.7	−156.3	107.0
1GCR/−0025−	L	Q	P	Y	5.5		T	T	T	−52.1	−41.8	−57.9	−35.2
1GCR/−0026−	Q	P	Y	F	5.8	T	T	T	t	−57.9	−35.2	−90.2	−24.6
1GCR/−0047−	R	P	N	Y	6.5	E	T	T	T	−65.5	170.1	68.1	30.1
1GCR/−0048−	P	N	Y	Q	5.9	T	T	T	E	68.1	30.1	63.4	47.8
1GCR/−0095−	R	D	D	F	6.4	S	t	T	T	−64.4	158.0	68.4	29.5
1GCR/−0096−	D	D	F	R	6.0	t	T	T	t	68.4	29.5	55.9	36.0
1GCR/−0109−	C	P	S	L	6.4	B	S	h	H	−85.3	−9.6	−155.8	105.9
1GCR/−0136−	M	P	S	Y	6.2	E	T	T	T	−66.4	159.5	63.2	35.6
1GCR/−0137−	P	S	Y	R	6.2	T	T	T	E	63.2	35.6	68.6	39.6

12 records selected. (approx 3.8 seconds CPU time)

Fig. 9. Query used to extract the β-turns in γ crystallin from the AMINO ACID table. The table must be joined to itself twice so that the internal ϕ and ψ angles can be extracted, hence the use of 'a.' and 'b.' in the query. AMINOID is the unique identifier for each residue, N, S, S, S hold the one-letter codes for residues $i, i+1, i+2, i+3$. CADP3 is the distance between the C-alpha atoms of residues i and $i+3$. M, M, M, M are the assigned secondary structures of residues $i \ldots i+3$. PHIP1, PSIP1, PHIP2, PSIP2 are the ϕ and ψ angles of residues $i+1$ and $i+2$.

number to each connection, corresponding to the number of intervening strands in the sheet, and an 'X' if the two strands lie parallel so that the connecting loop 'crosses over' the sheet (cross-over connection).

For each strand in the protein the STRANDS table holds the 'topological linkage number' for the connection to the next strand in the sequence. Thus this table could, for example, be used to extract all examples of beta-hairpins from the database. This can be achieved in a few seconds, whereas until now such information has had to be extracted manually by examining each structure on a computer graphics terminal (e.g. Sibanda & Thornton 1985). The SHEETS table holds similar information about

```
SQL>   run
  1    SELECT aminoidi, namei, nameip1, nameip2, namee,
  2    cadist, phiip1, psiip1, phiip2, psiip2,
  3    class, type
  4    FROM turns
  5*   WHERE brookid = '1GCR' and class = 'BETA'
```

AMINOIDI	N	N	N	N	CADIST	PHIIP1	PSIIP1	PHI IP2	PSIIP2	CLASS	TYPE
1GCR/−0008−	D	R	G	F	6.5	−77.3	168.2	66.2	24.3	BETA	IV
1GCR/−0009−	R	G	F	Q	6.0	66.2	24.3	69.2	33.2	BETA	IV
1GCR/−0022−	C	P	N	L	6.5	−66.7	−24.7	−156.3	107.0	BETA	IV
1GCR/−0025−	L	Q	P	Y	5.5	−52.1	−41.8	−57.9	−35.2	BETA	IV
1GCR/−0026−	Q	P	Y	F	5.8	−57.9	−35.2	−90.2	−24.6	BETA	I
1GCR/−0047−	R	P	N	Y	6.5	−65.5	170.1	68.1	30.1	BETA	IV
1GCR/−0048−	P	N	Y	Q	5.9	68.1	30.1	63.4	47.8	BETA	IV
1GCR/−0095−	R	D	D	F	6.4	−64.4	158.0	68.4	29.5	BETA	IV
1GCR/−0096−	D	D	F	R	6.0	68.4	29.5	55.9	36.0	BETA	IV
1GCR/−0109−	C	P	S	L	6.4	−85.3	−9.6	−155.8	105.9	BETA	IV
1GCR/−0136−	M	P	S	Y	6.2	−66.4	159.5	63.2	35.6	BETA	IV
1GCR/−0137−	P	S	Y	R	6.2	63.2	35.6	68.6	39.6	BETA	IV

12 records selected. (approx 1.3 seconds CPU time)

Fig. 10. Query used to extract the β-turns in gamma crystallin directly from the TURNS table. AMINOIDI is the unique identifier for the initial residue. NAMEI, NAMEIP1, NAMEIP2, NAMEE are the one-letter codes for residues i, $i + 1$, $i + 2$, $i + 3$ in the turn. PHIIP1, PSIIP1, PHIIP2, PSIIP2 are the ϕ and ψ angles of the central two residues. CLASS holds the type of turn – all the turns extracted are β-turns. TYPE indicates the turn-type classified according to the central ϕ and ψ angles (Richardson 1981).

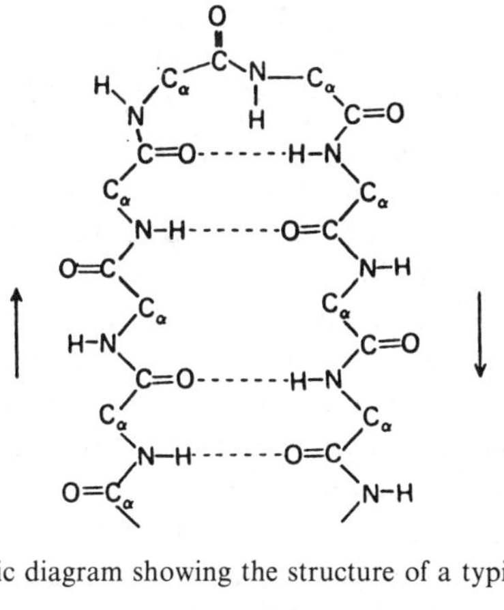

Fig. 11. Schematic diagram showing the structure of a typical beta hairpin.

connections for each β sheet, and can be used to extract structural motifs involving more than two strands. For example, the eight-stranded barrel topology first observed in triose phosphate isomerase can be defined by the following string of connections:

'1X,1X,1X,1X,1X,1X,1X' representing 8 adjacent parallel strands. The table also holds the sequential numbers for each of the strands (numbered from 1 for the first strand in the protein). These are written in the order in which they occur in the sheet, so that '1, 2, 3, 4, 5, 6, 7, 8' would indicate that this sheet is composed of the first eight strands in the protein with the above topology. A search for all closed sheets (barrels) with this topology would extract all the structures related to this one.

6.   IDITIS — A SPECIALISED DATABASE SYSTEM FOR PROTEIN STRUCTURES

After some years of experience in using proprietary products such as Oracle it is clear that traditional relational database management systems have many inbuilt limitations which inhibit their use for protein structures. The main problem is that the order of rows within a table is undefined, whereas proteins consist of ordered lengths of connected amino acids and atoms, for example in an α helix. To represent this ordered information in RDBMSs, various strategies have been devised. Explicit logical numbering schemes can be used in conjunction with self-join operations as described previously, or with external programs. Unfortunately this process cannot be made transparent to the user. Extra fields of information which duplicate previous and subsequent entries can also be used, for example the incorporation of 10 extra columns containing the amino acid sequence at position $i-5$, $i-4 \ldots i+5$. This environmental information is then available on a single row and can be accessed easily. These practices are cumbersome in use and inefficient in reality both in terms of speed and disk space, and are perhaps the biggest hurdle to overcome when designing relational protein structure databases. In addition, as the volume of data in the databases has increased, so too has the mean number of hits (database entries matching the search criteria) returned from a particular query. An integrated strategy is required to process, classify, and visualize these ever longer lists of database hits.

A radically new approach to the interaction and analysis of data is required if databases are to play a major role in protein research in the future. In response to this challenge a new RDBMS system (IDITIS) has been designed. The objectives of the system were quite clear. It had to provide RDBMS functionality, have SQL compatibility, be quicker and more efficient, and recognize order based information, thereby eliminating relational 'fixes' such as extra redundancy, explicit logical numbering, and redundant joining. In addition the system must be extremely portable and run on microcomputers, but remain configurable to exploit the full potential of larger machines. We aimed to provide the framework for a flexible protein engineering specific database which can be used as an effective research tool.

The IDITIS system has been implemented in C. The software is completely portable with the exception of isolated system specific modules which are relevant only to the system upon which the software is running, and should be easily ported to other operating systems such as UNIX. When transferring to larger virtual memory machines IDITIS can be optimized to use virtual memory preferentially to disk.

The high-level query language SQL itself is the main obstacle to order based querying in traditional RDBMSs, as there is no provision for specification of relationships such as next or previous row except by inefficient artificial constructs as discussed above. Order Based SQL (OBSQL) was developed within IDITIS to be a form of the query language which was compatible with standard SQL, but which could also cope with order based queries. Within IDITIS all rows have a connectivity determined by their logical row numbers (LRN).

Order is specified in OBSQL by the use of column offsets which can be specified in the SELECT and WHERE clauses of a query. The offsets are enclosed by square brackets [ ] which follow the column name. Within the brackets a single integer, or two integers separated by a colon, represent the offsets required. For example SEQ[-2:2] would mean the values in column SEQ from row i-2 to $i + 2$ where i is the fundamental row of the query. The following OBSQL query (Fig. 12) would be used to extract information on the residues involved in a β-turn (as described before). This is much more elegant and simpler for the user.

```
1 > SELECT AMINOID, SEQ[:3], CADIS, PH1[1], PSI[1],
2 > PHI[2], PSI[2]
3 > FROM AMINO
4 > WHERE BROOKID = '1GCR' AND CADIST < 7.0
5 > AND STRK[1] ! = 'H' AND STRK[1] ! = 'G'
6 > AND STRK[2] ! = 'H' AND STRK[2] ! = 'G'
```

Fig. 12 OBSQL query to extract all β-turns in γ-crystallin

IDITIS is a stand-alone RDBMS, and a protein specific front end, called 3-D SCAN, has also been written. This allows a high level of interaction with the data, which is essential for the database to function as a proper analysis tool. For example the user can instigate fuzzy sequence and structural searches using predefined or specified sets. There will also be secondary structural vector representations and scans, C-alpha and torsional geometry searches, generation of coordinates for fragments in the hit list, and fragment superpositions. Eventually, clustering and classification of hit lists using pre-existing homologous family structure alignments will be possible.

7. APPLICATIONS

The applications of the protein structure database can be described under four main headings:

> Dictionary/Atlas of Protein Structure
> Analysis of Structural Features
> Aid to knowledge-based prediction of structure from sequence
> Tool to help design successful protein engineering experiments

Some examples of such applications are given below.

7.1   Dictionary/atlas of protein structure

We have used the Oracle database to extract information on many different features some of which are listed below:

RESIDUE DATA:-   *cis*-peptides, proline residues, side-chain conformations, D- and L-amino acids (chirality), errors in structures

SECONDARY STRUCTURE FEATURES:- β-turn, ψ-loops

INTERACTIONS:-   zinc binding sites, proteinase inhibitor loops, disulphide bridges, salt bridges

7.2   Analysis of structural features

The Oracle version of the database provides a good robust dictionary with fast access times. In addition it includes calculation of statistical quantities and generation of histograms. We have used these facilities widely in several analyses of different types of feature.

At the simplest residue level we have analysed the influence of prolines on protein

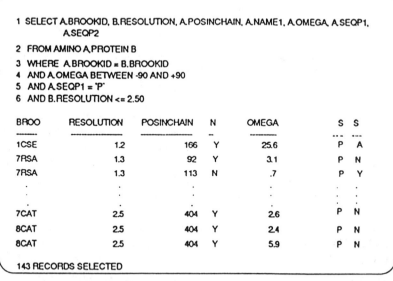

Fig. 13. Query used to extract all the *cis* peptides which occur before a proline residue in protein structures determined to a resolution ≤ 2.5 Å. (Figure taken from MacArthur & Thornton 1991).

conformation (MacArthur & Thornton 1991). For example the query in Fig. 13 was used to extract all *cis*-peptides which occur before a proline residue. In total we found 143 examples, but many of these were homologous, leaving only 58 independent X-cisPro, that is, 5.7% of prolines. We found a preference for tyrosine (Fig. 14) in the

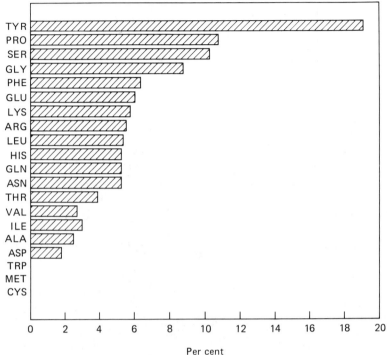

% Amino acid in χ − cisPROLINE

Per cent

Fig. 14. Amino acid preferences for residues preceding a *cis* proline. The histogram shows for each residue (X) the percentage of X-Pro which occur as X-*cis*-Pro. (Figure obtained from M. MacArthur).

X position with almost 20% of Tyr–Pro dipeptides in the database adopting a *cis*-peptide linkage. Previous NMR data for small peptides also suggested a preference for bulky groups before a *cis*-peptide linkage. The database was also used to extract proline patterns (such as X-Pro–Pro-X and Pro-X-Pro) and to investigate their structures. From these data were constructed Table 2 which summarizes the strong influence of such proline patterns on secondary structure.

Considering higher orders of structure, we have extracted information on the relative frequencies of the different connections between consecutive beta strands within a sheet. The results are shown in the histogram in Fig. 15. It can clearly be seen that the most favoured topology for two consecutive strands in the same sheet is the β hairpin described earlier. Figure 16 shows some examples of the ψ loop structures defined by an antiparallel connection between two non-adjacent strands with a 'topological linkage number' of 2. Once these motifs have been identified automatically from the database they can be plotted by using a separate program (HERA, Hutchinson & Thornton 1990) as shown in the figure. In contrast to the hairpins, which occur very frequently, the ψ loops form a select group containing only 8 non-homologous examples.

We have also used the database to look at the accuracy of protein coordinates.

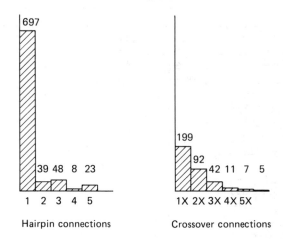

Fig. 15. Histograms showing the frequencies of occurrence of hairpin and crossover connections between strands.

Table 2. Secondary structure of proline pairs separated by other residues. Percentages in helix and strand are for examples where both prolines occur within the same secondary structure (taken from MacArthur & Thornton 1991)

	Number	Helix ($\alpha\alpha$) %	Strand %	Other %
-P-	1021	27	11	62
-PP-	37	3	0	97
-PXP-	39	8	0	92
-PXXP-	47	0	2	98
-PXXXP-	64	0	0	100
-PXXXXP-	47	0	6	94
-PXXXXXP-	45	2	2	96

For example we have considered the distortions at the α carbon atom which can lead to D-amino acids, rather than the obligatory L form. Such distortions are flagged in the database, and we found 29 examples of such non-allowed conformations in around 93 000 residues. Some proteins (for example deer hemoglobin (1HDS) and tomato bushy stunt virus (2TBV)) include several examples, which are suggestive of low resolution data and poor refinement.

Such analyses of structural features need to include consideration of sequence homology, especially if one is considering statistical significance. Currently, it is only possible to exclude the effects of homologous proteins by taking only one example from each family (e.g. one serine proteinase from the 12 structures in the Brookhaven Data Bank). However, we are hoping to include an automatic clustering of structurally equivalent features in homologous proteins and to allow the user to choose different criteria for acceptance.

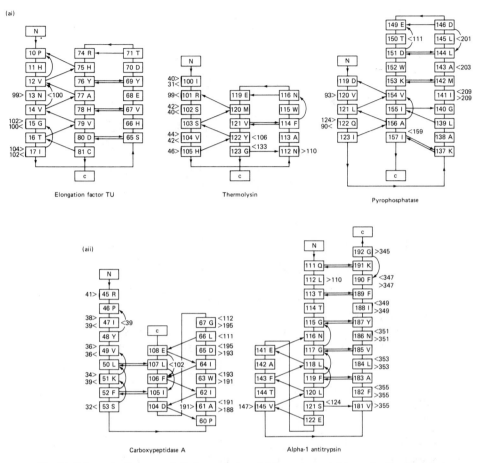

Fig. 16. Schematic diagrams of all the examples of ψ loops extracted from the Brookhaven Data Bank. (a) Single ψ loops with topological linkage numbers (i) '+2, −1' from elongation factor TU (1ETU), thermolysin (7TLN) and pyrophospatase (1PYP), (ii) '+2, −1X' from carboxypeptidase (5CPA) and α₁-antitrypsin (6API).

7.3   Knowledge-based prediction

The database can be used as an aid to knowledge-based prediction either in secondary structure prediction or homology modelling. It can provide the data by which such predictions are made. For example, the homology based method of Levin et al. (1986) for secondary structure prediction requires tables of sequences and secondary structure assignments. These can be generated by the database.

Similarly, in modelling one protein on the basis of a homologous structure, the loops often change radically and the whole database can be used as a source of loop conformers with fixed-end constraints. In this application the matrix of Cα separations is searched to locate putative loops of a fixed length and end-point separation, and possibly including some sequence requirements. Having constructed a hit list of loops from the database, these can then be modelled onto the framework in order to choose

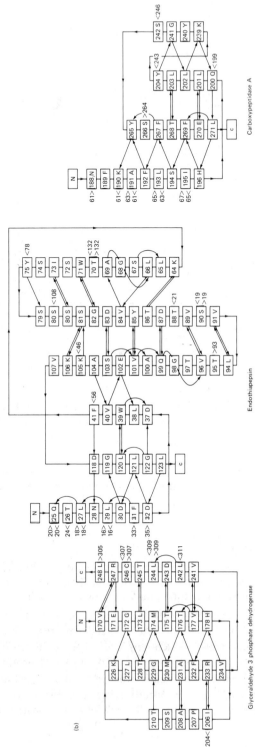

Fig. 16. (b) Double ψ-loops from glyceraldehyde 3-phosphate dehydrogenase (3GPD), endothiapepsin (4APE) and carboxypeptidase (5CPA). The other aspartic proteinases have a topology similar to endothiapepsin. (Figure taken from Hutchinson & Thornton (1990)).

```
Select all examples where a PRO in beta sheet conformation
has been inserted in the aspartic proteases.

1  SELECT ANUM1 "P1APR",ANUM2 "P2APP",ANUM3 "P4APE",
2  RTYP1,RTYP2,RTYP3," ",SSTRC1,SSTRC2,SSTRC3
3  FROM APALIGN
4  WHERE (RTYP1<>'P' OR RTYP2<>'P' OR RTYP3<>'P') AND
5  (( RTYP1='P' AND SSTRC1='E')
6  OR (RTYP2='P' AND SSTRC2='E')
7* OR (RTYP3='P' AND SSTRC3='E'))

   P1APR P2APP P4APE  R R R       S S S
   ----- ----- -----  - - ---     - - -
      7     7     3    P T T       E E E
     10    10     6    D P P       E E E
     20    20    17    Q P P       E E E
    187   183   183    P G A       E E E
    227   222   224    P D P       E T T
    251   248   249    S D P       E E
    259   255   256    P D S       E E E
    322   321   325    P P S       E E B

   8 records selected.
```

Fig. 17. Query and response using a table of structurally aligned protein families in the data base. The table APALIGN holds the structural alignment of the aspartyl protease family: rhizopuspepsin (1APR), penicillopepsin (2APP) and endothiapepsin (4APE) with coordinates aligned from Brookhaven. The columns are labelled as follows: P1APR, P2APP, and P4APE columns hold structurally equivalent residue numbers, so that each row represents a residue position in the family alignment. R, R, R are the respectiv sequences associated with the three residue numbers, and S, S, S the corresponding secondary structural assignments. (Figure taken from Thornton & Gardner (1989)).

the most likely candidate.

Statistical information on preferred conformers may also be valuable when building side chains onto a backbone framework. For example, most residues in an α helix tend to avoid the g- ($\chi_1 = 60°$) conformation, as found by McGregor *et al.* (1987) by using the database.

These prediction algorithms will remain separate from the database, but should integrate with it so that, as new coordinate sets become available, their parameters can be immediately updated to include all the new information.

7.4 Protein engineering experiments

In designing protein engineering experiments information currently available in the database should be used as a guide. For example the query in Fig. 17 could be used to assess the effects of changing a β strand residue to a proline. Information on disulphide geometry and best possible sites needs to be extracted and analysed in order to design additional disulphide bridges to increase protein stability (Pabo & Suchanek 1986). Similarly the knowledge base is crucial in more ambitious experiments to design in metal binding sites (e.g. Roberts *et al.* 1990). Currently, the database could be used to extract all such information, analyse it, and produce statistics on geometry and sequence preferences. Ideally we would like to include a 'front end' which could not only extract such information on specific structural features, but could also tell the experimenter the best sites on the target protein to perform the mutagenesis experiments.

8. CONCLUSIONS

As the number of protein structures increases, the use of databases such as that described here will become obligatory for both experimental biochemists and theoreticians. Ideally we want an open, user-friendly system which will allow flexible data input and output, and integration with other programs and the exponentially growing sequence database. Only such a system will allow the rapid updating and full use of available data which are necessary in any good laboratory. These data provide the essential information for tackling the protein folding problem, for designing novel proteins and peptides, and for understanding the plethora of protein sequences which will be generated over the next decade.

REFERENCES

Akrigg, D., Bleasby, A.J.M., Dix, N.I.M., Findlay, J.B.C., North, A.C.T., Parry-Smith, D., Wooten, J.C., Blundell, T.L., Gardner, S.P., Hayes, F.R.F., Islam, S.A., Sternberg, M.J.E., Thornton, J.M., Tickle, I.J., & Murray-Rust, P.M. (1988) *Nature* **335**, 745–746.

Bernstein, F.C., Koetzle, T.F., Williams, G.J.B., Meyer, E.F., Brice, M.D., Rodgers, J.R., Kennard, O., Shimanouchi, T., & Tasumi, M. (1977) *J. Mol. Biol.* **122**, 535–542.

Codd, E.F. (1970) *Commun. ACM* **13**, 377–387.

Eisenberg, D. & Hill, C.H. (1989) *TIBS* **14**, 260–264.

Efimov, A.V. (1986) *Mol. Biol. (USSR)* **20**, 250–260.

Ellis, R.J. (1990) *Seminars in Cell Biology* **1**, 1–9.

Hutchinson, E.G. & Thornton, J.M. (1990) *Proteins* **8**, 203–212.

Islam, S.A. & Sternberg, M.J.E. (1989) *Protein Engineering* **2**, 431–442.

IUPAC-IUB Commission on Biochemical Nomenclature (1970) *J. Biological Chemistry* **245**, 6489–6497.

IUPAC Commission on the Nomenclature of Organic Chemistry and IUPAC-IUB Commission of Biochemical Nomenclature (1975) *Biochemistry* **14**, 449–462.

Kabsch, W. & Sander C. (1983) *Biopolymers* **22**, 2577–2637.

Levin, J.M., Robson, B., & Garnier, J. (1986) *FEBS Lett.* **205**, 303–308.

MacArthur, M.W. & Thornton, J.M. (1991) *J. Mol. Biol.* **217** (in press).

McGregor, M.J., Islam, S.A., & Sternberg, M.J.E. (1987) *J. Mol. Biol.*, **198**, 295–310.

Pabo, C.O. & Suchanek, E.G. (1986) *Biochemistry* **25**, 5987–5991.

Priestle, J.P., Schar, H.P., & Grutter, M.G. (1988) *EMBO J.* **16**, 949–953.

Richards, F. (1991) *Scientific American*: January 1991, 34–41.

Richardson, J.S. (1981) *Adv. Protein Chem.* **34**, 167–339.

Roberts, V.A., Iverson, B.L., Iverson, S.A., Benkovic, S.J., Lerner, R.A., Getzoff, E.D., & Tainer, J.A. (1990) *Proc. Nat. Acad. Sci.* **87**, 6654–6658.

Sibanda, B.L. & Thornton, J.M. (1985) *Nature* **316**, 170–174.

Smith, D.K., Gardner, S.P., Hutchinson, E.G., & Thornton, J.M. (1991) manuscript in preparation.

Thornton, J.M. & Gardner, S.P. (1989) *TIBS* **14**, 300–304.

11

From modelling homologous proteins to prediction of structure

A. Sali, J.P. Overington, M.S. Johnson and T.L. Blundell
ICRF Unit of Structural Molecular Biology, Department of Crystallography,
Birkbeck College, University of London, Malet Street, London WC1E 7HX

1. INTRODUCTION

Divergent evolution has given rise to families of homologous proteins that differ in
sequence but adopt the same general fold. This provides an opportunity to learn
about the three-dimensional structures of proteins if their sequences have been defined
and at least one other member of the family has a structure defined by X-ray analysis
or nuclear magnetic resonance.

The first application recorded in the literature of this procedure was the construction
of a model for alpha-lactalbumin on the basis of the 3D structure of lysozyme
(Browne *et al.* 1969). Other applications included construction of models for relaxins
and insulin-like growth factors (Bedarkar *et al.* 1977, Blundell & Humbel 1980) for
review), various serine proteinases (Greer 1981) and aspartic proteinases such as
renin (Blundell *et al.* 1983). The advent of computerized techniques, particularly the
computer graphics program FRODO (see Jones & Thirup (1986) for references),
made the task of replacing sidechains and making insertions and deletions more
straightforward. However, modelling was rarely performed applying rigorous rules,
although some systematic procedures were suggested, for example for the use of loops
from homologous proteins (Greer 1981).

The challenge now is to learn from the experience of these often subjective and
usually interactive modelling procedures. We require an automated procedure that
uses the known structures and the rules obtained from them — the knowledge base.
It has been apparent for some time that such an approach can have very wide
applications for prediction of protein structure in general (see Blundell *et al.* 1987).
This arises because many protein sequences adopt the same general fold even when

there is no obvious evolutionary relationship. Recent structure determinations suggest that the majority of new structures comprise motifs or domains that have been previously identified in other, often functionally different proteins. For this reason it is important to develop general approaches that can be extended from modelling homologous structures with clear similarities in their sequences to the more difficult problem of protein prediction using weaker analogies between tertiary structures of proteins that may have little sequence similarity and no functional or evolutionary

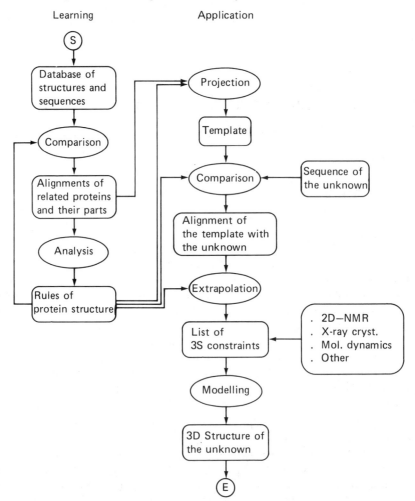

Fig. 1. Knowledge-based modelling of proteins.

relationship. Figure 1 shows a scheme that generalizes such approaches to modelling and provides an outline of our review.

We must first establish and formulate rules. We achieve this not only by analysing individual protein structures as they are defined by experiment, but also by comparing sequences and 3D structures. For this we need methods not only for aligning many sequences but also for comparing three-dimensional structures in order to establish equivalences within a family of proteins. The rules are then derived by careful, computerized analysis of the compared structures. This is the learning stage and it is summarized on the left-hand side of Fig. 1.

These rules can then be applied in two important ways shown on the right-hand side of Fig. 1. First, they are used to define all those sequences that can adopt each experimentally defined fold; this can be considered as a mapping from a 3D structure onto a 1D sequence. It is usually achieved through construction of a 'template', which summarizes knowledge about the family fold and is presented in a form suitable for comparison with the sequence of the 'unknown'. Secondly, when the alignment of sequence with the template has been achieved, the rules are used to map structural features to the sequence of the protein to be modelled.

In this review we emphasize our own approaches to modelling (Blundell *et al.* 1988; Sali *et al.* 1990). The most helpful learning set is that of homologous proteins; because there are fewer ambiguities in their comparisons, they provide a reliable source for the definition of rules but they remain a challenge for modelling. We describe new approaches that can be used in modelling more distantly related protein structures.

2. PROCEDURES FOR COMPARISON AND CLUSTERING OF PROTEIN SEQUENCES AND STRUCTURES

Our first task is to develop systematic ways of comparing and clustering protein structures.

The comparison of 3D structures often involves rigid-body least-squares superposition of the C_α positions (KenKnight, 1984, for review). Several homologous structures can be aligned (Sutcliffe *et al.*, 1987a) without bias to any one in the set in order to define a 'framework', which comprises a set of helices or strands that are conserved in the family. However, although dissimilar proteins usually retain the general arrangement of strands and helices, the differences in relative orientation and position may preclude their direct superposition (Chothia & Lesk, 1986; Hubbard & Blundell, 1987; Johnson *et al.* 1990a,b).

The extension of comparison methods to more dissimilar tertiary structures was addressed more than a decade ago (Eventoff & Rossmann, 1975; Matthews & Rossmann, 1985). The methods included information about mainchain direction in the alignment or based their comparisons on rigid body superposition of small parts of the whole structure. Our approach to protein comparison (Sali & Blundell, 1990; Z. Zhu, unpublished results), encoded in the program COMPARER, simultaneously employs a large number of protein features that were used individually in previous approaches. COMPARER can be used to obtain alignments of both sequence and three-dimensional structures. We first define the protein as an indexed string of elements that may exist at several levels in the protein hierarchical organization — residue, secondary structure, supersecondary structure, motif or domain. We then associate with every element features, either properties or relationships that indicate a common fold. Properties include element identity (for example, residue or secondary structure type), hydrophobicity, local conformation and solvent accessibility. Comparison of all such properties can be incorporated in a residue weight matrix and optimal alignment can then be derived using the dynamic programming approach. A similar approach based principally on intra-molecular distances has been described by Taylor & Orengo (1989).

At each level of the hierarchical structure of proteins, specific relationships such as hydrogen bonding interactions or packing relations that tend to be conserved in protein folds can also be used in our alignment procedure (Sali & Blundell 1990). However, a relationship affects more than one element in a sequence and this makes the conventional dynamic programming approach expensive in computer time. Instead we use simulated annealing to provide an initial set of equivalences based on relationships which are then introduced directly into the residue by residue weight matrix.

Figure 2 shows part of the alignment using COMPARER of the two domains of pepsins and the subunits of retroviral proteinases. These have only three residues that are identical in all the structures compared and the sequences vary from 99 to 170 amino acid residues in length. A direct multiple superposition equivalences very few residues and these are mainly in the active site region. In contrast the COMPARER alignment identifies all those strands and helices that have previously been considered equivalent on a more subjective basis and which have been shown to be common with the retroviral proteinases (see, for example, Lapatto et al. (1989)).

While extensive methodology for tree construction from protein sequences has been developed for the study of evolution (Doolittle 1989), the clustering of protein three-dimensional structures has been less studied. Rao et al. (1975) constructed dendrograms based on structural features alone to describe distant phylogenetic relationships among the mono-nucleotide and di-nucleotide binding proteins. We have shown that a useful structural pairwise distance metric can be defined from fractional topological equivalence and root mean square deviation as calculated by least squares superposition (Johnson et al. 1990a,b). This distance measure correlates well with the sequence metric. Recently we have extended this approach by reflecting additional structural and sequence features in the classification (Johnson et al. 1990a,b; Sali & Blundell 1990). Moreover, since these features can include relationships such as hydrogen bonding patterns, which are known to be conserved in evolution, structures that bear little similarity in other respects can be compared and classified at statistically significant levels. Figure 3 shows classifications of cytochrome c structures based on sequences and structures (Johnson et al. 1990a,b).

3. ESTABLISHING RULES FROM FAMILIES OF HOMOLOGOUS PROTEIN STRUCTURES

We have produced a database of alignments of three-dimensional structures obtained by COMPARER (Z. Zhu, A. Sali, J. Overington, T.L. Blundell). We have used this to derive a set of rules useful for modelling. For example, we can quantify the well-

```
                    180              190              200
                                                              90
HIV       - - p v N I I G - - - - - - - - - - - - - R̃ ñ L L T q I
2RSV      - - r g S̃ I L G - - - - - - - - - - - - - R̃ d̠ C L q g L
                    110
                    120              130                       140
4APE-N    s ĩ I D G L L G L A f s̃ t l Ñ̠t V s p t q q k T F F d̃ ñ A
2APP-N    t ñ Ñ̠D̠ G L L G L A F s̃ s i Ñ̠t V q p q̃ s q t̠ T F F d̃ t̠ V
2APR-N    - P Ñ̠D G L L G L G F d̃ t i T̠t̠ V r - - g V k T̃ P M d̃ Ñ L
PEP-N     - p F D̃ G I L G L A Ỹ p s i S̠̃ a s - - - g A t P V F D̃ Ñ L
CHY-N     - e̠ F D G I L G M A Ỹ p s̠ l A s̃ e - - - y S̃ i P V F D̃ Ñ M
4APE-C    - - g i Ñ̠ I F G - - - - - - - - - - - - - D̠ V A L K̃ A A
2APP-C    - - g f S I F G - - - - - - - - - - - - - D̠ I F L K̃ S̠ Q̃
2APR-C    - w g F A I I G - - - - - - - - - - - - - D̠ T̠ F L K̃ Ñ̠N̠
PEP-C     s g ẽ L W I L G - - - - - - - - - - - - - D̠ V F I R̃ q Y̠
CHY-C     - - q k Wi L G - - - - - - - - - - - - - D V F I R̃ Ẽ Y
                    β β β                           α α
                    300                             310
```

Fig. 2. Two sections of the alignment of sequences of aspartic proteinases achieved by comparing the three-dimensional structures using COMPARER (Sali & Blundell 1989). APE: endothiapepsin; APP: penicillopepsin; APR: rhizopuspepsin; PEP: hexagonal porcine pepsin; CHY: calf chymosin; RSV: Rous sarcoma virus proteinase; HIV: human immunodeficiency virus proteinase. The last letter refers to the amino (N) or carboxy (C) terminal domains of the pepsins. The coordinates of the three-dimensional structures were obtained from the PDB databank (Bernstein *et al.* 1977). The amino acid code is the standard one-letter code formatted using the following convention: *italic*, positive ϕ; UPPER CASE, solvent inaccessible residue; lower case, solvent accessible residue; **bold type**, hydrogen bond to mainchain amide; underline, hydrogen bond to mainchain carbonyl; tilde, sidechain–sidechain hydrogen bond.

known rule that solvent inaccessible residues tend to be among the more conserved residues in a family. Rules obtained from comparisons also include those that correlate an unknown sidechain dihedral angle with those dihedral angles for equivalent positions in related proteins (Summers *et al.* 1987; Sutcliffe *et al.* 1987b; Donnelly *et al.* 1990). Such correlations can be best represented as a multidimensional probability density table. This table has as many dimensions as there are features included in the analysis and every dimension has as many columns as the corresponding feature can assume. Elements in this table are then filled by simply counting the number of occurrences of the corresponding combination of features in the database of alignments

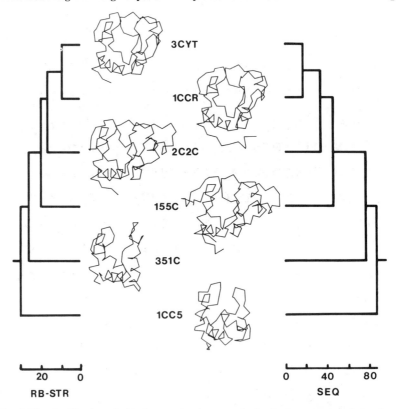

3CYT

1CCR

2C2C

155C

351C

1CC5

20   0   0   40   80
RB-STR   **SEQ**

Fig. 3. The classification of cytochrome structures on the basis of sequence and structure.
The tree was constructed by the program KITSCH from the PHYLIP package (1985).

where all the features including the 'unknown' are defined. Such rules can be used directly to obtain spatial constraints on the sequence of the unknown.

Rules for the substitution of amino acids in three-dimensional structures are derived in a similar way by counting how many times two residue types occur at structurally equivalent positions. We have constructed a number of residue substitution tables (Overington *et al.* 1990) in which only a subset of residues that have a certain structural environment are considered. For example, 20 by 20 substitution tables were built separately for inaccessible residues (Fig. 4(a)). Other structural features included in our analysis were local mainchain conformation (positive ϕ angle, α-helical, β-strand or other) and sidechain hydrogen-bonding to peptide groups (Fig. 4(b)) or other sidechains. These environment-dependent substitution tables are specific examples of the general multidimensional density table described above.

The environment-dependent substitution tables quantify the importance of individual structural features for the acceptance of amino acid mutations in evolution. For example, Fig. 4 shows that the substitution of polar residues such as aspartic acid, asparagine, glutamine, serine and threonine is strongly influenced by sidechain accessibility and hydrogen bonding. Large differences exist in the mutability pattern of the same residue type in different structural environments. Hydrogen-bonded and

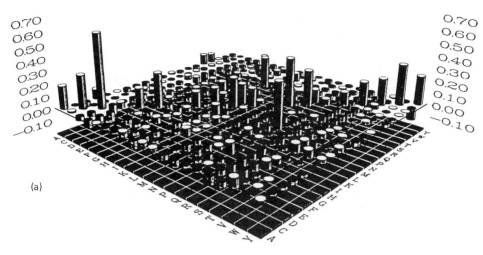

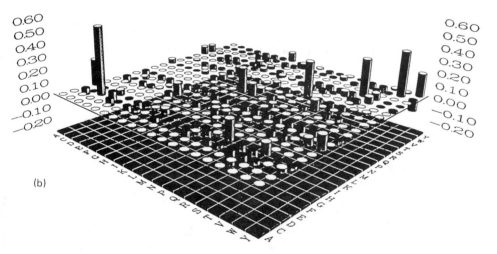

Fig. 4. Difference substitution tables for amino acids that occupy (a) solvent inaccessible and (b) solvent inaccessible and sidechain hydrogen-bonded to a mainchain carbonyl positions in globular proteins. The horizontal axis is that of an amino acid in such an environment in three-dimensional structure of a protein. The vertical axis is the amino acid type in an homologous protein at a topologically equivalent position defined by COMPARER.

inaccessible residues are among the most highly conserved residues in families of proteins. Their structural roles are relatively specific; as a result it is not easy to vary the amino acid type and also retain the important structural role. One specific case is shown in Fig. 2 where Thr 33 and Thr 216 of pepsin are conserved or conservatively varied to serine in all pepsin-like and retroviral proteinases. These buried residues play an important role in holding together the two subunits in retroviral proteinases and the two lobes in pepsins.

4. DERIVATION OF A SEQUENCE TEMPLATE FROM A 3D STRUCTURE OF A PROTEIN

Traditionally, templates have been constructed from the alignment of many sequences of often quite divergent structures (Doolittle 1989). This may allow identification of sequence fingerprints that are characteristic of the structure or function. Such templates can be used in the form of consensus sequences or mutability profiles to search out distantly related proteins in the sequence database. By defining Venn diagrams describing relatedness of amino acids, Taylor (1986) has increased the versatility of templates when few or only closely related structures are available.

One or more protein three-dimensional structures should also provide a basis for the construction of templates. Ponder & Richards (1987) have suggested such an algorithm for generating all sequences of amino acids and their sidechain conformations that are consistent with a particular fold. The tables described above can also be used to estimate the probability of substituting any amino acid at a particular position in a known three-dimensional structure. For each topologically equivalent position in each known structure, we use the tables to predict the variability of amino acid residues. This allows use of knowledge of the 3D structure to project constraints onto the 1D sequence or to construct the family template (Johnson, M.S., Overington, J. and Blundell, T.L., unpublished results). Such a template expressed in the form of a sequence can be used to align the family fold with the sequence to be modelled.

The templates of all known three-dimensional structures or families of structures including loops, motifs, domains and complete globular proteins should be precalculated so that a new sequence can be compared with them rather than with individual proteins. This will result in a better alignment of whole proteins or their parts and thereby extend the usefulness of knowledge-based or comparative modelling.

5. MODELLING 3D STRUCTURE

5.1 Composer

In the previous sections we have described procedures for comparison of protein three-dimensional structures. We have shown that comparisons of homologous families of proteins can give rise to rules. For example, we have described rules that relate the sidechain dihedral angle with the residue type at equivalent positions in homologous proteins and rules that predict the sequence variability at each position in the tertiary structure of a protein; there are many others. We shall now consider methods for constructing a model on the basis of such rules derived not only from comparison of related structures but also from the analyses of protein structures in general. The use of these rules depends very importantly on the alignment of the sequence of the protein to be modelled with the template for the family fold.

Most current methods depend on the assembly of rigid fragments (Jones & Thirup 1986; Blundell *et al.* 1987, 1988, Claessens *et al.* 1989). In our approach encoded in the program COMPOSER we first select the homologous structures that are most useful for construction of the model; this we do on the basis of the sequence and

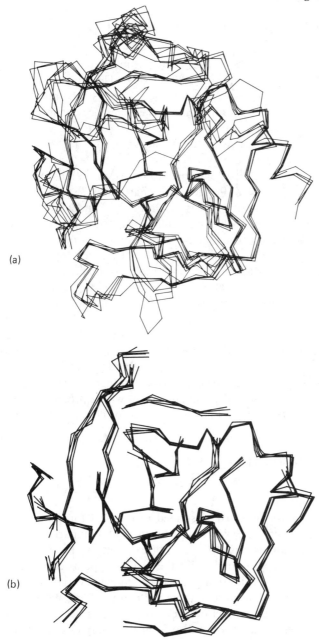

Fig. 5. Modelling the serine proteinase domain of tissue plasminogen activator from homologous serine proteinases by the program COMPOSER. (a) shows the superposition of the structures defined by X-ray analysis. (b) indicates the fragments in the structurally conserved regions that contribute towards generation of the framework shown in (c). Fragments, selected using rules from a broader database of structures, are used to model the structurally variable regions. The C_α atom positions of the complete model are shown in (d). Sidechains, not shown, are also generated by a set of rules derived from comparisons of known structures.

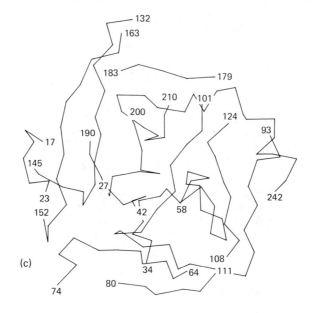

(c)

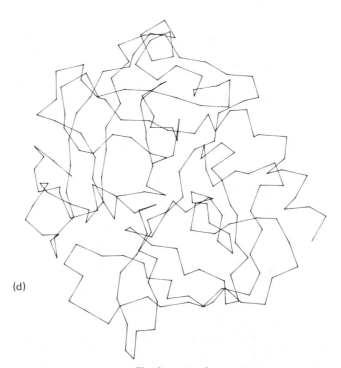

(d)

Fig. 5. *continued*

structure classification as described above (Johnson *et al.* 1990a,b). Three sets of fragments are selected:

(1) Fragments from the framework are defined by multiple least-squares superposition of the chosen structures (Sutcliffe *et al.* 1987a).
(2) Fragments for regions outside the framework are selected from the database of loop substructures using a distance filter in a similar way to Jones & Thirup (1986). The sequences of selected fragments are then compared to the sequence of the unknown using the environment-dependent substitution tables (McCleod, Thomas, Topham, Overington, Johnson and Blundell, 1990, work in progress). The top-ranking fragment is annealed onto the core using an optimization procedure (Eisenmenger, unpublished results) and checked for overlap with other parts of the model structure. If it is rejected on these grounds, the next ranking fragment is processed in the same way.
(3) Fragments of sidechains are selected by using a set of rules derived from the analysis of sidechain dihedral angles at topologically equivalent positions in homologous structures (Sutcliffe *et al.* 1987b). The 1200 rules derived from this analysis include one for each of the 20 by 20 amino acid replacements in each of the three secondary structure types (α-helix, β-strand or irregular). Where there is no applicable rule, the most probable conformation is chosen from a rotamer library, and where there is more than one prediction, the one closest to the median of all predictions is chosen. See also Sumners *et al.* (1987) for a related approach.

Finally, the model is energy minimized to remove small inconsistencies such as steric clashes. This modelling procedure is very successful where the known structures cluster around that to be predicted and where the percentage sequence identity to the unknown is high (greater than 40%). For example, in a model building of porcine trypsin from four other structurally known serine proteinases, the root mean square difference between the model and the known structure is 0.60 Å for the 150 residues defined in the framework. Similarly, 80% of sidechain conformations are correctly predicted for closely homologous structures. In all cases the accuracy of the prediction decreases very quickly as the sequence identity between the known and unknown decreases. For these cases a different approach is essential.

5.2 Modeller

New modelling techniques are required that are not restricted by a rigid body model of protein structure. These are best defined in terms of distance constraints in a similar way to the methods of interpreting NMR data like those of Braun & Go (1985) and Havel *et al.* (1983) but which also allow simultaneous inclusion of different types of information and rules into the derivation of the model (Sali *et al.* 1990).

The alignment of the sequence with the template is used to derive a list of spatial constraints, most of which can be expressed as distance constraints. For example, if two equivalent positions in the alignment of known structures are always hydrogen bonded, we can assume that the same hydrogen bond exists in the unknown structure

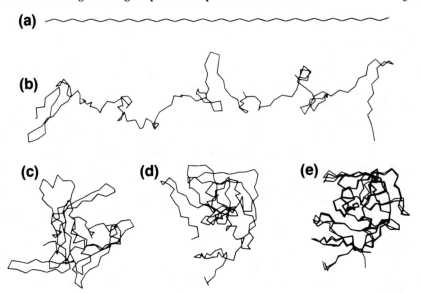

Fig. 6. Generation of a model of a domain of endothiapepsin using rules from homologous aspartic proteinases and from protein 3D structures in general expressed as distance constraints. (a) is the extended chain, (b) shows the influence of mainly local constraints, (c) and (d) are intermediate structures, and (e) is the final structure compared with that experimentally defined.

as well. This represents a distance constraint on the atoms involved in the hydrogen bond.

The most precise description of each constraint on the distance between two atoms treats the distance as a random variable associated with its probability density function. For example, there is a Gaussian probability density function for a length of a chemical bond. Likewise, an estimate of a certain C_α–C_α distance from an equivalent distance in an homologous protein can also be described as a Gaussian probability density function with the mean equal to the known distance and standard deviation proportional to the similarity between proteins and the magnitude of the distance. The probability density function for a sidechain dihedral angle is trimodal with the peaks corresponding to t, g + and g − conformations and their relative magnitudes depending on the particular residue type and the values of equivalent dihedral angles in related known structures (Sali *et al.* 1990).

The goal is then to use the list of spatial constraints on the structure of the protein to construct the three-dimensional model for the protein that will minimize the violations of these constraints. We achieve this by optimization of the molecular probability density function for the whole protein.

In general, every structural feature can be constrained by several knowledge sources. For example, a distance between a particular pair of C_α atoms may be constrained by information from several homologous proteins and also by van der Waals criteria. In such cases we obtain the probability density function for the given feature as a combination of individual probability density functions. The protein three-dimensional structure is uniquely determined if a sufficiently large number of its spatial features are specified. Obviously, the most probable structure of the molecule as a whole is the one that maximizes the product of all feature probability density functions. So the problem of predicting the structure of the molecule using the knowledge-based approach is transformed into finding the optimum of the complicated function.

The optimization is performed in Cartesian coordinate space using a combination of conjugate gradients and simulated annealing minimization to make the best use of the speed of the former and large radius of convergence of the latter (Sali *et al.* 1990). Additionally, the variable target function (Braun & Go 1985) approach is applied to speed up the program and increase the radius of convergence.

A model for the amino-terminal lobe of endothiapepsin (Fig. 6) obtained by our optimization program has a root mean square deviation to the crystallographically determined structure of 0.76 Å although only $C_\alpha - C_\alpha$ and sidechain dihedral constraints were used.

6. CONCLUSIONS

Knowledge-based or comparative modelling, most often in its simplest form of modelling by homology, is now widely used by biochemists. This reflects the steady advancement in the field including the automation of the algorithms and development of integrated systems synthesizing such diverse tools as databases of sequences and structures (Akrigg *et al.* 1988, Thornton & Gardner 1989), interactive molecular graphics, molecular dynamics and energy minimization together with methods for pattern recognition, comparison and clustering. It also reflects the steady advance in the numbers of sequences and structures defined experimentally.

In this article we have concentrated on a description of our own modelling procedures and those that are closely related. An alternative rule-based approach, which has been developed for predicting protein structures where no obvious homology or analogy is apparent, has been developed by Cohen and his collaborators.

The modelling techniques described here are firmly based on the progress and success of experiment. As a consequence we can expect that the next decade will bring a closer integration of modelling techniques with experimental analyses using crystallography, 2D NMR, image reconstruction in electron microscopy, epitope mapping and cross-linking, which have contributed so much to our understanding of complex protein structures and assemblies. The great challenge will be to unify all techniques for determination or prediction of protein structure into a single protocol making the best use of all available information about the structure of a given protein, regardless of whether it is directly based on experiment, on the broader knowledge base, on empirical force potentials or intuition.

ACKNOWLEDGEMENTS

A.S. was supported by an ORS Awards Scheme, the Research Council of Slovenia, the J. Stefan Institute and Merck, Sharp and Dohme. M.S.J. is funded by the American

Cancer Society and J.P.O. by Pfizer and SERC. We are grateful to the Imperial Cancer Research Fund, the SERC and the EEC for general financial support.

Note. This chapter was written in 1990 and therefore more recent references are not included.

REFERENCES

Argos, P. (1987) *J. Mol. Biol.* **193**, 385–396.

Bedarker, B., Turnell, W.G., Schwabe, C. & Blundell, T.L. (1977) *Nature* **270**, 449–451.

Blundell, T.L. & Humbel, R.E. (1980) *Nature* **287**, 781–787.

Blundell, T.L., Sibanda, B.L. & Pearl, L. (1983) *Nature* **304**, 273–275.

Blundell, T.L., Sibanda, B.L., Sternberg, M.J. & Thornton, J.M. (1987) *Nature* **326**, 347–352.

Blundell, T.L., Carney, D., Gardner, S., Hayes, F., Howlin, B., Hubbard, T. & Overington, J. (1988) *Eur. J. Biochem.* **172**, 513–520.

Browne, W.J., North, A.C.T., Phillips, D.C., Brew, K., Vanaman, T.C. & Hill, R.L. (1969) *J. Mol. Biol.* **42**, 65–86.

Chothia, C. & Lesk, A.M. (1986) *EMBO J.* **5**, 823–826.

Claessens, M., Cutsem, E.V., Lasters, I. & Wodak, S. (1989) *Prot. Eng.* **2**, 335–345.

Doolittle, R. (1989) *TIBS* **14**, 244–245.

Eventoff, W. & Rossmann, M.G. (1975) *Crit. Rev. Biochem.* **3**, 111–140.

Greer, J. (1981) *J. Mol. Biol.* **153**, 1027–1042.

Havel, T.F., Kuntz, I.D. & Crippen, G.M. (1983) *Bull. Math. Biol.* **45**, 665–720.

Hubbard, T.J.P. & Blundell, T.L. (1987) *Prot. Eng.* **1**, 159–171.

Johnson, M.S., Sutcliffe, M.J. & Blundell, T.L. (1990a) *J. Mol. Evol.* **30**, 43–59.

Johnson, M.S., Sali, A. & Blundell, T.L. (1990b) *Meth. Enzymol.* **783**, 670–690.

Jones, T.H. & Thirup, S. (1986) *EMBO J.* **5**, 819–822.

KenKnight, C.E. (1984) *Acta Cryst.* **A40**, 708–712.

Lapatto, R., Blundell, T.L., Hemmings, A., Overington, J., Wilderspin, A., Wood, S., Merson, J.R., Whittle, P.J., Danley, D.E., Geoghegan, K.F., Hawrylik, S.J., Lee, S.E., Scheld, K.G. & Hobart, P.M. (1989) *Nature* **342**, 299–302.

Matthews, B.W. & Rossmann, M.G. (1985) *Meth. Enzymol.* **115**, 397–420.

Needleman, S.B. & Wunsch, C.D. (1970) *J. Mol. Biol.* **48**, 443–453.

Overington, J., Johnson, M.J., Sali, A. & Blundell, T.L. (1990) *Proc. Roy. Soc. B.* **241**, 132–145.

Ponder, J.W. & Richards, F.M. (1987) *Proteins*, 775–791.

Sali, A. & Blundell, T.L. (1990) *J. Mol. Biol.* **212**, 403–428.

Sali, A., Donnelly, D. & Blundell, T.L. (1990) unpublished results.

Sibanda, B.L., Blundell, T.L. & Thornton, J.M. (1989) *J. Mol. Biol.* **206**, 759–777.

Summers, N.L., Carson, W.D. & Karplus, M. (1987) *J. Mol. Biol.* **196**, 175–198.

Sutcliffe, M.J., Haneef, I., Carney, D. & Blundell, T.L. (1987a) *Prot. Eng.* **1**, 377–384.

Sutcliffe, M.J., Hayes, F.R.F. & Blundell, T.L. (1987b) *Prot. Eng.* **1**, 385–392.

Taylor, W.R. & Orengo, C.A. (1989) *J. Mol. Biol.* **208**, 1–22.
Thornton, J.M. & Gardner, S. (1989) *TIBS* **14**, 300–304.

Index